International Agency For Research On Cancer

The International Agency for Research on Cancer (IARC) was established in 1965 by the World Health Assembly, as an independently financed organization within the framework of the World Health Organization. The headquarters of the Agency are in Lyon, France.

The Agency conducts a programme of research concentrating particularly on the epidemiology of cancer and the study of potential carcinogens in the human environment. Its field studies are supplemented by biological and chemical research carried out in the Agency's laboratories in Lyon and, through collaborative research agreements, in national research institutions in many countries. The Agency also conducts a programme for the education and training of personnel for cancer research.

The publications of the Agency contribute to the dissemination of authoritative information on different aspects of cancer research. A complete list is printed at the back of this book. Information about IARC publications, and how to order them, is also available via the Internet at: **http://www.iarc.fr/**

Note to the Reader

Anyone who is aware of published data that may influence any consideration in these *Handbooks* is encouraged to make the information available to the Unit of Chemoprevention, International Agency for Research on Cancer, 150 Cours Albert Thomas, 69372 Lyon Cedex 08, France

Although all efforts are made to prepare the *Handbooks* as accurately as possible, mistakes may occur. Readers are requested to communicate any errors to the Unit of Chemoprevention, so that corrections can be reported in future volumes.

Contents

Aspirin

List of participants

Volume 1. Non-steroidal Anti-inflammatory Drugs

Lyon, 2–8 April 1997

H.O. Adami[1]
Department of Cancer Epidemiology
University Hospital
S75 185 Uppsala
Sweden

V.A. Alexandrov
Laboratory of Preclinical Studies
Petrov Institute of Oncology
68 Leningradskaya Str. Pesochny-2
St Petersburg 189646
Russian Federation

J.A. Baron
Dartmouth Medical School
7927 Strasenburgh
Hanover
NH 03755-3861
USA

R. Benamouzig
Hôpital Avicenne
125 rue de Stalingrad
93000 Bobigny
France

J. Burn
Department of Human Genetics
19/20 Claremont Place
University of Newcastle upon Tyne NE2 4AA
United Kingdom

A. Castonguay
Laboratory of Cancer Etiology and Chemoprevention
Laval University
531, Bld des Prairies
Quebec
G1K 7P4 Canada

R.N. DuBois
Department of Medicine,
Vanderbilt University Medical Center
Nashville
TN 37232-2279, USA

D.L. Earnest
Department of Gastroenterology
University of Arizona
Tucson
AZ 85724
USA

P. Greenwald
Division of Cancer Prevention and Control
Department of Health & Human Services
National Institutes of Health
National Cancer Institute
Bethesda
MD 20892
USA

M.R. Griffin
Department of Preventive Medicine and Medicine
Vanderbilt University
Nashville
TN 37232-2637
USA

E.T. Hawk
Chemoprevention Branch
National Cancer Institute
Bethesda
MD 20892
USA

Y. Konishi
Department of Oncological Pathology
Cancer Center
Nara Medical University
840 Shijo-cho, Kashihara
Nara 634
Japan

M.J. Langman
Queen Elizabeth Medical Centre
University Road West
Edgbaston
Birmingham B15 2TT
United Kingdom

---

[1] As of August 1997, Karolinska Institute, Box 281, S-71 77
Stockholm, Sweden

J. Little
Epidemiology Unit
Department of Medicine and Therapeutics
University of Aberdeen
Polwarth Building
Foresterhill
Aberdeen AB25 2ZD
United Kingdom

M. Marselos
Department of Pharmacology
Medical School
University of Ioannina
Ioannina 45110
Greece

A.B. Miller *(Chairman)*
Early Detection Branch
National Cancer Institute
6130 Executive Blvd
Bethesda
MD 20892-734
USA

B.S. Reddy
American Health Foundation,
Division of Nutritional Carcinogenesis
1 Dana Road
Valhalla
NY 10595
USA

B. W. Stewart *(Vice-Chairman)*
Children's Leukaemia & Cancer Research Centre
The Prince of Wales Children's Hospital
University of New South Wales
High Street
Randwick NSW 2031
Australia

M.J. Thun
Epidemiology & Surveillance Research
American Cancer Society
1599 Clifton Road NE
Atlanta
GA 30329-4251
USA

M.D. Waters
Health Effects Research Laboratory
US Environmental Protection Agency
MD-51A, Research Triangle Park
NC 27711
USA

G. Winde
University of Münster
Waldeyer St. 1
48129 Münster
Germany

Observer:

G. Latta
Support Aspirin Prevention
Consumer Care Europe
Bayer AG
51368 Leverkusen
Bayerwerk
Germany

Secretariat:

P. Boffetta
M. Friesen
E. Heseltine *(Editor)*
V. Krutovskikh
C. Malaveille
D. McGregor
G. Morgan
H. Ohshima
E. Riboli
J. Rice
J. Siemiatycki
H. Vainio *(Responsible Officer)*
J. Wilbourn

Technical Assistance:

B. Geoffre
M. Lézère
A. Meneghel
D. Mietton
S. Ruiz
J. Mitchell
S. Reynaud
J. Thévenoux

Unable to attend: L.J. Marnett, A.B. Hancock Jr Memorial Laboratory for Cancer Research,Vanderbilt University, Nashville, TN 37232-0146, USA. **B. Rigas,**10, Karkavistsa Street,15452 Psyhiko, Athens, Greece. **G.D. Stoner,** Division of Environmental Health Sciences, School of Public Health, Ohio State University, Columbus, OH 43210, USA

Preamble to the IARC *Handbooks of Cancer Prevention*

The prevention of cancer is one of the key objectives of the International Agency for Research on Cancer (IARC). This may be achieved by avoiding exposures to known cancer-causing agents, by increasing host defence through immunization or chemoprevention, or by modifying lifestyle. The aim of the *IARC Monographs* programme is to evaluate carcinogenic risks of human exposure to chemical, physical and biological agents, providing a scientific basis for national or international decisions on avoidance of exposures. The aim of the series of the *IARC Handbooks of Cancer Prevention* is to evaluate scientific information on agents and interventions that may reduce the incidence of or mortality from cancer. This preamble is divided into two parts. The first addresses the general scope, objectives and structure of the *Handbooks*. The second describes the procedures for evaluating chemopreventive agents.

Part One

Scope
Prevention strategies embrace chemical, immunological, dietary and behavioural interventions that may retard, block or reverse carcinogenic processes or reduce underlying risk factors. The term 'chemoprevention' is used to refer to interventions with pharmaceuticals, vitamins, minerals and other chemicals to reduce cancer incidence. The *IARC Handbooks* address the efficacy, safety and mechanisms of cancer-preventive strategies and the adequacy of the available data, including those on timing, dose, duration and indications for use.

Prevention strategies can be applied across a continuum of: (1) the general population; (2) subgroups with particular predisposing host or environmental risk factors, including genetic susceptibility to cancer; (3) persons with precancerous lesions; and (4) cancer patients at risk for second primary tumours. Use of the same strategies or agents in the treatment of cancer patients to control the growth, metastasis and recurrence of tumours is considered to be patient management, not prevention, although data from clinical trials may be relevant when making a *Handbooks* evaluation.

Objective
The objective of the *Handbooks* programme is the preparation of critical reviews and evaluations of evidence on the cancer-preventive and other relevant properties of a wide range of potential cancer-preventive agents and strategies by international working groups of experts. The resulting *Handbooks* may also indicate where additional research is needed.

The *Handbooks* may assist national and international authorities in devising programmes of health promotion and cancer prevention and in making benefit–risk assessments. The evaluations of IARC working groups are scientific judgements about the available evidence for cancer-preventive efficacy and safety. No recommendation is given with regard to national and international regulation or legislation, which are the responsibility of individual governments and/or other international authorities. No recommendations for specific research trials are made.

IARC Working Groups
Reviews and evaluations are formulated by international working groups of experts convened by the IARC. The tasks of each group are: (1) to ascertain that all appropriate data have been collected; (2) to select the data relevant for the evaluation on the basis of scientific merit; (3) to prepare accurate summaries of the data to enable the reader to follow the reasoning of the Working Group; (4) to evaluate the significance of the available data from human studies and experimental models on cancer-preventive activity, carcinogenicity and other beneficial and adverse effects; and (5) to evaluate data relevant to the understanding of mechanisms of action.

Working Group participants who contributed to the considerations and evaluations within a particular *Handbook* are listed, with their addresses, at the beginning of each publication. Each participant serves as an individual scientist and not as a representative of any organization, government or industry. In addition, scientists nominated by national and international agencies, industrial associations and consumer and/or environmental organizations may be invited as observers. IARC staff involved in the preparation of the *Handbooks* are listed.

Working procedures

Approximately 13 months before a working group meets, the topics of the *Handbook* are announced, and participants are selected by IARC staff in consultation with other experts. Subsequently, relevant clinical, experimental and human data are collected by the IARC from all available sources of published information. Representatives from producer or consumer associations may assist in the preparation of sections on production and use as appropriate.

About eight months before the meeting, the material collected is sent to meeting participants to prepare sections for the first drafts of the *Handbooks*. These are then compiled by IARC staff and sent, before the meeting, to all participants of the Working Group for review. There is an opportunity to return the compiled specialized sections of the draft to the experts, inviting preliminary comments, before the complete first draft document is distributed to all members of the Working Group.

Data for *Handbooks*

The *Handbooks* do not necessarily cite all of the literature on the agent or strategy being evaluated. Only those data considered by the Working Group to be relevant to making the evaluation are included. In principle, meeting abstracts and other reports that do not provide sufficient detail upon which to assess their quality should be avoided.

With regard to data from toxicological, epidemiological and experimental studies and from clinical trials, only reports that have been published or accepted for publication in the openly available scientific literature are reviewed by the Working Group. In certain instances, government agency reports that have undergone peer review and are widely available are considered. Exceptions may be made on an ad-hoc basis to include unpublished reports that are in their final form and publicly available, if their inclusion is considered pertinent to making a final evaluation. In the sections on chemical and physical properties, on production, on use, on analysis and on human exposure, unpublished sources of information may be used.

Criteria for selection of topics for evaluation

Agents, classes of agents and interventions to be evaluated in the *Handbooks* are selected on the basis of one or more of the following criteria.

- The available evidence suggests potential for significantly reducing the incidence of cancers.
- There is a substantial body of human, experimental, clinical and/or mechanistic data suitable for evaluation.
- The agent is in widespread use and of putative protective value, but of uncertain efficacy and safety.
- The agent shows exceptional promise in experimental studies but has not been used in humans.
- The agent is available for further studies of human use.

Part Two

Evaluation of cancer-preventive agents

A wide range of findings must be taken into account before a particular agent can be recognized as preventing cancer. On the basis of experience from the *IARC Monographs* programme, a systematized approach to data presentation is adopted for *Handbooks* evaluations.

1.   Chemical and physical characteristics of the agent

The Chemical Abstracts Services Registry Number, the latest Chemical Abstracts Primary Name, the IUPAC Systematic Name and other definitive information (such as genus and species of plants) are given as appropriate. Information on chemical and physical properties and, in particular, data relevant to identification, occurrence and biological activity are included. A description of technical products of chemicals includes trade names,

Outline of data presentation scheme for evaluating chemopreventive agents

1. **Chemical and physical characteristics**

2. **Occurrence, production, use, analysis and human exposure**
   - 2.1 Occurrence
   - 2.2 Production
   - 2.3 Use
   - 2.4 Analysis
   - 2.5 Human exposure

3. **Metabolism, kinetics and genetic variation**
   - 3.1 Human studies
   - 3.2 Experimental models
   - 3.3 Genetic variation

4. **Cancer-preventive effects**
   - 4.1 Human studies
   - 4.2 Experimental models
     - 4.2.1 Experimental animals
     - 4.2.2 *In vitro* models
   - 4.3 Mechanisms of chemoprevention

5. **Other beneficial effects**

6. **Carcinogenicity**
   - 6.1 Humans
   - 6.2 Experimental animals

7. **Other toxic effects**
   - 7.1 Adverse effects
     - 7.1.1 Humans
     - 7.1.2 Experimental animals
   - 7.2 Genetic and related effects
     - 7.2.1 Humans
     - 7.2.2 Experimental models

8. **Summary of data**
   - 8.1 Chemistry, occurrence and human exposure
   - 8.2 Metabolism and kinetics
   - 8.3 Cancer-preventive effects
     - 8.3.1 Humans
     - 8.3.2 Experimental animals
     - 8.3.3 Mechanism of action
   - 8.4 Other beneficial effects
   - 8.5 Carcinogenicity
     - 8.5.1 Humans
     - 8.5.2 Experimental animals
   - 8.6 Toxic effects
     - 8.6.1 Humans
     - 8.6.2 Experimental animals

9. **Recommendations for research**

10. **Evaluation**
   - 10.1 Cancer-preventive activity
     - 10.1.1 Humans
     - 10.1.2 Experimental animals
   - 10.2 Overall evaluation

relevant specifications and available information on composition and impurities. Some of the trade names given may be those of mixtures in which the agent being evaluated is only one of the ingredients.

2. Occurrence, production, use, analysis and human exposure

2.1 Occurrence

Information on the occurrence of an agent or mixture in the environment is obtained from data derived from the monitoring and surveillance of levels in occupational environments, air, water, soil, foods and animal and human tissues. When available, data on the generation, persistence and bioaccumulation of the agent are included. For mixtures, information is given about all agents present.

2.2 Production

The dates of first synthesis and of first commercial production of a chemical or mixture are provided; for agents that do not occur naturally, this information may allow a reasonable estimate to be made of the date before which no human use of, or exposure to, the agent could have occurred. The dates of first reported occurrence of an exposure are also provided. In addition, methods of synthesis used in past and present commercial production and methods of production that may give rise to different impurities are described.

2.3   Use

Data on production, international trade and uses and applications are obtained for representative regions. Some identified uses may not be current or major applications, and the coverage is not necessarily comprehensive. In the case of drugs, mention of their therapeutic applications does not necessarily represent current practice, nor does it imply judgement as to their therapeutic efficacy.

2.4   Analysis

An overview of current methods of analysis or detection is presented. Methods for monitoring human exposure are also given, when available.

2.5   Human exposure

Human uses of, or exposure to, the agent are described. If an agent is used as a prescribed or over-the-counter pharmaceutical product, then the type of person receiving the product in terms of health status, age, sex and medical condition being treated are described. For nonpharmaceutical agents, particularly those taken because of cultural traditions, the characteristics of use or exposure and the relevant populations are described. In all cases, quantitative data, such as dose-response data, are considered to be of special importance.

3.   Metabolism, kinetics and genetic variation

In evaluating the potential utility of a suspected chemopreventive agent or strategy, a number of different properties, in addition to direct effects upon cancer incidence, are described and weighed. Furthermore, as many of the data leading to an evaluation are expected to come from studies in experimental animals, information that facilitates interspecies extrapolation is particularly important; this includes metabolic, kinetic and genetic data. Whenever possible, quantitative data, including information on dose, duration and potency, are considered.

Information is given on absorption, distribution (including placental transfer), metabolism and excretion in humans and experimental animals. Kinetic properties within the target species may affect the interpretation and extrapolation of dose–response relationships, such as blood concentrations, protein binding, tissue concentrations, plasma half-lives and elimination rates. Comparative information on the relationship between use or exposure and the dose that reaches the target site may be of particular importance for extrapolation between species. Studies that indicate the metabolic pathways and fate of the agent in humans and experimental animals are summarized, and data on humans and experimental animals are compared when possible. Observations are made on interindividual variations and relevant metabolic polymorphisms. Data indicating long-term accumulation in human tissues are included. Physiologically based pharmacokinetic models and their parameter values are relevant and are included whenever they are available. Information on the fate of the compound within tissues and cells (transport, role of cellular receptors, compartmentalization, binding to macromolecules) is given.

Genotyping will be used increasingly, not only to identify subpopulations at increased or decreased risk for cancers but also to characterize variation in the biotransformation of, and responses to, chemopreventive and chemotherapeutic agents.

This subsection can include effects of the compound on gene expression, enzyme induction or inhibition, or pro-oxidant status, when such data are not described elsewhere. It covers data obtained in humans and experimental animals, with particular attention to effects of long-term use and exposure.

4.   Cancer-preventive effects

4.1   Human studies

Types of studies considered. Human data are derived from experimental and non-experimental study designs and are focused on cancer, precancer or intermediate biological end-points. The experimental designs include randomized controlled trials and short-term experimental studies; non-experimental designs include cohort, case–control and cross-sectional studies.

Cohort and case–control studies relate individual use of, or exposure to, the agents under study to the occurrence or prevention of cancer in individuals and provide an estimate of relative risk (ratio of incidence or mortality in those exposed to incidence or mortality in those not exposed) as the main measure of association. Cohort and case–control studies follow an observational approach, in which the use of, or exposure to, the agent is not controlled by the investigator.

Intervention studies are experimental in design — that is, the use of, or exposure to, the agent is assigned by the investigator. The intervention study or clinical trial is the design that can provide the strongest and most direct evidence of a protective or preventive effect; however, for practical and ethical reasons, such studies are limited to observation of the effects among specifically defined study subjects of interventions of 10 years or fewer, which is relatively short when compared with the overall lifespan.

Intervention studies may be undertaken in individuals or communities and may or may not involve randomization to use or exposure. The differences between these designs is important in relation to analytical methods and interpretation of findings.

In addition, information can be obtained from reports of correlation (ecological) studies and case series; however, limitations inherent in these approaches usually mean that such studies carry limited weight in the evaluation of a preventive effect.

Quality of studies considered. The *Handbooks* are not intended to summarize all published studies. It is important that the Working Group consider the following aspects: (1) the relevance of the study; (2) the appropriateness of the design and analysis to the question being asked; (3) the adequacy and completeness of the presentation of the data; and (4) the degree to which chance, bias and confounding may have affected the results.

Studies that are judged to be inadequate or irrelevant to the evaluation are generally omitted. They may be mentioned briefly, particularly when the information is considered to be a useful supplement to that in other reports or when it is the only data available. Their inclusion does not imply acceptance of the adequacy of the study design, nor of the analysis and interpretation of the results, and their limitations are outlined.

Assessment of the cancer-preventive effect at different doses and durations. The Working Group gives special attention to quantitative assessment of the preventive effect of the agent under study, by assessing data from studies at different doses. The Working Group also addresses issues of timing and duration of use or exposure. Such quantitative assessment is important to clarify the circumstances under which a preventive effect can be achieved, as well as the dose at which a toxic effect has been shown.

Criteria for a cancer-preventive effect. After summarizing and assessing the individual studies, the Working Group makes a judgement concerning the evidence that the agent in question prevents cancer in humans. In making their judgement, the Working Group considers several criteria for each relevant cancer site.

Evidence of protection derived from intervention studies of good quality is particularly informative. Evidence of a substantial and significant reduction in risk, including a dose–response relationship, is more likely to indicate a real effect. Nevertheless, a small effect, or an effect without a dose–response relationship, does not imply lack of real benefit and may be important for public health if the cancer is common.

Evidence is frequently available from different types of studies and is evaluated as a whole. Findings that are replicated in several studies of the same design or using different approaches are more likely to provide evidence of a true protective effect than isolated observations from single studies.

The Working Group evaluates possible explanations for inconsistencies across studies, including differences in use of, or exposure to, the agent, differences in the underlying risk for cancer and metabolism and genetic differences in the population.

The results of studies judged to be of high quality are given more weight. Note is taken of both the applicability of preventive action to several cancers and of possible differences in activity, including contradictory findings, across cancer sites.

Data from human studies (as well as from experimental models) that suggest plausible mechanisms for a cancer-preventive effect are important in assessing the overall evidence.

The Working Group may also determine whether, on aggregate, the evidence from human studies is consistent with a lack of preventive effect.

4.2 Experimental models

4.2.1 Experimental animals

Animal models are an important component of chemopreventive research. They provide a means of identifying effective compounds, of carrying out fundamental investigations into their mechanisms of action, of determining how they can be used optimally, of evaluating toxicity and, ultimately, of providing an information base for developing intervention trials in humans. Models that permit evaluation of the effects of chemopreventive agents on the occurrence of cancer in most major organ sites are available. Major groups of animal models include: those in which carcinogenesis is produced by the administration of chemical or physical carcinogens; those involving genetically engineered animals; and those in which tumours develop spontaneously. Most chemopreventive agents investigated in such studies can be placed into one of three categories: compounds that prevent molecules from reaching or reacting with critical target sites (blocking agents); compounds that decrease the sensitivity of target tissues to carcinogenic stimuli; and compounds that prevent evolution of the neoplastic process (suppressing agents). There is increasing interest in the use of combinations of agents as a means of improving efficacy and minimizing toxicity. Animal models are useful in evaluating such combinations. The development of optimal strategies for human intervention trials can be facilitated by the use of animal models that mimic the neoplastic process in humans.

Specific factors to be considered in such experiments are: (1) the temporal requirements of administration of the chemopreventive agents; (2) dose–response effects; (3) the site-specificity of a chemopreventive action; and (4) the number and structural diversity of carcinogens whose action can be reduced by the agent being evaluated. Other types of studies include experiments in which the end-point is not cancer but a defined preneoplastic lesion or tumour-related, inter-medi-

ate biomarker. An important variable in the evaluation of the cancer-preventive response is the time and the duration of the administration of the chemopreventive agent in relation to any carcinogenic treatment, or in transgenic or other experimental models in which no carcinogen is administered. Furthermore, concurrent administration of a chemopreventive agent may result in a decreased incidence of tumours in a given organ and an increase in another organ of the same animal. Thus, in these experiments it is important that multiple organs be examined.

For all these studies, the nature and extent of impurities or contaminants present in the chemopreventive agent or agents being evaluated are given when available. For experimental studies of mixtures, consideration is given to the possibility of changes in the physicochemical properties of the test substance during collection, storage, extraction, concentration and delivery. Chemical and toxicological interactions of the components of mixtures may result in nonlinear dose–response relationships.

As certain components of commonly used diets for experimental animals are themselves known to have chemopreventive activity, particular consideration should be given to the interaction between the diet and the apparent effect of the agent being studied. Likewise, restriction of diet may be important. The appropriateness of the diet given relative to the composition of human diets may be commented on by the Working Group.

Qualitative aspects. An assessment of the experimental prevention of cancer involves several considerations of qualitative importance, including: (1) the experimental conditions under which the test was performed (route and schedule of exposure, species, strain, sex and age of animals studied, duration of the exposure, and duration of the study); (2) the consistency of the results, for example across species and target organ(s); (3) the stage or stages of the neoplastic process, from preneoplastic lesions and benign tumours to malignant neoplasms, studied and (4) the possible role of modifying factors.

Considerations of importance to the Working Group in the interpretation and evaluation of a particular study include: (1) how clearly the agent was defined and, in the case of mixtures, how adequately the sample composition was reported; (2) the composition of the diet and the stability of the agent in the diet; (3) whether the source, strain and quality of the animals was reported; (4) whether the dose and schedule of treatment with the known carcinogen were appropriate in assays of combined treatment; (5) whether the doses of the chemopreventive agent were adequately monitored; (6) whether the agent(s) was absorbed, as shown by blood concentrations; (7) whether the survival of treated animals was similar to that of controls; (8) whether the body and organ weights of treated animals were similar to those of controls; (9) whether there were adequate numbers of animals, of appropriate age, per group; (10) whether animals of each sex were used, if appropriate; (11) whether animals were allocated randomly to groups; (12) whether appropriate respective controls were used; (13) whether the duration of the experiment was adequate; (14) whether there was adequate statistical analysis; and (15) whether the data were adequately reported. If available, recent data on the incidence of specific tumours in historical controls, as well as in concurrent controls, are taken into account in the evaluation of tumour response. The observation of effects on the occurrence of lesions presumed to be preneoplastic or the emergence of benign or malignant tumours may in certain instances aid in assessing the mode of action of the presumed chemopreventive agent. Particular attention is given to assessing the reversibility of these lesions and their predictive value in relation to cancer development.

Quantitative aspects. The probability that tumours will occur may depend on the species, sex, strain and age of the animals, the dose of carcinogen (if any), the dose of the agent, and the route and duration of exposure. A decreased incidence and/or decreased multiplicity of neoplasms in adequately designed studies provides evidence of a chemopreventive effect. A dose-related decrease in incidence and/or multiplicity further strengthens this association.

Statistical analysis. Major factors considered in the statistical analysis by the Working Group include the adequacy of the data for each treatment group: (1) the initial and final effective numbers of

animals studied and the survival rate; (2) body weights; and (3) tumour incidence and multiplicity. The statistical methods used should be clearly stated and should be the generally accepted techniques refined for this purpose. In particular, the statistical methods should be appropriate for the characteristics of the expected data distribution and should account for interactions in multifactorial studies. Consideration is given as to whether the appropriate adjustments were made for differences in survival.

4.2.2 In-vitro models

Cell systems *in vitro* contribute to the early identification of potential chemopreventive agents and to elucidation of mechanistic aspects. A number of assays in prokaryotic and eukaryotic systems are used for this purpose. Evaluation of the results of such assays includes consideration of: (1) the nature of the cell type used; (2) whether primary cell cultures or cell lines (tumorigenic or nontumorigenic) were studied; (3) the appropriateness of controls; (4) whether toxic effects were considered in the outcome; (5) whether the data were appropriately summated and analysed; (6) whether appropriate quality controls were used; (7) whether appropriate concentration ranges were used; (8) whether adequate numbers of independent measurements were made per group; and (9) the relevance of the end-points, including inhibition of mutagenesis, morphological transformation, anchorage-independent growth, cell–cell communication, calcium tolerance and differentiation.

4.3 Mechanisms of chemoprevention

Data on mechanisms can be derived from both human and experimental systems. For a rational implementation of chemopreventive measures, it is essential not only to assess protective end-points but also to understand the mechanisms by which the agents exert their anticarcinogenic action. Information on the mechanisms of chemopreventive agents can be inferred from relationships between chemical structure and biological activity, from analysis of interactions between agents and specific molecular targets, from studies of specific end-points *in vitro*, from studies of the inhibition of tumorigenesis *in vivo* and the efficacy of modulating intermediate biomarkers, and from human studies. Therefore, the Working Group takes account of mechanistic data in making the final evaluation of chemoprevention.

Several classifications of mechanisms have been proposed, as have several systems for evaluating them. Chemopreventive agents may act at several distinct levels. Their action may be: (1) extracellular, for example, inhibiting the uptake or endogenous formation of carcinogens, or forming complexes with, diluting and/or deactivating carcinogens; (2) intracellular, for example, trapping carcinogens in non-target cells, modifying transmembrane transport, modulating metabolism, blocking reactive molecules, inhibiting cell replication or modulating gene expression or DNA metabolism; or (3) at the level of the cell, tissue or organism, for example, affecting cell differentiation, intercellular communication, proteases, signal transduction, growth factors, cell adhesion molecules, angiogenesis, interactions with the extracellular matrix, hormonal status and the immune system.

Many chemopreventive agents are known or suspected to act by several mechanisms, which may operate in a coordinated manner and allow them a broader spectrum of anticarcinogenic activity. Therefore, multiple mechanisms of action are taken into account in the evaluation of chemoprevention.

Beneficial interactions, generally resulting from exposure to inhibitors that work through complementary mechanisms, are exploited in combined chemoprevention. Because organisms are naturally exposed not only to mixtures of carcinogenic agents but also to mixtures of protective agents, it is also important to understand the mechanisms of interactions between inhibitors.

5.   Other beneficial effects

This section contains mainly background information on preventive activity. Use is described in Section 2.3. An expanded description is given, when appropriate, of the efficacy of the agent in the maintenance of a normal healthy state and the treatment of particular diseases. Information on the mechanisms involved in these activities is described. Reviews, rather than individual studies, may be cited as references.

The physiological functions of agents such as vitamins and micronutrients can be described

briefly, with reference to reviews. Data on the therapeutic effects of drugs approved for clinical use are summarized.

6.   Carcinogenicity

Some agents may have both carcinogenic and anti-carcinogenic activities. If the agent has been evaluated within the *IARC Monographs on the Evaluation of Carcinogenic Risks to Humans*, that evaluation is accepted, unless significant new data have appeared that may lead the Working Group to reconsider the evidence. When a re-evaluation is necessary or when no carcinogenic evaluation has been made, the procedures described in the Preamble to the *IARC Monographs on the Evaluation of Carcinogenic Risks to Humans* are adopted as guidelines.

7.   Other toxic effects

Toxic effects are of particular importance in the case of agents that may be used widely over long periods in healthy populations. Data are given on acute and chronic toxic effects, such as organ toxicity, increased cell proliferation, immunotoxicity and adverse endocrine effects. If the agent occurs naturally or has been in clinical use previously, the doses and durations used in chemopreventive trials are compared with intakes from the diet, in the case of vitamins, and previous clinical exposure, in the case of drugs already approved for human use. When extensive data are available, only summaries are presented; if adequate reviews are available, reference may be made to these. If there are no relevant reviews, the evaluation is made on the basis of the same criteria as are applied to epidemiological studies of cancer. Differences in response as a consequence of species, sex, age and genetic variability are presented when the information is available.

Data demonstrating the presence or absence of adverse effects in humans are included; equally, lack of data on specific adverse effects is stated clearly.

Findings in humans and experimental animals are presented sequentially under the headings 'Toxic and other adverse effects' and 'Genetic and related effects'.

The section 'Toxic and other adverse effects' includes information on immunotoxicity, neurotoxicity, cardiotoxicity, haematological effects and toxicity to other target organs. Specific case reports in humans and any previous clinical data are noted. Other biochemical effects thought to be relevant to adverse effects are mentioned. The reproductive and developmental effects described include effects on fertility, teratogenicity, fetotoxicity and embryotoxicity. Information from nonmammalian systems and *in vitro* are presented only if they have clear mechanistic significance.

The section 'Genetic and related effects' includes results from studies in mammalian and nonmammalian systems *in vivo* and *in vitro*. Information on whether DNA damage occurs via direct interaction with the agent or via indirect mechanisms (e.g. generation of free radicals) is included, as is information on other genetic effects such as mutation, recombination, chromosomal damage, aneuploidy, cell immortalization and transformation, and effects on cell–cell communication. The presence and toxicological significance of cellular receptors for the chemopreventive agent are described.

The adequacy of epidemiological studies of toxic effects, including reproductive outcomes and genetic and related effects in humans, is evaluated by the same criteria as are applied to epidemiological studies of cancer. For each of these studies, the adequacy of the reporting of sample characterization is considered and, where necessary, commented upon. The available data are interpreted critically according to the end-points used. The doses and concentrations used are given, and, for *in vitro* experiments, mention is made of whether the presence of an exogenous metabolic system affected the observations. For in vivo studies, the route of administration and the formulation in which the agent was administered are included. The dosing regimens, including the duration of treatment, are also given. Genetic data are given as listings of test systems, data and references; bar graphs (activity profiles) and corresponding summary tables with detailed information on the preparation of genetic activity profiles are given in appendices. Genetic and other activity in humans and experimental mammals is regarded as being of greater relevance than that in other organisms. The in-vitro experiments providing these data must be carefully evaluated, since there are many trivial reasons why a response to one agent may be modified by the addition of another.

Structure–activity relationships that may be relevant to the evaluation of the toxicity of an agent are described.

Studies on the interaction of the suspected chemopreventive agent with toxic and subtoxic doses of other substances are described, the objective being to determine whether there is inhibition or enhancement, additivity, synergism or potentiation of toxic effects over an extended dose range.

Biochemical investigations that may have a bearing on the mechanisms of toxicity and chemoprevention are described. These are carefully evaluated for their relevance and the appropriateness of the results.

8. Summary of data

In this section, the relevant human and experimental data are summarized. Inadequate studies are generally not summarized; such studies, if cited, are identified in the preceding text.

8.1 Chemistry, occurrence and human exposure

Human exposure to an agent is summarized on the basis of elements that may include production, use, occurrence in the environment and determinations in human tissues and body fluids. Quantitative data are summarized when available.

8.2 Metabolism and kinetics

Data on metabolism and kinetics in humans and in experimental animals are given when these are considered relevant to the possible mechanisms of chemoprotective, carcinogenic and toxic activity.

8.3 Cancer-preventive effects

8.3.1 Humans

The results of relevant studies are summarized, including case reports and correlation studies when considered important.

8.3.2 Experimental animals

Data relevant to an evaluation of cancer-preventive activity in experimental models are summarized. For each animal species and route of administration, it is stated whether a change in the incidence of neoplasms or preneoplastic lesions was observed, and the tumour sites are indicated. Negative findings are also summarized. Dose–response relationships and other quantitative data may be given when available.

8.3.3 Mechanism of action

Data relevant to the mechanisms of cancer-preventive activity are summarized.

8.4 Other beneficial effects

When beneficial effects other than cancer prevention have been identified, the relevant data are summarized.

8.5 Carcinogenicity

Normally, the agent will have been reviewed and evaluated within the *IARC Monographs* programme, and that summary is used with the inclusion of more recent data, if appropriate.

8.5.1 Humans

The results of epidemiological studies that are considered to be pertinent to an assessment of human carcinogenicity are summarized. When relevant, case reports and correlation studies are also summarized.

8.5.2 Experimental animals

Data relevant to an evaluation of carcinogenic effects in animal models are summarized. For each animal species and route of administration, it is stated whether a change in the incidence of neoplasms or preneoplastic lesions was observed, and the tumour sites are indicated. Negative findings are also summarized. Dose–response relationships and other quantitative data may be mentioned when available.

8.6 Toxic effects

Adverse effects in humans are summarized, together with data on general toxicological effects and cytotoxicity, receptor binding and hormonal and immunological effects. The results of investigations on the reproductive, genetic and related effects are summarized. Toxic effects are summarized for whole animals, cultured mammalian cells and non-mammalian systems. When available, data for humans and for animals are compared.

Structure–activity relationships are mentioned when relevant to toxicity.

9. Recommendations for research

During the evaluation process, it is likely that opportunities for further research will be identified. This is clearly stated, with the understanding that the areas are recommended for future investigation. It is made clear that these research opportunities are identified in general terms on the basis of the data currently available.

10. Evaluation

Evaluations of the strength of the evidence for cancer-preventive activity and carcinogenicity from studies in humans and experimental models are made, using standard terms. These terms may also be applied to other beneficial and adverse effects, when indicated. When appropriate, reference is made to specific organs and populations.

It is recognized that the criteria for these evaluations, described below, cannot encompass all factors that may be relevant to an evaluation of cancer-preventive activity. In considering all the relevant scientific data, the Working Group may assign the agent, or other intervention to a higher or lower category than a strict interpretation of these criteria would indicate.

10.1 Cancer-preventive activity

These categories refer to the strength of the evidence that an agent prevents cancer. The evaluations may change as new information becomes available.

Evaluations are inevitably limited to the cancer sites, conditions and levels of exposure and length of observation covered by the available studies. An evaluation of degree of evidence, whether for a single agent or a mixture, is limited to the materials tested, as defined physically, chemically or biologically. When the agents evaluated are considered by the Working Group to be sufficiently closely related, they may be grouped together for the purpose of a single evaluation of degree of evidence.

Information on mechanisms of action is taken into account when evaluating the strength of evidence in humans and and in experimental animals, as well as in assessing the consistency of results between studies in humans and experimental models.

10.1.1   Cancer-preventive activity in humans

The evidence relevant to prevention in humans is classified into one of the following four categories.

- *Sufficient evidence of cancer-preventive activity*
  The Working Group considers that a causal relationship has been established between use of the agent and the prevention of human cancer in studies in which chance, bias and confounding could be ruled out with reasonable confidence.
- *Limited evidence of cancer-preventive activity*
  The data suggest a reduced risk for cancer with use of the agent but are limited for making a definitive evaluation either because chance, bias or confounding could not be ruled out with reasonable confidence or because the data are restricted to intermediary biomarkers of uncertain validity in the putative pathway to cancer.
- *Inadequate evidence of cancer-preventive activity*
  The available studies are of insufficient quality, consistency or statistical power to permit a conclusion regarding a cancer-preventive effect of the agent, or no data on the prevention of cancer in humans are available.
- *Evidence suggesting lack of cancer-preventive activity*
  Several adequate studies of use or exposure are mutually consistent in not showing a preventive effect.

The strength of the evidence for any carcinogenic activity is assessed in parallel. Both cancer-preventive activity and carcinogenicity are identified and, when appropriate, tabulated, by organ site. The evaluation also cites the population subgroups concerned, specifying ages, sex, genetic or environmental predisposing risk factors and the presence of precancerous lesions.

10.1.2   Cancer-preventive activity in experimental animals

Evidence for prevention in experimental animals is classified into one of the following categories.

- *Sufficient evidence of cancer-preventive activity*
  The Working Group considers that a causal relationship has been established between the agent and a decreased incidence and/or multiplicity of neoplasms.
- *Limited evidence of cancer-preventive activity*
  The data suggest a preventive effect but are limited for making a definitive evaluation because, for example, the evidence of prevention is restricted to a single experiment, the agent decreases the incidence and/or multiplicity only of benign neoplasms or lesions of uncertain neoplastic potential or there is conflicting evidence.
- *Inadequate evidence of cancer-preventive activity*
  The studies cannot be interpreted as showing either the presence or absence of a preventive effect because of major qualitative or quantitative limitations (unresolved questions regarding the adequacy of the design, conduct or interpretation of the study), or no data on prevention in experimental animals are available.
- *Evidence suggesting lack of cancer-preventive activity*
  Adequate evidence from conclusive studies in several models shows that, within the limits of the tests used, the agent does not prevent cancer.

10.2   Overall evaluation

Finally, the body of evidence is considered as a whole, and summary statements are made that encompass the effects of the agents in humans with regard to cancer-preventive activity, carcinogenicity and other beneficial and adverse effects, as appropriate.

General Remarks

1. Introduction

The history of non-steroidal anti-inflammatory drugs (NSAIDs) can be traced to ancient Egypt, where an extract of willow bark was used to treat inflammation (Vane *et al.*, 1990; Wright, 1993). The active component of the extract was subsequently identified as the glucoside of salicyl alcohol. Hydrolysis of the carbohydrate moiety produces salicyl alcohol, which can be oxidized to salicylic acid, the actual anti-inflammatory agent. Severe gastric side-effects associated with oral use of sodium salicylate prompted synthesis of its *ortho*-acetyl derivative for use as a possible pro-drug, i.e. a pharmacologically inactive precursor that is converted *in vivo* to an active drug, by metabolism or other physiologically active processes (Vane *et al.*, 1990). In fact, acetylsalicylic acid is anti-inflammatory, analgesic and antipyretic but also ulcerogenic. Acetylsalicylic acid was synthesized in 1897 and was mass produced from 1899 by the German company Bayer for the treatment of fever and rheumatism under the commercial name 'Aspirin®[1]'. Subsequently, new, important pharmacological activities have been reported that have been the subject of much basic and clinical investigation. A number of other anti-inflammatory agents have been developed over the past 50 years (Frölich, 1997). These fall into six distinct classes, listed in Table 1.

In the 1970s, Bennett and Del Tacca (1975) and others observed that certain human cancers, including those in the colon and rectum, produced more prostaglandin E_2 than did surrounding normal tissue. They suggested that tumours that overproduce certain prostaglandins promote their own growth and spread. As NSAIDs inhibit prostaglandin synthesis, this theory gave rise to a series of experimental studies in rodents to test whether high doses of these compounds would inhibit or prevent the growth of colon cancers. Most of the NSAIDs tested effectively inhibited colorectal tumours in rats and mice. Whereas these early studies assessed the broad hypothesis that inhibition of prostaglandin synthesis would inhibit the occurrence or progression of neoplasia, subsequent studies have revealed the probable mechanistic complexity of these processes.

NSAIDs are currently understood to function primarily through a reduction in prostaglandin synthesis by inhibiting the enzyme prostaglandin endoperoxide synthase. This polypeptide enzyme contains both cyclooxygenase and peroxidase activities. It occurs as two isoforms, designated isoforms 1 and 2, which are referred to as cyclooxygenase (COX-1 and COX-2) in the current literature and in this volume. When the term COX is used alone, it denotes a generic property that is conserved in the two isoforms.

Table 1. Some commonly available, conventional non-steroidal anti-inflammatory drugs

Anthranilic acid derivatives
    Flufenamic acid, mefanamic acid
Indomethacin and related derivatives
    Indomethacin, sulindac
Oxicams
    Isoxicam, piroxicam
Phenylalkanoic acid and related derivatives
    Alclofenac, diclofenac, fenclofenac, flurbiprofen, ibuprofen, ketaprofen, naproxen
Pyrazole derivatives
    Azapropazone, dipyrone, oxyphenbutazone, phenylbutazone
Salicylates
    Aspirin, benzorylate, diflunisal, salicylamide, sodium salicylate

---

[1] Aspirin is a protected trade name of Bayer Company in more than 70 countries

1.1 Observational studies of colorectal cancer

Studies of the effect of NSAIDs on the risk for colorectal cancer initially evolved independently of experimental work on the mechanism of action of these drugs. Kune *et al.* (1988) reported a negative association between the incidence of colorectal cancer and use of aspirin, and reductions of lesser magnitude with the use of other NSAIDs. The potential cancer-preventive activity of aspirin was then evaluated in other epidemiological studies (Gann *et al.*, 1993; Greenberg *et al.*, 1993; Suh *et al.*, 1993; Thun *et al.*, 1993). These are described in the chapter on aspirin.

Studies of cancer occurrence in patients with rheumatoid arthritis in Finland (Isomäki *et al.*, 1978; Laakso *et al.*, 1986) and Sweden (Gridley *et al.*, 1993) were motivated by concern that use of NSAIDs might increase the risk for gastric cancer and that chronic immune stimulation due to rheumatoid arthritis might cause lymphatic or haematopoietic cancers.

1.2 Studies in experimental animals

When the findings in humans were published, there was an extant literature on inhibition of colorectal carcinogenesis by NSAIDs in rodent models (Kudo *et al.*, 1980; Pollard & Luckert, 1980; Narisawa *et al.*, 1981; Pollard & Luckert, 1981a,b; Narisawa *et al.*, 1983; Pollard & Luckert, 1983; Pollard *et al.*, 1983; Narisawa *et al.*, 1984; Pollard & Luckert, 1984; Birkenfeld *et al.*, 1987; Reddy *et al.*, 1987; Moorghen *et al.*, 1988; Reddy *et al.*, 1990; Rao *et al.*, 1991; Reddy *et al.*, 1992). Most of these studies are based on inhibition of tumours induced at particular sites by appropriate chemical carcinogens. Their results suggest that rodent models may be useful for evaluating the chemopreventive activity of NSAIDs and for investigating their mechanisms of action. All of the experimental studies involved single compounds and are thus discussed in the individual chapters.

1.3 Drugs considered

The present volume contains evaluations of the cancer-preventive activity of four specific NSAIDs, together with other relevant findings. The drugs covered are aspirin, indomethacin, sulindac and piroxicam. These NSAIDs were selected because of the amount and nature of the information available on possible cancer-preventive activity. In some studies, NSAIDs or NSAIDs apart from aspirin were addressed as a class. As for many years aspirin was the most commonly used NSAID, studies on NSAIDs in general are covered in that chapter; those on NSAIDs other than aspirin are summarized in the chapter on sulindac. The cancer-preventive activity of NSAIDs as a class was not evaluated.

2. Colorectal cancer

2.1 Descriptive epidemiology

Cancers of the large bowel (colon and rectum) are the third most frequent cancers in the world in people of each sex, after cancers of the lung and stomach in males and after those of the breast and cervix in females. In developed countries, colorectal cancer ranks second; the age-standardized rates are about four times higher than those in developing countries. Thus, about two-thirds of the estimated annual total of 677 000 new cases in 1985 occurred in the developed world, which includes only one-quarter of the world's population (Parkin *et al.*, 1993).

2.2 Biology of colorectal cancer in humans

Malignant tumours are understood to arise from normal cells as a consequence of a multistep process marked by the successive evolution of cell populations with progressively altered growth characteristics. Colorectal cancer is perceived as exemplifying this hypothesis particularly well, because certain intermediate stages in tumour growth are recognized. Aberrant crypt foci are considered to be early preneoplastic lesions that are observed consistently in the colonic mucosa of patients with colorectal cancer (Pretlow *et al.*, 1992). Evidence that several inhibitors of aberrant crypt foci reduce the risk for colorectal tumours in experimental animals suggests that induction of these foci could be used to evaluate new agents for potential preventive properties against colorectal cancer.

Adenomatous colonic polyps are perceived as marking an early stage of cancer development. Patients with an autosomal dominant condition, familial adenomatous polyposis, characterized by the development of hundreds to thousands of polyps, are at greatly increased risk of colorectal cancer and are offered prophylactic colectomy in early adulthood (Burn *et al.,* 1994; Mills *et al.,* 1997). Mutations in the *APC* gene underlie this phenotype and are demonstrable in the earliest stages of most sporadic cases of colon cancer (Powell *et al.,* 1992; Kinzler & Vogelstein, 1996).

There is good evidence that chronic inflammation predisposes to the development of cancer at various sites. Examples (reviewed by Gordon & Weitzman, 1993) include the associations of urinary bladder cancer with schistosomiasis, stones or in-dwelling catheters left for long periods; oesophageal cancer subsequent to reflux oesophagitis or Barrett's oesophagus; pancreatic cancer subsequent to chronic pancreatitis; gastric cancer following gastritis due to *Helicobacter pylori* and cancer of the gall-bladder subsequent to cholecystitis. The corresponding observation for colorectal cancer is primarily an increased risk in patients suffering from long-standing, extensive inflammatory diseases such as ulcerative colitis. Interestingly, a drug structurally similar to aspirin, aminosalicylate, is used in the treatment of this condition.

The molecular basis of malignant transformation mainly involves the activation of genes that are not usually expressed in normal cells (oncogenes) and loss or mutation of genes associated with the control of cell growth (tumour suppressor genes). Colorectal cancer represents the most comprehensive relationship between genetic changes and successive morphological changes marking the development of malignant tumours. Vogelstein and Kinzler (1993) identified the activation of particular oncogenes, including *ras*, and the loss of particular tumour suppressor genes, including *APC* and *p53*, with various stages in tumour growth: development of hyperplastic lesions, growth of adenomas and development of carcinomas (Fig. 1). Most of the genes that have been associated with the development of colorectal cancer are involved in the control of cell growth and/or the maintenance of genomic stability (Table 2).

ras proto-oncogenes have been the subject of studies relevant to the cancer-preventive activity of some NSAIDs. Thus, recent evidence suggests that activation of *ras* proto-oncogenes, coupled with the loss or inactivation of suppressor genes,

induces the malignant phenotype in colonic cells. *ras* proto-oncogenes are functionally related to 21-kDa proteins, ras p21, which are anchored to the cytoplasmic face of the plasma membrane and are believed to function as molecular switches in transmembrane signalling events of cell growth and differentiation (Forrester *et al.,* 1987). By far the most frequent *ras* activation has been observed in codons 12 and 13 of *K-ras*, occurring at a frequency of about 30% in lung adenocarcinomas (Rodenhuis & Slebos, 1992), 40–60% in those in the colon (Burmer *et al.,* 1991) and over 90% in those in the pancreas (Almoguera *et al.,* 1988).

Hereditary non-polyposis colon cancer is an autosomal dominant or recessive condition characterized by the development of multiple cancers at an early age, predominantly in the proximal colon. As adenomas do not occur in large numbers, this syndrome can be distinguished from familial adenomatous polyposis (Jass & Stewart, 1992). Single gene abnormalities leading to hereditary non-polyposis colon cancer may underlie 5–10% of cases of colorectal cancer. The two genes in which causative mutations occur most commonly, *hMLH1* and *hMSH2*, belong to a group responsible for the detection and repair of mismatch mutations during DNA replication (Fishel *et al.,* 1993; Papadopoulos *et al.,* 1994).

Despite the general correlations that have been made between particular genes and the development of carcinomas of the colon, marked heterogeneity is seen between individuals and within tumour cell populations. Thus, some malignant tumours may have only a subset of the genetic changes generally associated with their particular pathological stage. Likewise, although understanding of tumour growth in terms of cellular evolution is widely if not universally accepted, it is not certain that all malignant cancers of the colon develop along this pathway.

2.3 Experimental studies

Knowledge of the cancer-preventive effects of NSAIDs is derived largely from a range of experimental studies. Primary among these are investigations involving administration of these agents to rats and mice treated with chemicals known to cause colon cancer, such as dimethylhydrazine, methylazoxymethanol and azoxymethane. A

Figure 1. Changes that occur during the evolution of a typical colorectal carcinoma in a model of tumour progression in which independent steps are required, leading to the activation of at least one proto-oncogene, coupled with the successive loss of several tumour suppressor genes.

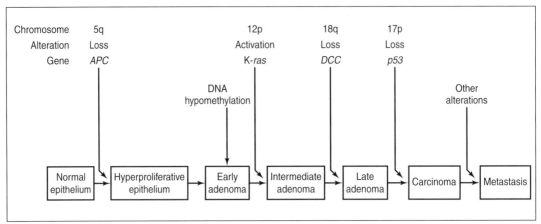

Adapted from Vogelstein & Kinzler (1993)

Table 2. Genes altered in colon cancer

Gene	Chromosome	Tumours with mutations (%)	Class	Action
hMSH2	2	15	Tumour suppressor	DNA repair
K-ras	12	50	Oncogene	Intracellular signalling molecule
Cyclins	Various	4	Oncogene	Regulation of cell cycle
neu/HER2	17	2	Oncogene	Growth factor receptor
myc	8	2	Oncogene	Regulation of gene activity
APC	5	> 70	Tumour suppressor	Regulation of gene activity
DCC	18	> 70	Tumour suppressor	Differentiation signal
p53	17	> 70	Tumour suppressor	Regulation of cell cycle arrest and apoptosis

Adapted from Marx (1993), Vogelstein & Kinzler (1994) and Fazeli et al. (1997)

number of specific tumours, such as those of the colon, urinary bladder and kidney, induced in rodents by carcinogens are known to mimic the histopathological development of the corresponding human cancers. These 'model' systems are therefore used in various aspects of cancer research. The relevance of animal models for human colorectal cancer is indicated by the occurrence in both of the adenoma–carcinoma sequence and by the similarity of histopathological appearance; furthermore, mutations in the *ras* oncogene at codons 12 and 13 are found in colorectal tumours from both humans and experimental animals. Many of the relevant studies are predicated on administration of the maximum tolerated dose (MTD) of an agent, which is defined as the highest dose that causes no more than a 10% weight decrement in comparison with appropriate controls and does not induce mortality or any clinical signs of toxicity that would be predicted to shorten the natural lifespan of the animal.

Experimental models of colorectal cancer have also provided information on the early stages of tumour growth. Thus, aberrant crypt foci have been recognized as early indicators of tumour development in experimental animals (McLellan et al., 1991; Rao et al., 1993; Wargovich et al., 1995), and several models of familial adenomatous polyposis exist in which a mouse strain carries different mutations in the *Apc* gene. The first of these was the Min mouse (Moser et al., 1990; Su et al., 1992; Moser et al., 1993). The Min/+ mouse carries a fully penetrant dominant mutation at codon 850 of the murine *Apc* gene and develops adenomas throughout the intestinal tract, mostly in the small intestine, without treatment by a carcinogen. The phenotypic expression of an *Apc* mutation in the Min/+ mouse is thus different from that of humans with familial adenomatous polyposis, in whom adenomas are found exclusively in the colon and duodenum. Nevertheless, this model has been used to study the chemopreventive properties of several NSAIDs. A molecular basis for the association between inflammation and the growth of colonic polyps has also been demonstrated. Studies of mice carrying an *Apc* mutation which were cross-bred with animals with a disrupted *Cox-2* gene demonstrated that induction of *Cox-2* is an early, rate-limiting step in adenoma formation (Oshima et al., 1996). Adenomas taken from Min/+ mice have a high level of *Cox-2* expression (Williams et al., 1996).

Cell culture systems have also been used to study the possible chemopreventive activity of NSAIDs. Much of the work was carried out with cultured intestinal epithelial cells and colon cancer cell lines. Such studies have shown both prostaglandin-dependent and -independent effects of parent compounds and, in some instances, their metabolites. When interpreting the results of these studies, it is vital to consider the experimental context in which they were generated, particularly with regard to the concentration of the agent and the specific model used. For example, many of the non-prostaglandin effects of NSAIDs shown in these systems may occur only at concentrations of the agent that are unachievable under physiological conditions *in vivo*. In addition, human colorectal tumour cells represent a late stage in the adenoma–carcinoma sequence; therefore, any observed effects may not represent the true mechanism (Kargman et al., 1995).

NSAIDs cause apoptosis when applied to *v-src*-transformed chicken embryo fibroblasts (Lu et al., 1995). This study was the first to indicate that cells that overexpress *Cox-2* may be somewhat resistant to programmed cell death and that this can be reversed by addition of an NSAID.

Few nontransformed intestinal epithelial cell lines are available for in-vitro studies. Cell lines have successfully been derived from the rat small intestine and placed in continuous culture, and several groups have evaluated the mechanisms for growth control of the rat intestinal epithelial-1 (RIE-1) cell line (DuBois et al., 1995). Sulindac sulfide can inhibit mitogenesis of these cells in culture. Additionally, these cells express the inducible Cox-2 enzyme after treatment with cytokines and growth factors (DuBois et al., 1994). The increased expression of Cox-2 alters their apoptotic phenotype and makes them resistant to programmed cell death (Tsujii & DuBois, 1995).

3. Pharmacological action of non-steroidal anti-inflammatory drugs

3.1 Synthesis and action of prostaglandins
Central to the understanding of the pharmacology of NSAIDs is the effect of these agents on prostaglandin synthesis (see the box for explanation of relevant terms).

COX catalyses the biosynthesis of prostaglandins and thromboxanes, which are bioactive lipids that play a role in a broad range of physiological and pathophysiological processes (Hamberg & Samuelsson, 1967; Needleman et al., 1986). COX has two enzymatic activities, a cyclooxygenase activity that oxygenates arachidonic acid to a hydroperoxy endoperoxide, prostaglandin G_2, and a peroxidase that reduces prostaglandin G_2 to the hydroxy endoperoxide, prostaglandin H_2 (Ohki et al., 1979).

NSAIDs act by binding tightly at the cyclooxygenase active site, preventing combination of the enzyme with arachidonic acid (Picot et al., 1994; Loll et al., 1995, 1996). Aspirin is unique among the NSAIDs in that it covalently modifies the protein by transferring its acetyl group to a serine hydroxyl group at the cyclooxygenase active site (Van Der Ouderaa et al., 1980). The acetylation is irreversible, so that aspirin treatment permanently disables COX until it is regenerated. All of the other NSAIDs bind reversibly to the protein. All of the commercially available NSAIDs, including aspirin, inhibit both COX-1 and COX-2 although the extent of inhibition differs (Meade et al., 1993;

Terms used in describing prostaglandin synthesis	
COX-1	Cyclooxygenase-1, a physiologically expressed enzyme that can convert arachidonic acid into prostaglandins and thromboxanes. Also called prostaglandin H synthase-1
COX-2	Cyclooxygenase-2, an inducible enzyme that is often up-regulated at sites of inflammation. Also called prostaglandin H synthase-2
Prostaglandin	A class of physiologically produced substances with effects such as vasodilatation (e.g. prostaglandin E_2) and vasoconstriction (prostaglandin F_2), which are believed to play an important role in the process of inflammation
Prostanoids	Any of several complex fatty acids 20 carbons in length, derived from arachidonic acid and containing an internal 5- or 6-carbon ring. Include prostaenoic acid, prostaglandins and thromboxanes
Eicosanoids	Physiologically active substances derived from arachidonic acid, e.g. prostaglandins, leukotrienes and thromboxane
Autocoid	Chemical produced by one type of cell which affects the functioning of different cells in the same region
Arachidonic acid	An unsaturated fatty acid essential in nutrition; the biological precursor of prostaglandins, thromboxanes and leukotrienes
Thromboxane	A series of compounds formed directly from prostaglandins; the name is derived from their physiological effect on platelet aggregation
Lipoxygenase	An enzyme that can convert arachidonic acid and other unsaturated fatty acids into leukotrienes
Leukotriene	Lipoxygenase enzyme product with postulated role in inflammation and allergy; differs structurally from the related prostanoids by the absence of a central ring

Laneuville *et al.*, 1994; O'Neill *et al.*, 1994; Gierse *et al.*, 1995).

The emphasis in this volume is mainly on prostaglandins, since inhibition of their synthesis is known to be a common mechanisms of action of NSAIDs (Vane, 1971); however, other metabolites of arachidonic acid, such as the leukotrienes and lipoxins, may also affect tumorigenesis (Marnett, 1992). Furthermore, other eicosanoids such as eicosopentanoic acid, may also be metabolized by cyclooxygenases and peroxidases to prostaglandins (Fig. 2).

COX-1 is expressed constitutively in a number of cell types and tissues, including gastric mucosa (Williams & DuBois, 1996). In contrast, *COX-2* belongs to a class of genes referred to as 'immediate early' or 'early growth response' genes, which are expressed rapidly and transiently after stimulation of cultured cells by growth factors, cytokines and tumour promoters (Nathans *et al.*, 1988; Herschman, 1991); *COX-2* expression is thus increased in inflammatory cells and at sites of inflammation (Masferrer *et al.*, 1994). It is also increased in malignant colorectal epithelial cells, fibroblasts and tumour vascular endothelium (Sano *et al.*, 1995).

The identification of two different forms of COX and their differential tissue distribution raised the possibility that selective COX inhibitors could be developed that would modulate the catalytic activity of only one of the forms. For example, one might expect COX-2-selective inhibitors to be anti-inflammatory and analgesic but to lack the gastrointestinal complications that are responsible for the dose-limiting toxicity of the currently available NSAIDs (DeWitt *et al.*, 1993).

3.2 Prostaglandins and human tumours

Numerous reports published over the past two decades provide overwhelming evidence of a significant association between prostaglandins and carcinogenesis (Jaffe, 1974; Lupulescu, 1978a,b; Karmali, 1980; Honn *et al.*, 1981). Increased levels of prostaglandins, most notably E_2, have been detected in many malignant tumours. Prostaglandins stimulate tumour growth and dramatically increase DNA and RNA synthesis in cancer cells (Lupulescu, 1975, 1977, 1978b). They presumably act as co-carcinogens by enhancing the rate of tumour progression (Lupulescu, 1978a). The finding that prostaglandins bind to nuclear chromatin and alter DNA synthesis further supports the hypothesis that they are tumour promoters (Lupulescu, 1980).

Increased levels of prostaglandins E_2, $F_{2\alpha}$ and all prostaglandins have been documented in medullary carcinoma of the thyroid (Williams *et al.*, 1968), ganglioneuroma, neuroblastoma, phaeochromocytoma, carcinoids (Sandler *et al.*,

Figure 2. Biosynthesis of eicosanoids

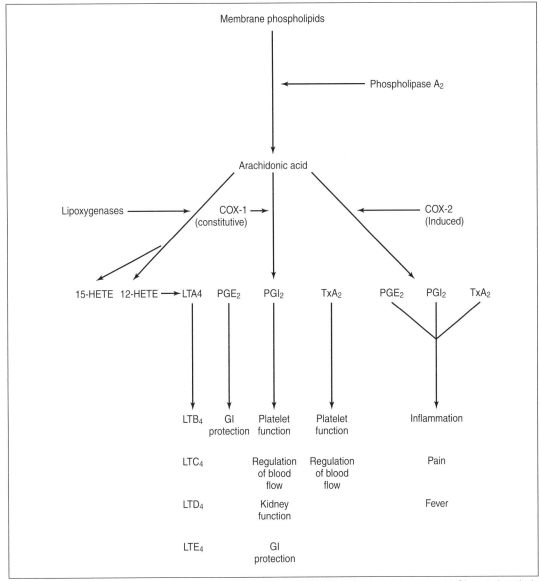

COX, cyclooxygenase; PG, prostaglandin; LT, leukotriene; Tx, thromboxane; HETE, hydroeicosatetraenoic acid; GI, gastrointestinal

1968), Kaposi's sarcoma (Bhana *et al.*, 1971), renal-cell carcinoma (Cummings & Robertson, 1977), lung cancer (Sandler *et al.,* 1968; Hubbard *et al.*, 1988), oesophageal carcinomas (Botha *et al.*, 1986), squamous-cell carcinomas of the head and neck (El Attar & Lin, 1987), breast cancers (Bennett *et al.*, 1977a, 1979) and colorectal cancers (Jaffe, 1974; Bennett & Del Tacca, 1975; Bennett *et al.*, 1977b; Lange *et al.*, 1985; Rigas *et al.*, 1993). In later studies, arachidonate, the substrate from which prostanoids are derived (Bennett *et al.*, 1987) and other eicosanoid metabolites were measured in various tumours (Dreyling *et al.*, 1986; Shimakura &

Boland, 1992; Marnett, 1992; Ghosh & Myers, 1996).

In some tumours, the concentrations of prostaglandins measured in homogenized samples of tissue or in venous blood draining from the tumour correlate with its size and/or invasiveness. Narisawa et al. (1990) observed that the level of prostaglandin E_2 in blood from human colorectal cancers was higher when the cancers were large or locally invasive. Similarly, Klapan et al. (1992) related plasma prostaglandin E_2 concentrations to the invasiveness of head-and-neck cancers. Several studies have shown that breast nodules contain more total prostanoids when they are malignant, and even more when they are metastatic or associated with shorter survival (Bennett et al., 1977a, 1979, Rolland et al., 1980).

The physiology of eicosanoids is complicated, however, in that the same autocoid may have opposite effects in different organs. For example, prostaglandin E_2 inhibits tumour growth in gastric KATO III and AGS carcinoma cell lines (Nakamura et al., 1991; Shimakura & Boland, 1992), yet appears to promote tumorigenesis at other sites. Such organ specificity may be analogous to the protective function of prostaglandin E_2 in the human stomach (Miller, 1983), despite its contribution to inflammation elsewhere.

It is also uncertain whether tumour epithelial cells or inflammatory cells are important producers of prostaglandins. Only one of three human colorectal cancer cell lines (adenocarcinomas and carcinomas) produced detectable eicosanoid levels in a survey by Hubbard et al. (1988). Tissue-fixed macrophages produce prostaglandin E_2 in colorectal cancers (Maxwell et al., 1990), and nonmalignant fibrous tissue was associated with increased prostaglandin synthesis in colorectal mucosa (Bennett et al., 1977b).

The conclusion that the increased activity of COX-2 and its prostaglandin products plays a direct role in tumorigenesis is suggested by a number of observations.

It has been demonstrated that COX-2 expression is greater in human colorectal adenocarcinomas than in adjacent normal colonic mucosa (Eberhart et al., 1994; Gustafson-Svärd et al., 1996; Kutchera et al., 1996), and it increases progressively from 40–50% in colorectal adenomas to 85–90% in carcinomas (Eberhart et al., 1994). These

findings have been confirmed by other investigators, who have shown elevated levels of COX-2 protein in colorectal tumours by western blotting (Kargman et al., 1995) and immunohistochemical staining (Sano et al., 1995). COX-2 is found in some (Caco-2, LoVo) but not all (LS123, SW480) cell lines of human colorectal cancers (Hecht et al., 1995). Experiments conducted on transfected colon tumour cells indicate that overexpression of COX-2 may be due partially to abnormal constitutive transcription of the COX-2 promoter (Kutchera et al., 1996). There are markedly elevated levels of Cox-2 messenger RNA and protein in colonic tumours that develop in rodents after treatment with a carcinogen (DuBois et al., 1996a) and in adenomas taken from Min mice (Williams et al., 1996). These observations of elevated Cox-2 expression in three different models of colorectal carcinogenesis have led to the hypothesis that COX-2 expression is causally related to colorectal tumorigenesis. A recent study demonstrated a 40–49% reduction in aberrant crypt formation in carcinogen-treated rats that were given a selective Cox-2 inhibitor (Reddy et al., 1996). Another report provides genetic evidence that directly links Cox-2 expression to intestinal tumorigenesis (Oshima et al., 1996; Prescott & White, 1996). In this study, mice lacking the Apc gene were generated, which developed hundreds of tumours per intestine. When these mice were bred with mice lacking Cox-2, there was an 80–90% reduction in tumour multiplicity in the homozygous null offspring. These results point to two important findings: (i) Cox-2 may act as a tumour promoter in the intestine, and (ii) increased levels of Cox-2 expression may result directly from disruption of the Apc gene (Prescott & White, 1996). These results clearly demonstrate that COX-2 is a feasible target for future strategies for the prevention and treatment of colorectal cancer.

Although there is strong evidence that inhibition of COX (especially, COX-2) contributes to the ability of NSAIDs to inhibit the development of colorectal cancer, the mechanisms by which COX expression contributes to tumorigenesis are unclear. Prostaglandins and thromboxane, the products of arachidonic acid oxygenation via the cyclooxygenase pathway, have diverse biological effects, including stimulation of cell proliferation, suppression of the immune response and alteration of haemodynamic properties (Marnett, 1992). Overexpression of *Cox-2* in rat intestinal epithelial cells induces a delay in G_1 and renders them resistant to the induction of apoptosis by sodium butyrate (Tsujii & DuBois, 1995; DuBois *et al.*, 1996b). Each prostaglandin and thromboxane has a specific *trans*-membrane, G-protein-linked receptor coupled to an intracellular signalling pathway. Thus, there are multiple mechanisms by which the products formed from COX could enhance the growth of transformed colonic epithelial cells.

3.3 Alternative mechanisms
3.3.1 Mechanisms independent of prostaglandins
Several lines of evidence indicate that the mechanism of action of NSAIDs is not mediated by prostaglandins. Their ability to inhibit growth and block cell differentiation has been shown in several tumour cell lines (Santoro *et al.*, 1976; Tutton & Barkla, 1980; Karmali, 1983). Furthermore, prostaglandin-induced inhibition of DNA synthesis has been reported (Craven *et al.*, 1983). In another investigation, the concentrations of NSAIDs that inhibited the growth of human fibroblasts and rat hepatoma cell lines were poorly correlated with the levels reported in other studies (DeMello *et al.*, 1980). Other reports suggest that NSAIDs induce apoptosis in colon tumour cells, including some lines that do not express COX or make prostaglandin (Elder *et al.*, 1996; Hanif *et al.*, 1996). Thus, NSAIDs may exert their chemopreventive effects on colon tumour cells by a combination of prostaglandin-dependent and -independent mechanisms.

Other possible actions include alternative facilitation of the formation of hydroxy eicosatetranoic acid (see Fig. 2), reduction of phosphodiesterase and protein kinase activity and modulation of immune and angiogenic responses (Benamouzig *et al.*, 1997). The high levels of salicylic acid in plants have been shown to be related to the induction of apoptosis in response to infection (Hunt *et al.*, 1996). At the site of invasion of a pathogen in plants, programmed cell death is the primary response in order to localize the disease. In addition, plants possess an inducible resistance mechanism, which is dependent upon accumulation of salicylic acid (Delaney *et al.*,

1994). This system enhances apoptosis at other sites in response to the same infectious agent. A study in the Netherlands demonstrated negligible quantities of salicylic acid in the current western diet, presumably as a result of agricultural control of plant pathogens (Janssen *et al.*, 1996).

The accumulation of genetic mutations in specific tissues appears to play an important role in malignant transformation. One well-known directly acting mutagen and lipid peroxidation product, malondialdehyde, can be generated by the cyclooxygenase pathway via enzymatic and non-enzymatic degradation of prostaglandin H_2 and also by lipid peroxidation of polyunsaturated fatty acids (Hamberg & Samuelsson, 1967; Mukai & Goldstein, 1976; Diczfalusy *et al.*, 1977). The mutagenicity of malondialdehyde has been demonstrated in several bacterial and mammalian systems (Mukai & Goldstein, 1976; Basu & Marnett, 1983), and its carcinogenic potential has been documented in rats (Spalding, 1988). Moreover, in human colorectal tumours, elevated levels of malondialdehyde were significantly correlated with prostaglandin E_2 concentrations (Hendricks *et al.*, 1994). Thus, prevention of malondialdehyde-induced mutagenesis may be yet another indirect mechanism relevant to the cancer-preventive action of NSAIDs.

3.3.2 Effects on non-cancerous tissues
Any link between up-regulated COX expression in cancerous tissue and the initial development of that cancer is unclear. However, COX-2 is also up-regulated in inflammatory tissues, and there is good evidence that inflammation due to, for example, *Helicobacter* gastritis and ulcerative colitis, is associated with cancer development. In the latter case, any reduction in the risk for colorectal cancer by aminosalicylate may thus be related to suppression of inflammatory activity rather than to an intrinsic effect on cell behaviour (Mulder *et al.*, 1996). It remains to be determined whether pharmacological down-regulation of induced COX-2 in inflamed tissues would interfere with any propensity to develop cancer. In this context, it should be noted that nitric oxide, another inflammatory mediator, may be involved in multistage carcinogenesis (Ohshima & Bartsch, 1994), and nitric oxide appears to activate COX enzymes (Salvemini *et al.*, 1993).

3.3.3 Cytochrome P450

A further possible mechanism is through inhibition of cytochrome P450 monooxygenase activity. Activation of the carcinogen 4-(methylnitrosamino)-1-(3-pyridyl)-1-butanone by some NSAIDs has been claimed to occur through inhibition of this enzyme (Bilodeau *et al.*, 1995).

Co-oxidation of xenobiotics through a COX-mediated mechanism has been the subject of several recent reviews (Eling *et al.*, 1990; Marnett, 1990; Smith *et al.*, 1991). While the possibility was raised that this pathway represents an alternative to the cytochrome P450 metabolizing enzymes, it is now generally accepted that it does not play a significant role in systemic drug metabolism; however, data linking urinary bladder cancer to the oxidation of aromatic amines in this tissue (Rice *et al.*, 1985) suggest that COX plays a role in producing tissue-specific carcinogens (Marnett, 1990).

A wide variety of potential environmental carcinogens, including polycyclic aromatic hydrocarbons, hydrazine, aromatic amines and phenols, are oxidized through the peroxidase activity of COX (Boyd & Eling, 1987; Reed, 1988; Schlosser *et al.*, 1989; Eling *et al.*, 1990; Smith *et al.*, 1991). Co-production of active oxygen species such as superoxide anions, hydrogen peroxide and hydroxyl radicals which are known to damage cellular DNA, may contribute to tumour initiation and promotion (Ames *et al.*, 1993; Gordon & Weitzman, 1993). Indeed, the peroxidase-generating activity of COX has been implicated in the toxicity of several xenobiotics, including benzene (Gaido & Weirda, 1987; Pirozzi *et al.*, 1989). COX catalyses conversion of the benzene metabolite hydroquinone into reactive oxygen products that accumulate in bone marrow and damage DNA (Lewis *et al.*, 1988).

4. Adverse effects

Many studies have shown that NSAIDs at doses used for the treatment of arthritis increase the risk for ulcer complications by two- to five-fold (Gabriel *et al.*, 1991; Bollini *et al.*, 1992; Henry *et al.*, 1996). It has been estimated in several populations that 15–35% of all ulcer complications are due to these drugs (Somerville *et al.*, 1986; Griffin *et al.*, 1988, 1991; Henry *et al.*, 1991; Laporte *et al.*, 1991; Gutthann *et al.*, 1994; Langman *et al.*,

1994). In the United States alone, there are an estimated 24 000 hospitalizations and 2600 deaths annually among patients with rheumatoid arthritis (Fries *et al.*, 1991a).

The rates of hospital deaths associated with peptic ulcer disease are 2–10% (Laporte *et al.*, 1991; Savage *et al.*, 1993; Garcia Rodriquez & Jick, 1994; Gutthann *et al.*, 1994), the higher estimates being those for older populations. The rate of fatal complications in elderly NSAID users is close to 1 per 1000 person-years of NSAID use; it is higher for those with additional risk factors such as a prior history of ulcer disease.

Variations in both the dose and duration of use of NSAIDs and in host factors are important in determining the rates of disease for individuals. Initial use and use of higher doses have been associated with higher risks for adverse effects (Griffin *et al.*, 1991). In a large meta-analysis (Henry *et al.*, 1996), most of the 12 NSAIDs evaluated were statistically indistinguishable with regard to the risk for ulcer complications; however, some were consistently associated with higher rates of such complications in individual studies. Henry *et al.* attempted to find a ranking order that best summarized the sequence of risks observed. In this analysis, with 1 being the most and 12 the least toxic, aspirin ranked 5.

The combination of NSAIDs and oral corticosteroids increased the risk for ulcer complications by 13–15 times that of non-users of either drug, such that older persons using this combination of drug have a hospitalization rate for ulcers of 5–6% per year (Piper *et al.*, 1991; Gutthann *et al.*, 1994).

Fries *et al.* (1991b) based a toxicity index for NSAIDs on the frequency and severity of a variety of adverse events among 2747 patients with rheumatoid arthritis receiving 11 different NSAIDs. The signs and symptoms (including rashes, oedema, central nervous system symptoms and gastrointestinal symptoms) were weighted to develop a score for each NSAID. This score was also adjusted for a large number of potentially confounding variables, including age, sex, other drug use and other measures of co-morbidity and disability. Aspirin (mean dose, 2415 mg) had the lowest adjusted toxicity score; sulindac (379 mg) and piroxicam (19 mg) had intermediate scores, with ranks of 5 and 6, respectively; and indomethacin (100 mg) had the highest score. The latter was heavily influenced by central nervous system symptoms, whereas the ranking of the other NSAIDs was influenced more strongly by gastrointestinal symptoms and complications.

NSAID treatment has been associated with stricture, acute bleeding, perforation and chronic inflammatory lesions in both the small and large bowel (Langman *et al.*, 1985; Ravi *et al.*, 1986; Bjarnason *et al.*, 1987a,b; Kaufmann & Taubin, 1987; Rampton, 1987; Banerjee, 1989). NSAIDs also cause dose-dependent increases in the frequency and severity of dyspepsia, haemorrhage and perforation. Death may ensue (Griffin *et al.*, 1988; Guess *et al.*, 1988; Gabriel *et al.*, 1991; Griffin *et al.*, 1991; Garcia-Rodriquez *et al.*, 1992; Smalley *et al.*, 1995). Symptoms in the upper gastrointestinal tract are common and are a frequent reason both for withdrawal of NSAIDs and for concomitant treatment with H_2 receptor antagonists, antacids, sucralfate or misoprostol (Hogan *et al.*, 1994; Smalley *et al.*, 1996).

Gastrointestinal lesions may result from the drug's direct action on the mucosa through oxygen radical-mediated lipid peroxidation and the subsequent accumulation of lipoxygenase and leukotriene products resulting from the shift of the arachidonic acid cascade into the 5-lipoxygenase pathway (Lippmann, 1974; Gaffney & Williamson, 1979; Cronen *et al.*, 1982; Ligumsky *et al.*, 1983; Flower *et al.*, 1985; Lippton *et al.*, 1987; Meyers *et al.*, 1991; Kapui *et al.*, 1993; Yoshikawa *et al.*, 1993; Zahavi *et al.*, 1995; Elliot *et al.*, 1996; Rioux & Wallace, 1996; Takeuchi *et al.*, 1996).

Although the gastrointestinal adverse effects of NSAIDs form by far the commonest and most important variety, there is a range of others. They include toxic hepatitis, blood dyscrasias, skin disorders, interstitial nephritis and cystitis. In general, these are rare and in some cases appear to be largely restricted to particular drugs.

4.1 Ulceration

Host factors that increase the rate of serious ulcer disease include older age (Garcia Rodriguez & Jick, 1994; Gutthann *et al.*, 1994), history of prior ulcer, gastrointestinal haemorrhage, dyspepsia and previous intolerance to NSAIDs (Fries *et al.*, 1991; Garcia Rodriguez & Jick,

1994; Gutthann *et al.*, 1994; Silverstein *et al.*, 1995), use of corticosteroids (Fries *et al.*, 1991a; Piper *et al.*, 1991; Garcia Rodriguez & Jick, 1994; Gutthann *et al.*, 1994), use of anticoagulants (Shorr *et al.*, 1993; Garcia Rodriguez *et al.*, 1994) and various measures of poorer health (Fries *et al.*, 1991a; Griffin *et al.*, 1991; Silverstein *et al.*, 1995).

4.1.1 Age

Hospitalizations for ulcer disease have been reported to be fewer than 1 per 1000 annually in most populations under the age of 60 years (Schoon *et al.*, 1989; Steering Committee of the Physicians' Health Study Research Group, 1989; Henry & Robertson, 1993; Johnson *et al.*, 1994a; Garcia Rodriguez & Jick, 1994). The rates increase with age, however, so people aged 65 years and older have incidences of 2–6 per 1000 (Laporte *et al.*, 1991; Garcia Rodriguez *et al.*, 1992; Graves & Kozak, 1992; Henry & Robertson, 1993; Shorr *et al.*, 1993; Smalley *et al.*, 1995). The higher absolute rate of ulcer complications associated with age has been observed consistently (Fries *et al.*, 1991a; Garcia Rodriguez *et al.*, 1992; Garcia Rodriguez & Jick, 1994; Gutthann *et al.*, 1994; Lanza *et al.*, 1995; Silverstein *et al.*, 1995).

For persons 65 years and older enrolled in the Tennessee Medicaid programme, the annual number of hospitalizations for ulcer was approximately 4 per 1000 person-years among non-users and 17 per 1000 among NSAID users (Smalley *et al.*, 1995). Because the rate of ulcer disease is much higher in older persons, multiplying this relatively high rate by a factor of 4 has a much greater impact than for populations with a low baseline rate. For patients with rheumatoid arthritis treated with NSAIDs, the incidence of hospitalization or death from acute gastrointestinal events increased from 3 to 19 to 42 per 1000 person–years of use among patients aged < 63, 63–75 and > 75 years, respectively (Fries *et al.*, 1991a).

4.1.2 History of ulcer disease

In most studies, NSAID use by patients with a past history of ulceration, haemorrhage or dyspepsia was associated with a lower relative risk than for patients without such a history (Henry *et al.*, 1996). The risk for ulcer complication in patients who both used NSAIDs and had a history of ulcer disease was 14–17 times that of patients who had neither of these factors (Garcia Rodriguez & Jick, 1994; Gutthann *et al.*, 1994).These relative risks are consistent with annual rates of hospitalization or death from gastrointestinal disease of 4–8% in a cohort of arthritis patients with both these factors (Fries *et al.*, 1991b).

4.1.3 Helicobacter pylori

Helicobacter pylori and NSAIDs are the major independent causes of both gastric and duodenal ulcers (Borody *et al.*, 1991; Nensey *et al.*, 1991; Borody *et al.*, 1992). Although *H. pylori* infection may not increase the risk for NSAID-associated ulcers (Graham *et al.*, 1991; Loeb *et al.*, 1992), *H. pylori* infection identifies persons with a past history and a higher risk for ulcer disease. Persons with both of these factors have a much higher rate of ulcer disease than those with neither of these factors (Martin *et al.*, 1989). It remains plausible that eradication of *H. pylori* in people with proven ulcer disease (current or past) would reduce the risk for NSAID-induced gastroduodenal ulceration and bleeding.

4.1.4 Corticosteroids

Oral corticosteroids, even at relatively low doses have been reported to double the rate of serious ulcer disease (Fries *et al.*, 1991a; Piper *et al.*, 1991; Garcia Rodriguez & Jick, 1994; Gutthann *et al.*, 1994). The combination of NSAIDs and oral corticosteroids increases the risk for ulcer complication by 13–15 times that of non-users of either drug, such that older persons using this combination of drugs have a hospitalization rate for ulcer of 5–6% per year (Piper *et al.*, 1991; Gutthann *et al.*, 1994).

4.1.5 Anticoagulants

Anticoagulants have no known or postulated ulcerogenic effect, yet they have a profound effect on bleeding. In the outpatient setting, these drugs increase the risk for upper gastrointestinal bleeding by three- to sixfold (Garcia Rodriguez & Jick, 1994; Shorr *et al.*, 1993). The combination of NSAIDs and anticoagulants greatly increases the rate of such complications, such that older person using this combination have a rate of hospitalization for upper gastrointestinal haemorrhage of about 3% per year (Shorr *et al.*, 1993).

4.2 Asthma

About 10% of adults with asthma develop acute, idiosyncratic bronchoconstriction after ingesting aspirin and other NSAIDs (Fischer *et al.*, 1994; Staton *et al.*, 1996). Often called 'aspirin-sensitive' asthma, this condition can be precipitated by currently available NSAIDs (Szczeklik, 1994). The symptoms begin within 15 min to 4 h (usually 1 h) after NSAID ingestion, and may include rhinorrhoea, conjunctival irritation, scarlet flushing of the head and neck and severe, even life-threatening asthma. The respiratory symptoms may continue beyond discontinuation of NSAIDs.

4.3 Drug interactions

Drug interactions may result in inhibition of drug metabolism or displacement of protein binding. Battellino *et al.* (1990) used the elimination rate of antipyrine to estimate the ability of a subject to biotransform drugs metabolized mainly through the oxidative reactions of the cytochrome P450 system. They found that antipyrine metabolism was impaired by concurrent administration of piroxicam. Therefore, drugs may accumulate and become toxic when piroxicam is administered simultaneously with steroid hormones or other compounds metabolized by the mixed-function oxidase system. Increased cytochrome P450 content and aryl hydrocarbon hydroxylase activity have been observed under such conditions (Mostafa *et al.*, 1990). Long-term administration of piroxicam may thus affect the intensity and duration of action of environmental carcinogens that are metabolized by the cytochrome P450-dependent monooxygenase system.

NSAIDs interact with many drugs, as reviewed by Verbeeck (1990; see also Table 3). A number of drugs, including warfarin, diazepam and ibuprofen, may competitively displace piroxicam from its serum albumin binding (Matsuyama *et al.* 1987; Brée *et al.*, 1990). The activities of lithium, methotrexate and, to a lesser extent cyclosporin may be affected by concomitant administration of an NSAID. Interaction with oral anticoagulants, oral antihyperglycaemic agents and the anticonvulsants phenytoin and valproic acid (sodium valproate) could lead to increased NSAID levels in blood. This is potentially dangerous, since high systemic concentrations of NSAIDs may reach the stomach and kidney and mediate toxicity.

Table 3. Therapeutic agents that can interact with non-steroidal anti-inflammatory drugs

Adsorbent antidiarrhoeal drugs

Antacids

Antihypertensive drugs

Cholestyramine

Cimetidine

Cisapride

Cyclosporin

Digoxin

Domperidone

Famotidine

Lithium

Methotrexate

Metoclopramide

Mucoprotective agents

Phenytoin

Ranitidine

Valproic acid

Warfarin

From Said & Foda (1989); Verbeeck (1990); Milligan *et al.* (1993); Brouwers & de Smet (1994); Koytchev *et al.* (1994); Combe *et al.* (1995); Mené *et al.* (1995)

Interactions with digoxin are most likely to occur in the elderly, newborns and patients with renal impairment. Piroxicam can interact with antico-agulant coumarin drugs, can influence thrombo-cyte aggregation and can enhance bleeding, espe-cially in patients with risk factors such as advanced age, chronic or acute peptic ulcer and use of corticosteroids.

NSAIDs have been shown to antagonize the action of most antihypertensive agents, so that their doses must be increased; however, concomi-tant administration of NSAIDs often prevents optimal control of blood pressure, particularly among black and elderly patients (Mené *et al.*, 1995). Piroxicam and indomethacin had the most marked effects and sulindac and aspirin the least (Johnson *et al.*, 1994b). The mechanism of the interaction is unknown.

4.4   Taking account of toxic effects

The strength of the evidence for the value of individual NSAIDs in preventing colorectal cancer will necessarily vary according to the intensity and breadth of searches for the benefi-cial effects obtainable with individual agents, of comparisons between agents and of examinations and comparisons of toxic effects. Although NSAIDs have many common structural features and anti-inflammatory, analgesic and antipyretic properties, they can differ notably with regard to the doses normally employed, their clinical phar-macological and pharmacokinetic characteristics and their toxicity.

Although the choice of a conventional NSAID should be among those for which there is the best evidence of efficacy and lack of toxicity, such information is not yet available. Most of the epi-demiological studies addressed NSAIDs as a class or separated only aspirin and non-aspirin NSAIDs, and most of the clinical studies, mainly in patients with familial adenomatous polyposis, investigated sulindac. Although some studies indicate large differences between NSAIDs in their toxicity to the upper gastrointestinal tract, these findings may reflect anti-inflammatory potency and dosage rather than any intrinsic difference in toxicity. Investigations in experimental animals are of limited value for making a choice, as opposed to demonstrating effects and elucidating mechanisms, as few cross-comparisons can be made and direct application of the findings to humans cannot be assumed.

4.5   Mitigating side-effects

Alternative strategies for minimizing toxicity include the co-administration of agents such as hyposecretory drugs, which can reduce the risk for peptic ulceration, and use of more selective NSAIDs which inhibit COX-2.

A range of drugs, including histamine H_2 antag-onists, proton pump inhibitors and synthetic prostaglandins, have been shown to reduce, to varying degrees, the risk for developing an ulcer during concurrent use of NSAIDs. Each has potential benefits and risks (Wallace, 1997). Histamine H_2 antagonists are more effective in reducing the frequency of duodenal than gastric ulceration (Ehsanullah *et al.*, 1988). Potency and dosage may partly explain this divergence, since famotidine at high doses appears to be more effec-tive than ranitidine in diminishing the risk for gastric ulcer (Taha *et al.*, 1996). Concern about the potential hazards of long-term use of H_2 antagonists now appears to be unfounded (Johnson *et al.*, 1996).

Proton pump inhibitors can prevent both gastric and duodenal ulceration (Scheiman *et al.*, 1994), but good evidence of long-term safety is lacking. The intense inhibition of acid output associated with use of drugs like omeprazole has been associated with a clear elevation of serum gastrin levels, and correlations have been noted between serum gastrin concentration and propensity for colon cancer (Watson *et al.*, 1995). Synthetic prostaglandins such as the prostaglandin E_1 analogue, misoprostil, have licensed indications in the prevention of damage to the upper gastrointestinal tract caused by NSAIDs. Instituting treatment with synthetic prostaglandins while at the same time evaluating whether suppression of their production by NSAIDs is useful would, however, be aberrant.

Newer NSAIDs which, to a greater or lesser degree, inhibit only COX-2 activity are particularly interesting because they could reduce upper gastrointestinal damage, which is probably dependent on suppression of COX-1. These newer drugs cannot, however, be assumed to be free of toxicity. Chemopreventive strategies may imply years of treatment of individuals many of whom may not have developed the disease under scrutiny. Detailed consideration of overall risk–benefit relationships will thus be important.

5. Recommendations for research

In comparison with many areas of research, investigation of chemoprevention is at an early stage. Not surprisingly, therefore, the research needs with regard to NSAIDs are similar to those for other types of chemopreventive agents. The current evidence is strong enough to indicate that NSAIDs as a group have properties that make them potentially important chemotherapeutic agents; however, there are significant gaps in knowledge, which are summarized below.

Most studies in experimental animals have been conducted with varying protocols and doses and have involved various agents. As a consequence, firm evidence for the relative potency of individual NSAIDs is lacking. In tissue culture, unrealistically high concentrations of NSAIDs have often been used to achieve effects, and in experimental animals attempts have not always been made to match the drug levels to those that might be attained in humans. There is a general deficiency of evidence about the levels achieved, whether in plasma, target tissues or colorectal tumours. Information on the levels achieved will be particularly important when the xenobiotic in question undergoes significant enterohepatic circulation. Finally, individual biomarkers such as cell proliferation as a measure of apoptosis or proliferation have not been applied consistently as surrogate end-points.

In epidemiological studies, there is a general lack of evidence on which to base an evaluation of the possible beneficial effects of individual non-aspirin NSAIDs. Such evidence may be obtainable within existing databases which hold information on drug usage and clinical outcomes, such as Medicard in the USA and the General Practitioner Research Database in the United Kingdom. Secondly, there is a relative lack of information on the possible benefits of NSAIDs against cancers outside the colon and rectum; again, this may be obtainable within the existing databases.

Clinical trials of cancer-preventive agents necessarily take many years to achieve results, and it is important that they be well designed and executed. In order to enhance quality and to minimize duplication of effort, it would be sensible to maintain a register of current studies, including sufficient detail for a realistic evaluation.

One feature of trials is likely to be the inclusion of aims to minimize drug toxicity. This design feature may require factorial methods and the inclusion of other promising chemopreventive agents, such as vitamin D and its analogues, in the hope that multiplicative actions can be obtained with reduced general toxicity. It is also noteworthy that slow-release NSAID preparations, which might reduce the general toxicity and delivery of the drug to the colon, could be of special value, although evidence of reduced gastric toxicity is limited.

Similar questions about the specificity, sensitivity and positive predictive value of surrogate end-points and biomarkers arise in clinical trials and experimental studies.

Randomized trials have been acknowledged as the means of providing unequivocal information about the efficacy of chemopreventive agents. The design of further trials of NSAIDs will be influenced greatly by experimental indications of which agents are best subject to evaluation in this way. At the same time, it is becoming evident that the extended period required for certain chemopreventive agents to exert an effect makes study by randomized trial awkward. Observational studies may be the only adequate vehicle for such long-term investigations in low-risk populations.

6. Procedures used

In general, the content of the chapters in this Handbook is as indicated in the Preamble. The only known use of these agents is as pharmaceutical drugs. Accordingly, 'Use' is covered in Section 2.3, and Section 2.5 is concerned only with exposure as a consequence of taking the drug. The sections on 'Other beneficial effects' address the action of these drugs on cardiovascular health, and no attempt was made to summarize findings on the anti-inflammatory, antipyretic or analgesic effects of these agents.

A limited number of studies are reasonably characterized as involving use of NSAIDs for treatment, rather than prevention, of malignant disease, e.g. administration of a drug to patients with malignant gastric cancer. Such studies were not included.

The definition of 'sufficient evidence of cancer-preventive activity' in humans caused concern to members of the Working Group, because the level of certainty that a causal relationship has been established between the use of an agent and the prevention of human cancer must be higher for chemoprevention than for treatment in order to justify the use of an agent. A particular difficulty that the Working Group faced was to determine whether the available studies sufficed to rule out chance, bias or confounding with reasonable confidence, in the absence of long-term randomized trials specifically designed to test for putative cancer-preventive activity. The underlying problem is that administration of an agent to healthy people in order to prevent a relatively rare event will result in many opportunities for harm that substantially outweigh the benefits. Although this difficult is addressed in the overall evaluation of each agent, it necessarily influenced members of the Working Group in reaching their conclusions about the weight of the evidence.

7. References

Almoguera, C., Shibata, D., Forrester, K., Martin, J., Arnheim, N. & Perucho, M. (1988) Most human carcinomas of the exocrine pancreas contain mutant c-K-*ras* genes. *Cell*, **53**, 549–554

Ames, B.N., Shigenaga, M.K. & Hagen, T.M. (1993) Oxidants, antioxidants, and the degenerative diseases of aging. *Proc. natl Acad. Sci. USA*, **90**, 7915–7922

Banerjee, A.K. (1989) Enteropathy induced by non-steroidal antiinflammatory drugs. Often subclinical, but may mimic Crohn's disease. *Br. med. J.*, **298**, 1539–1540

Basu, A.K. & Marnett, L.J. (1983) Unequivocal demonstration that malondialdehyde is a mutagen. *Carcinogenesis*, **4**, 331–333

Battellino, L.J., Dorronsoro de Cattoni, S.T. & Ragagnin, C. (1990) Impairment of human antipyrine metabolism by piroxicam. *Can. J. Physiol. Pharmacol.*, **68**, 711–717

Benamouzig, R., Chaussade, S., Little, J., Muñoz, N., Rantureau, J. & Couturier, D. (1997) [Aspirin, nonsteroidal anti-inflammatory agents and colon carcinogenesis.] *Gastroenterol. clin. biol.*, **21** (in press) (in French)

Bennett, A. & Del Tacca, M. (1975) Proceedings: Prostaglandins in human colonic carcinoma. *Gut*, **16**, 409

Bennett, A., Charlier, E.M., McDonald, A.M., Simpson, J.S., Stamford, I.F. & Zebro, T. (1977a) Prostaglandins and breast cancer. *Lancet*, **ii**, 624–626

Bennett, A., Tacca, M.D., Stamford, I.F. & Zebro, T. (1977b) Prostaglandins from tumours of human large bowel. *Br. J. Cancer*, **35**, 881–884

Bennett, A., Berstock, D.A., Raja, B. & Stamford, I.F. (1979) Survival time after surgery is inversely related to the amounts of prostaglandins extracted from human breast cancers. *Br. J. Pharmacol.*, **66**, 451P

Bennett, A., Civier, A., Hensby, C.N., Melhuish, P.B. & Stamford, I.F. (1987) Measurement of arachidonate and its metabolites extracted from human normal and malignant gastrointestinal tissues. *Gut.*, **28**, 315–318

Bhana, D., Hillier, K. & Karim, S.M. (1971) Vasoactive substances in Kaposi's sarcoma. *Cancer*, **27**, 233–237

Bilodeau, J.F., Wang, M., Chung, F.L. & Castonguay, A. (1995) Effecs of nonsteroidal antiinflammatory drugs on oxidative pathways in A/J mice. *Free Radical Biol. Med.*, 18, 47–54

Birkenfeld, S., Zaltsman, Y.A., Krispin, M., Zakut, H., Zor, U. & Kohen, F. (1987) Antitumor effects of inhibitors of arachidonic acid cascade on experimentally induced intestinal tumors. *Dis. Colon Rectum*, 30, 43–46

Bjarnason, I., Zanelli, G., Smith, T., Prouse, P., Williams, P., Smethurst, P., Delacey, G., Gumpel, M.J. & Levi, A.J. (1987a) Nonsteroidal antiinflammatory drug-induced intestinal inflammation in humans. *Gastroenterology*, 93, 480–489

Bjarnason, I., Zanelli, G., Prouse, P., Smethurst, P., Smith, T., Levi, S., Gumpel, M.J. & Levi, A.J. (1987b) Blood and protein loss via small intestinal inflammation induced by non-steroidal antiinflammatory drugs. *Lancet*, ii, 711–714

Bollini, P., Garcia Rodriguez, L.A., Perez Gutthann, S. & Walker, A.M. (1992) The impact of research quality and study design on epidemiologic estimates of the effect of nonsteroidal anti-inflammatory drugs on upper gastrointestinal tract disease. *Arch. intern. Med.*, 152, 1289–1295

Borody, T.J., George, L.L., Brandl, S., Andrews, P., Ostapowicz, N., Hyland, L. & Devine, M. (1991) *Helicobacter pylori*-negative duodenal ulcer. *Am. J. Gastroenterol.*, 86, 1154–1157

Borody, T.J., Brandl, S., Andrews, P., Jankiewicz, E. & Ostapowicz, N. (1992) *Helicobacter pylori*-negative gastric ulcer. *Am. J. Gastroenterol.*, 87, 1403–1406

Botha, J.H., Robinson, K.M., Ramchurren, N., Reddi, K. & Norman, R.J. (1986) Human esophageal carcinoma cell lines: Prostaglandin production, biological properties, and behavior in nude mice. *J. natl Cancer Inst.*, 76, 1053–1056

Boyd, J.A. & Eling, T.E. (1987) Prostaglandin H synthase-catalyzed metabolism and DNA binding by 2-naphthylamine. *Cancer Res.*, 47, 4007–4014

Brée, F., Urien, S., Nguyen, P., Riant, P., Albengres, E. & Tillement, J.P. (1990) A re-evaluation of the HSA-piroxicam interaction. *Eur. J. Drug Metab. Pharmacokinet.*, 15, 303–307

Brouwers, J.R. & de Smet, P.A. (1994) Pharmacokinetic–pharmacodynamic drug interactions with nonsteroidal anti-inflammatory drugs. *Clin. Pharmacokinet.*, 27, 462–485

Burn, J., Chapman, P.D. & Eastham, E.J. (1994) Familial adenomatous polyposis. *Arch. Dis Child.*, 71, 103–105

Combe, B., Edno, L., Lafforgue, P., Bologna, C., Bernard, J.C., Acquaviva, P., Sany, J. & Bressolle, F. (1995) Total and free methotrexate pharmacokinetics, with and without piroxicam, in rheumatoid arthritis patients. *Br. J. Rheumatol.*, 34, 421–428

Craven, P.A., Saito, R. & DeRubertis, F.R. (1983) Role of local prostaglandin synthesis in the modulation of proliferative activity of rat colonic epithelium. *J. clin. Invest.*, 72, 1365–1375

Cronen, P.W., Nagaraj, H.S., Janik, J.S., Groff, D.B., Passmore, J.C. & Hock, C.E. (1982) Effect of indomethacin on mesenteric circulation in mongrel dogs. *J. pediatr. Surg.*, 17, 474–478

Cummings, K.B. & Robertson, R.P. (1977) Prostaglandin: Increased production by renal cell carcinoma. *J. Urol.*, 118, 720–723

Delaney, T.P., Uknes, S., Vernooij, B., Friedrich, L., Weymann, K., Negrotto, D., Gaffney, T., Gut-Rella, M., Kesmann, H., Ward, E. & Ryals, J. (1994) A central role of salicylic acid in plant disease resistance. *Science*, 266, 1247

DeMello, M.C.F., Bayer, B.M. & Beaven, M.A. (1980) Evidence that prostaglandins do not have a role in the cytostatic action of anti-inflammatory drugs. *Biochem. Pharmacol.*, 29, 311–318

DeWitt, D.L., Meade, E.A. & Smith, W.L. (1993) PGH synthase isoenzyme selectivity: The potential for safer nonsteroidal antiinflammatory drugs. *Am. J. Med.*, 95, 40S–44S

Dicztalusy, U., Falardeau, P. & Hammarstrom, S. (1977) Conversion of prostaglandin endoperoxides to C-17 hydroxy acids catalyzed by human platelet thromboxane synthase. *FEBS Lett.*, 84, 271–274

Dreyling, K.W., Hoppe, U., Peskar, B.A., Morgenroth, K., Kozuschek, W. & Peskar, B.M. (1986) Leukotriene synthesis by human gastrointestinal tissues. *Biochim. biophys. Acta*, 878, 184–193

DuBois, R.N., Tsujii, M., Bishop, P., Awad, J.A., Makita, K. & Lanahan, A. (1994) Cloning and characterization of a growth factor-inducible cyclooxygenase gene from rat intestinal epithelial cells. *Am. J. Physiol.*, 266, G822–G827

DuBois, R.N., Bishop, P.R., Graves-Deal, R. & Coffey, R.J. (1995) Transforming growth factor α regulation of the two zinc finger-containing immediate early response genes in intestine. *Cell Growth Differentiation*, 6, 523–529

DuBois, R.N., Radhika, A., Reddy, B.S. & Entingh, A.J. (1996a) Increased cyclooxygenase-2 levels in carcinogen-induced rat colonic tumors. *Gastro-enterology*, 110, 1259–1262

DuBois, R.N., Shao, J.Y., Tsujii, M., Sheng, H. & Beauchamp, R.D. (1996b) G_1 delay in cells overexpressing prostaglandin endoperoxide synthase-2. *Cancer Res.*, 56, 733–737

Eberhart, C.E., Coffey, R.J., Radhika, A., Giardiello, F.M., Ferrenbach, S. & DuBois, R.N. (1994) Up-regulation of cyclooxygenase 2 gene expression in human colorectal adenomas and adenocarcinomas. *Gastroenterology*, 107, 1183–1188

Ehsanullah, R.S.B., Page, M.C., Tildesly, G. & Wood, J.R. (1988) Prevention of gastroduodenal damage induced by non-steroidal anti-inflammatory drugs: Controlled trial of ranitidine. *Br. med. J.*, 297, 1017–1021

El Attar, T.M. & Lin, H.S. (1987) Prostaglandin synthesis by squamous carcinoma cells of head and neck, and its inhibition by non-steroidal anti-inflammatory drugs. *J. oral Pathol.*, 16, 483-487

Elder, D.J.E., Hague, A., Hicks, D.J. & Paraskeva, C. (1996) Differential growth inhibition by the aspirin metabolite salicylate in human colorectal tumor cell lines: Enhancedapoptosis in carcinoma and in vitro-transformed adenoma relative to adenoma cell lines. *Cancer Res.*, 56, 2273–2276

Eling, T.E., Thompson, D.C., Foureman, G.L., Curtis, J.F. & Hughes, M.F. (1990) Prostaglandin H synthase and xenobiotic oxidation. *Ann. Rev. Pharmacol. Toxicol.*, 30, 1–45

Elliott, S.L., Ferris, R.J., Giraud, A.S., Cook, G.A., Skerjo, M.V. & Yeomans, N.D. (1996) Indomethacin damage to rat gastric mucosa is markedly dependent on luminar pH. *Clin. exp. Pharmacol. Physiol.*, 23, 432–434

Fazeli, A., Dickinson, S.L., Hermiston, M.L., Righe, R.V., Steen, R.G., Small, C.G., Stoeckli, E.T., Keino-Masu, K., Masu, M., Rayburn, H., Simons, J., Bronson, R.T., Gordon, J.I., Tessier-Lavigne, M. & Weinberg, R.A. (1997) Phenotype of mice lacking functional (deleted in colorectal cancer) DCC gene. *Nature*, 386, 796–804

Fischer, A.R., Rosenberg, M.A., Lilly, C.M., Callery, J.C., Rubin, P., Cohn, J., White, M.V., Igarashi, Y., Kaliner, M.A., Drazen, J.M. *et al.* (1994) Direct evidence for a role of the mast cell in the nasal response to aspirin in aspirin-sensitive asthma. *J. Allergy clin. Immunol.*, 94, 1046–1056

Fishel, R., Lescoe, M.K., Rao, M.R.S., Copeland, N.G., Jenkins, N.A., Garber, J., Kane, M. & Kolodner, R. (1993) The human mutator gene homolog MSH2 and its association with hereditary nonpolyposis colon cancer. *Cell*, 75, 1027–1038

Flower, R.J., Moncada, S., Vane, J.R., Gilman, A.G., Goodman, L.S., Rall, J.W. & Murad, F. eds (1985) *The Pharmacological Basis of Therapeutics*, 7th Ed., New York, MacMillan Publishing Co., pp. 674–715

Forrester, K., Almoguera, C., Han, K., Grizzle, W.E. & Perucho, M. (1987) Detection of high incidence of *K-ras* oncogenes during human colon tumorigenesis. *Nature*, 327, 298–303

Fries, J.F., Williams, C.A., Bloch, D.A. & Michel, B.A. (1991a) Nonsteroidal anti-inflammatory drug-associated gastropathy: Incidence and risk factor models. *Am. J. Med.*, 91, 213–222

Fries, J.F., Williams, C.A. & Bloch, D.A. (1991b) The relative toxicity of nonsteroidal antiinflammatory drugs. *Arthritis Rheum.*, 34, 1353–1360

Frölich, J.C. (1997) A classification of NSAIDs according to the relative inhibition of cyclooxygenase isoenzymes. *TIPS*, 18, 30–34

Gabriel, S.E., Jaakkimainen, L. & Bombardier, C. (1991) Risk for serious gastrointestinal complications related to use of nonsteroidal anti-inflammatory drugs. A meta-analysis. *Ann. intern. Med.*, 115, 787–796

Gaffney, G.R. & Williamson, H.E. (1979) Effect of indomethacin and meclofenamate on canine mesenteric and celiac blood flow. *Res. Commun. Chem. Pathol. Pharmacol.*, 25, 165–168

Gaido, K.W. & Wierda, D. (1987) Suppression of bone marrow stromal cell function by benzene and hydroquinone is ameliorated by indomethacin. *Toxicol. appl. Pharmacol.*, 89, 378–390

Gann, P.H., Manson, J.E., Glynn, R.J., Buring, J.E. & Hennekens, C.H. (1993) Low dose aspirin and incidence of colorectal tumors in a randomized trial. *J. natl Cancer Inst.*, 85, 1220–1224

Garcia Rodriguez, L.A. & Jick, H. (1994) Risk of upper gastrointestinal bleeding and perforation associated with individual non-steroidal anti-inflammatory drugs [published erratum appears in *Lancet* 1994, 343, 1048]. *Lancet, 343*, 769–772

Garcia Rodriguez, L.A., Walker, A.M. & Perez Gutthann, S. (1992) Nonsteroidal antiinflammatory drugs and gastrointestinal hospitalizations in Saskatchewan: A cohort study. *Epidemiology, 3*, 337–342

Garcia Rodriguez, L.A., Williams, R., Derby, L.E., Dean, A.D. & Jick, H. (1994) Acute liver injury associated with nonsteroidal anti-inflammatory drugs and the role of risk factors. *Arch. intern. Med., 154*, 311–316

Ghosh, J. & Myers, C.E. Jr (1996) Modulation of prostate cancer cell growth and invasion by arachidonic acid: Involvement of the metabolites of 5 lipoxygenase pathway (Abstract). *Proc. Am. Assoc. Cancer Res., 37*, 4111

Gierse, J.K., Hauser, S.D., Creely, D.P., Koboldt, C., Rangwala, S.H., Isakson, P.C. & Seibert, K. (1995) Expression and selective inhibition of the constitutive and inducible forms of human cyclooxygenase. *Biochem. J., 305*, 479–484

Gordon, L.I. & Weitzman, S.A. (1993) Inflammation and cancer. *Cancer J., 6*, 257–261

Graham, D.Y., Lidsky, M.D., Cox, A.M., Evans, D.J., Jr., Evans, D.G., Alpert, L., Klein, P.D., Sessoms, S.L., Michaletz, P.A. & Saeed, Z.A. (1991) Long-term nonsteroidal antiinflammatory drug use and *Helicobacter pylori* infection. *Gastroenterology, 100*, 1653–1657

Greenberg, E.R., Baron, J.A., Freeman, T.H., Mandel, J.S. & Haile, R. (1993) Reduced risk of large bowel adenomas among aspirin users. *J. natl Cancer Inst., 85*, 912–916

Graves, E.J. & Kozak, L.J. (1992) National Hospital Discharge Survey. *Vital Health Stat., 13*, 1–51

Gridley, G., McLaughlin, J.K., Ekbom, A., Klareskog, L., Adami, H.O., Hacker, D.G., Hoover, R. & Fraumeni, J.F. (1993) Incidence of cancer among patients with rheumatoid arthritis. *J. natl. Cancer Inst., 85*, 307–311

Griffin, M.R., Ray, W.A. & Schaffner, W. (1988) Nonsteroidal anti-inflammatory drug use and death from peptic ulcer in elderly persons. *Ann. intern. Med., 109*, 359–363

Griffin, M.R., Piper, J.M., Daugherty, J.R., Snowden, M. & Ray, W.A. (1991) Nonsteroidal anti-inflammatory drug use and increased risk for peptic ulcer disease in elderly persons. *Ann. intern. Med., 114*, 257–263

Guess, H.A., West, R., Strand, L.M., Helston, D., Lydick, E.G., Bergman, U. & Wolski, K. (1988) Fatal upper gastrointestinal hemorrhage or perforation among users and nonusers of nonsteroidal anti-inflammatory drugs in Saskatchewan, Canada 1983. *J. clin. Epidemiol., 41*, 35–45

Gustafson-Svärd, C., Lilja, I., Hallbook, O. & Sjödahl, R. (1996) Cyclooxygenase-1 and cyclooxygenase-2 gene expression in human colorectal adenocarcinomas and in azoxymethane induced colonic tumours in rats. *Gut, 38*, 79–84

Gutthann, S.P., Garcia Rodriguez, L.A. & Raiford, D.S. (1994) Individual non-steroidal anti-inflammatory drugs and the risk of hospitalization for upper gastrointestinal bleeding and perforation in Saskatchewan: A nested case–control study. *Pharmacoepidemiol. Drug Saf., 3*, S63

Hamberg, M. & Samuelsson, B. (1967) Oxygenation of unsaturated fatty acids by the vesicular gland of sheep. *J. biol. Chem., 242*, 5344–5354

Hanif, R., Pittas, A., Feng, Y., Koutsos, M.I., Qiao, L., Staiano-Coico, L., Shiff, S.I. & Rigas, B. (1996) Effects of nonsteroidal anti-inflammatory drugs on proliferation and on induction of apoptosis in colon cancer cells by a prostaglandin-independent pathway. *Biochem. Pharmacol., 52*, 237–245

Hecht, J.R., Rovai, L.E. & Herschman, H. (1995) Cyclooxygenase-2 expression and regulation in colonic mucosa, cancer and cell lines (Abstract). *Proc. Am. Assoc. Cancer Res., 36*, 598

Hendrickse, C.W., Kelly, R.W., Radley, S., Donovan, I.A., Keighley, M.R. & Neoptolemos, J.P. (1994) Lipid peroxidation and prostaglandins in colorectal cancer. *Br. J. Surg., 81*, 1219–1223

Henry, D. & Robertson, J. (1993) Nonsteroidal anti-inflammatory drugs and peptic ulcer hospitalization rates in New South Wales. *Gastroenterology, 104*, 1083–1091

Henry, D., Dobson, A., Turner, C., Hall, P., Forbes, C. & Patey, P. (1991) NSAIDs and risk of upper gastrointestinal bleeding. *Lancet, 337*, 730

Henry, D., Lim, L.L., Garcia Rodriguez, L.A., Perez Gutthann, S., Carson, J.L., Griffin, M., Savage, R., Logan, R., Moride, Y., Hawkey, C., Hill, S. & Fries, J.T. (1996) Variability in risk of gastrointestinal complications with individual non-steroidal anti-inflammatory drugs: Results of a collaborative meta-analysis. *Br. med. J.*, **312**, 1563–1566

Herschman, H.R. (1991) Primary response genes induced by growth factors and tumor promoters. *Ann. Rev. Biochem.*, **60**, 281–319

Hogan, D.B., Campbell, N.R., Crutcher, R., Jennett, P. & MacLeod, N. (1994) Prescription of nonsteroidal anti-inflammatory drugs for elderly people in Alberta. *Can. med. Assoc. J.*, **151**, 315–322

Honn, K.V., Bockman, R.S. & Marnett, L.J. (1981) Prostaglandins and cancer: A review of tumor initiation through tumor metastasis. *Prostaglandins*, **21**, 833–864

Hubbard, W.C., Alley, M.C., McLemore, T.L. & Boyd, M.R. (1988) Profiles of prostaglandin biosynthesis in sixteen established cell lines derived from human lung, colon, prostate, and ovarian tumors. *Cancer Res.*, **48**, 4770–4775

Hunt, M.D., Neuenschwander, U.H., Delaney, T.P., Weymann, K.B., Friedrich, L.B., Lawton, K.A., Steiner, H.Y. & Ryals, J.A. (1996) Recent advances in systemic acquired resistance research — A review. *Gene*, **179**, 89–95

Isomäki, H.A., Hakulinen, T. & Joutsenlahti, U. (1978) Excess risk of lymphomas, leukemia and myeloma in patients with rheumatoid arthritis. *J. chron. Dis.*, **31**, 691–696

Jaffe, B.M. (1974) Prostaglandins and cancer: An update. *Prostaglandins*, **6**, 453–461

Janssen, P.L. Hollman, P.C., Reichman, E., Venema, D.P., van Staveren, W.A. & Katan, M.B. (1996) Urinary salicylate excretion in subjects eating a variety of diets shows that amounts of bioavailable salicylates in foods are low. *Am. J. clin. Nutr.*, **64**, 743–747

Jass, J.R. & Stewart, J.M. (1992) Evolution of hereditary non-polyposis colorectal cancer. *Gut*, **33**, 783–786

Johnson, A.G., Seidemann, P. & Day, R.O. (1994a) NSAID-related adverse drug interactions with clinical relevance. An update. *Int. J. clin. Pharmacol. Ther.*, **32**, 509–532

Johnson, A.G., Nguyen, T.V. & Day, R.O. (1994b) Do nonsteroidal anti-inflammatory drugs affect blood pressure? A meta analysis. *Ann. intern. Med.*, **121**, 289–300

Johnson, A.G., Jick, S.S., Perera, D.R. & Jick, H. (1996) Histamine-2 receptor antagonists and gastric cancer. *Epidemiology*, **7**, 434–436

Kapui, Z., Boer, K., Rozsa, I., Blasko, G. & Hermecz, I. (1993) Investigations of indomethacin-induced gastric ulcer in rats. *Arzneimittel.-forsch.*, **43**, 767–771

Kargman, S.L., O'Neill, G.P., Vickers, P.J., Evans, J.F., Mancini, J.A. & Jothy, S. (1995) Expression of prostaglandin G/H synthase-1 and -2 protein in human colon cancer. *Cancer Res.*, **55**, 2556–2559

Karmali, R.A. (1980) Review: Prostaglandins and cancer. *Prostaglandins Med.*, **5**, 11–18

Karmali, R.A. (1983) Prostaglandins and cancer. *CA Cancer J. Clin.*, **33**, 322–332

Kaufmann, H.J. & Taubin, H.L. (1987) Nonsteroidal anti-inflammatory drugs activate quiescent inflammatory bowel disease. *Am. J. Med.*, **107**, 513–516

Kinzler, K.W. & Vogelstein, B. (1996) Lessons from hereditary colon cancer. *Cell*, **87**, 159–170

Klapan, I., Katic, V., Culo, F. & Cuk, V. (1992) Prognostic significance of plasma prostaglandin E concentration in patients with head and neck cancer. *J. Cancer Res. clin. Oncol.*, **118**, 308–313

Koytchev, R., Alken, R.G. & Gromnica Ihle, E. (1994) Serum concentration of piroxicam and inhibition of platelet aggregation in patients with rheumatoid arthritis and M. Bechterew. *Agents Actions*, **43**, 48–52

Kudo, T., Narisawa, T. & Abo, S. (1980) Antitumor activity of indomethacin on methylzoxy-methanol-induced large bowel tumors in rats. *Gann*, **71**, 260–264

Kune, G.A., Kune, S. & Watson, L.F. (1988) Colorectal cancer risk, chronic illnesses, operations, and medications: Case control results from the Melbourne Colorectal Cancer Study. *Cancer Res.*, **48**, 4399–4404

Kutchera, W., Jones, D.A., Matsunami, N., Gordon, J., McIntyre, T.M., Zimmerman, G.A., White, R.L. & Prescott, S.M. (1996) Prostaglandin H synthase 2 is expressed abnormally in human colon cancer. Evidence for a transcriptional effect. *Proc. natl Acad. Sci. USA*, **93**, 4816–4820

Laakso, M., Mutru, O., Isomäki, H. & Koota, K. (1986) Cancer mortality in patients with rheumatoid arthritis. *J. Rheumatol.*, **13**, 522–526

Laneuville, O., Breuer, D.K., DeWitt, D.L., Hla, T., Funk, C.D. & Smith, W.L. (1994) Differential inhibition of human prostaglandin endoperoxide H synthases-1 and -2 by nonsteroidal anti-inflammatory drugs. *J. Pharmacol. exp. Ther.*, **271**, 927–934

Lange, K., Simmet, T., Peskar, B.M. & Peskar, B.A. (1985) Determination of 15-keto-13,14-dihydro-prostaglandin E2 and prostaglandin D2 in human colonic tissue using a chemiluminescence enzyme immunoassay with catalase as labeling enzyme. *Adv. Prostaglandin Thromboxane Leukotriene Res.*, **15**, 35–38

Langman, M.J., Morgan, L. & Worrall, A. (1985) Use of anti-inflammatory drugs by patients admitted with small or large bowel perforations and haemorrhage. *Br. med. J.*, **290**, 347–349

Langman, M.J., Weil, J., Wainwright, P., Lawson, D.H., Rawlins, M.D., Logan, R.F., Murphy, M., Vessey, M.P. & Colin Jones, D.G. (1994) Risks of bleeding peptic ulcer associated with individual non-steroidal anti-inflammatory drugs [published erratum appears in *Lancet,* 1994, **343**]. *Lancet*, **343**, 1075–1078

Lanza, L.L., Walker, A.M., Bortnichak, E.A. & Dreyer, N.A. (1995) Peptic ulcer and gastrointestinal hemorrhage associated with nonsteroidal anti-inflammatory drug use in patients younger than 65 years. A large health maintenance organization cohort study. *Arch. intern. Med.*, **155**, 1371–1377

Laporte, J.R., Carne, X., Vidal, X., Moreno, V. & Juan, J. (1991) Upper gastrointestinal bleeding in relation to previous use of analgesics and non-steroidal anti-inflammatory drugs. Catalan Countries Study on Upper Gastrointestinal Bleeding. *Lancet,* **337**, 85–89

Lewis, J.G., Stewart, W. & Adams, D.O. (1988) Role of oxygen radicals in induction of DNA by metabolites of benzene. *Cancer Res.*, **48**, 4762–4765

Ligumsky, M., Golanska, E.M., Hansen, D.G. & Kauffman, G.L. (1983) Aspirin can inhibit gastric mucosal cyclo-oxygenase without causing lesions in rat. *Gastroenterology*, **84**, 756–761

Lippmann, W. (1974) Inhibition of indomethacin-induced gastric ulceration in the rat by perorally-administered synthetic and natural prostaglandin analogues. *Prostaglandins*, **7**, 1–10

Lippton, H.L., Armstead, W.M., Hyman, A.L. & Kadowitz, P.J. (1987) Characterization of the vasoconstrictor activity of indomethacin in the mesenteric vascular bed of the cat. *Prostaglandins Leukotrienes Med.*, **27**, 81–91

Loeb, D.S., Talley, N.J., Ahlquist, D.A., Carpenter, H.A. & Zinsmeister, A.R. (1992) Long-term nonsteroidal anti-inflammatory drug use and gastroduodenal injury: The role of *Helicobacter pylori*. *Gastroenterology,* **102**, 1899–1905

Loll, P.J., Picot, D. & Garavito, R.M. (1995) The structural basis of aspirin activity inferred from the crystal structure of inactivated prostaglandin H$_2$ synthase. *Nature Struct. Biol.*, **2**, 637–642

Loll, P.J., Picot, D., Ekabo, O. & Garavito, R.M. (1996) Synthesis and use of iodinated nonsteroidal antiinflammatory drug analogs as crystallographic probes of the prostaglandin H$_2$ synthase cyclooxygenase active site. *Biochemistry*, **35**, 7330–7340

Lu, X., Xie, W., Reed, D., Bradshaw, W.S. & Simmons, D.L. (1995) Nonsteroidal antiinflammatory drugs cause apoptosis and induce cyclooxygenases in chicken embryo fibroblasts. *Proc. natl Acad. Sci. USA*, **92**, 7961–7965

Lupulescu, A. (1975) Effect of prostaglandins on protein, RNA, DNA and collagen synthesis in experimental wounds. *Prostaglandins*, **10**, 573–579

Lupulescu, A.P. (1977) Cytologic and metabolic effects of prostaglandins on rat skin. *J. invest. Dermatol.*, **68**, 138–145

Lupulescu, A. (1978a) Enhancement of carcinogenesis by prostaglandins in male albino Swiss mice. *J. natl Cancer Inst.*, **61**, 97–106

Lupulescu, A. (1978b) Enhancement of carcinogenesis by prostaglandins. *Nature*, **272**, 634–636

Lupulescu, A. (1980) Heavy incorporation of 3H-prostaglandin F2 alpha in the neoplastic cells as revealed by autoradiographic studies. *Experentia*, **36**, 246–247

Marnett, L.J. (1990) Prostaglandin synthase-mediated metabolism of carcinogens and a potential role for peroxyl radicals as reactive intermediates. *Environ. Health Perspect.*, **88**, 5–12

Marnett, L.J. (1992) Aspirin and the potential role of prostaglandins in colon cancer. *Cancer Res.*, **52**, 5575–5589

Martin, D.F., Montgomery, E., Dobek, A.S., Patrissi, G.A. & Peura, D.A. (1989) *Campylobacter pylori*, NSAIDs, and smoking: Risk factors for peptic ulcer disease. *Am. J. Gastroenterol.*, **84**, 1268–1272

Marx, J. (1993) New colon gene discovered. *Science*, **260**, 751–752

Matsuyama, K., Sen, A.C. & Perrin, J.H. (1987) Binding of piroxicam to human serum albumin: Effect of piroxicam on warfarin and diazepam binding. *Pharm. Res.*, **4**, 355–357

Maxwell, W.J., Kelleher, D., Keating, J.J., Hogan, F.P., Bloomfield, F.J., MacDonald, G.S. & Keeling, P.W. (1990) Enhanced secretion of prostaglandin E2 by tissue-fixed macrophages in colonic carcinoma. *Digestion, ***47**, 160–166

McLellan, E.A., Medline, A. & Bird, R.P. (1991) Sequential analyses of the growth and morphological characteristics of aberrant crypt foci: Putative preneoplastic lesions. *Cancer Res.*, **51**, 5270–5274

Meade, E.A., Smith, W.L. & DeWitt, D.L. (1993). Differential inhibition of prostaglandin endoperoxide synthase (cyclooxygenase) isozymes by aspirin and other non-steroidal anti-inflammatory drugs. *J. Biol. Chem.*, **268**, 6610–6614

Mené, P., Pugliese, F. & Patrono, C. (1995) The effects of nonsteroidal anti-inflammatory drugs on human hypertensive vascular disease. *Semin. Nephrol.*, **15**, 244–252

Meyers, R.L., Alpan, G., Lin, E. & Clyman, R.I. (1991) Patent ductus arteriosus, indomethacin, and intestinal distension: Effects on intestinal blood flow and oxygen consumption. *Pediatr. Res.*, **29**, 569–574

Miller, T.A. (1983) Protective effects of prostaglandins against gastric mucosal damage: Current knowledge and proposed mechanisms. *Am. J. Physiol.*, **245**, G601–G623

Milligan, P.A., McGill, P.E., Howden, C.W., Kelman, A.W. & Whiting, B. (1993) The consequences of H2 receptor antagonist–piroxicam coadministration in patients with joint disorders. *Eur. J. clin. Pharmacol.*, **45**, 507–512

Mills, S.J., Chapman, P.D., Burn, J. & Gunn, A. (1997) Endoscopic screening and surgery for familial adenomatous polyposis: Dangerous delays. *Br. J. Surg.*, **84**, 774–777

Moorghen, M., Ince, P., Finney, K.J., Sunter, J.P., Appleton, D.R. & Watson, A.J. (1988) A protective effect of sulindac against chemically-induced primary colonic tumours in mice. *J. Pathol.*, **156**, 341–347

Moser, A.R., Pitot, H.C. & Dove, W.F. (1990) A dominant mutation that predisposes to multiple intestinal neoplasia in the mouse. *Science*, **247**, 322–324

Moser, A.R., Mattes, E.M., Dove, W.F., Lindstrom, M.J., Haag, J.D. & Gould, M.N. (1993) *Apc^{Min}*, a mutation in the murine *Apc* gene, predisposes to mammary carcinomas and focal alveolar hyperplasias. *Proc. natl Acad. Sci. USA*, **90**, 8977–8981

Mostafa, M.H., Sheweita, S.A. & Abdel Moneam, N.M. (1990) Influence of some anti-inflammatory drugs on the activity of aryl hydrocarbon hydroxylase and the cytochrome P450 content. *Environ. Res.*, **52**, 77–82

Mukai, F.H. & Goldstein, B.D. (1976) Mutagenicity of malondialdehyde, a decomposition product of peroxidized polyunsaturated fatty acids. *Science*, **191**, 868–869

Mulder, C.J.J., Fockens, P., Meijer, J.W.R., van der Heide, H., Wiltink, Ed H.H. & Tygat, G. N.J. (1996) Beclomethasone dipropionate (3 mg) versus 5 amino-salicylic acid (2 g) versus the combination of both (3 mg/2 mg) as retention enemas in active ulcerative proctitis. *Eur. J. Gastro-hepatol.*, **8**, 549–553

Nakamura, A., Yamatani, T., Fujita, T. & Chiba, T. (1991) Mechanism of inhibitory action of prostaglandins on the growth of human gastric carcinoma cell line KATO III. *Gastroenterology*, **101**, 910–918

Narisawa, T., Sato, M., Tani, M., Kudo, T., Takahashi, T. & Goto, A. (1981) Inhibition of development of methylnitrosourea-induced rat colon tumors by indomethacin. *Cancer Res.*, **41**, 1954–1957

Narisawa, T., Satoh, M., Sano, M. & Takahashi, T. (1983) Inhibition of initiation and promotion by *N*-methylnitrosourea-induced colon carcinogenesis in rats by non-steroid and anti-inflammatory agent indomethacin. *Carcinogenesis*, **4**, 1225–1227

Narisawa, T., Hermanek, P., Habs, M. & Schmähl, D. (1984) Reduction of carcinogenicity of N-nitrosomethylurea by indomethacin and failure of resuming effect of prostaglandin E_2 (PGE_2) against indomethacin. *J. Cancer Res. clin. Oncol.*, **108**, 239–242

Narisawa, T., Kusaka, H., Yamazaki, Y., Takahashi, M., Koyama, H., Koyama, K., Fukaura, Y. & Wakizaka, A. (1990) Relationship between blood plasma prostaglandin E2 and liver and lung metastases in colorectal cancer. *Dis. Colon Rectum,* **33**, 840–845

Nathans, D., Lau, L.F., Christy, B., Hartzell, S., Nakabeppu, Y. & Ryder, K. (1988) Genomic response to growth factors. *Cold Spring Harbor Symp. Quant. Biol.,* **53**, 893–900

Needleman, P., Turk, J., Jakschik, B.A., Morrison, A.R. & Lefkowith, J.B. (1986) Arachidonic acid metabolism. *Ann. Rev. Biochem.,* **55**, 69–102

Nensey, Y.M., Schubert, T.T., Bologna, S.D. & Ma, C.K. (1991) *Helicobacter pylori*-negative duodenal ulcer. *Am. J. Med.,* **91**, 15–18

Ohki, S., Ogino, N., Yamamoto, S. & Hayashi, O. (1979) Prostaglandin hydro-peroxidase, an integral part of prostaglandin endoperoxide synthetase from bovine vesicular gland microsomes. *J. biol. Chem.,* **254**, 829–836

Ohshima, H. & Bartsch, H. (1994) Chronic infections and inflammatory processes as cancer risk factors: Possible role of nitric oxide in carcinogenesis. *Mutat. Res.,* **305**, 253–264

O'Neill, G.P., Mancini, J.A., Kargman, S., Yergey, J., Kwan, M.Y., Falgueyret, J.P., Abramovitz, M., Kennedy, B.P., Ouellet, M., Cromlish, W. *et al.* (1994) Overexpression of human prostaglandin G/H synthase-1 and -2 by recombinant vaccinia virus: Inhibition by nonsteroidal anti-inflammatory drugs and biosynthesis of 15-hydroxy-eicosatetraenoic acid. *Mol. Pharmacol.,* **45**, 245–254

Ohshima, M., Dinchuk, J.E., Kargman, S., Oshima, H., Hancock, B., Kwong, E., Trzaskos, J.M., Evans, J.F. & Taketo, M.M. (1996) Suppression of intestinal polyposis in *Apc*[D761] knockout mice by inhibition of cyclooxygenase 2 (COX-2). *Cell,* **87**, 803–809

Parkin, D.M., Pisani, P. & Ferlay, J. (1993) Estimates of worldwide incidence of eighteen major cancers in 1985. *Int. J. Cancer,* **54**, 594–606

Papadopoulos, N. Nicolaides, N.C., Wei, Y.F., Ruben, S.M., Carter, K.C., Rosen, C.A., Haseltine, W.A., Fleischmann, R.D., Fraser, C.M., Adams, M.D. *et al.* (1994) Mutation of *mutL* homolog in hereditary colon cancer. *Science,* **263**, 1625–1629

Picot, D., Loll, P.J. & Garavito, R.M. (1994) The X-ray crystal structure of the membrane protein prostaglandin H$_2$ synthase-1. *Nature,* **367**, 243–249

Piper, J.M., Ray, W.A., Daughety, J.R. & Griffin, M.R. (1991) Corticosteroid use and peptic ulcer disease: Role of nonsteroidal anti-inflammatory drugs. *Ann. intern. Med.,* **114**, 735–740

Pirozzi, S.J., Renz, J.F. & Kalf, G.F. (1989b) The prevention of benzene-induced genotoxicity in mice by indomethacin. *Mutat. Res.,* **222**, 291–298

Pirozzi, S.J., Schlosser, M.J. & Kalf, G.F. (1989) Prevention of benzene-induced myelotoxicity and prostaglandin synthesis in bone marrow of mice by inhibitors of prostaglandin H synthase. *Immuno-pharmacology,* **18**, 39–55

Pollard, M. & Luckert, P.H. (1980) Indomethacin treatment of rats with dimethylhydrazine-induced intestinal tumors. *Cancer Treat. Rep.,* **64**, 1323–1327

Pollard, M. & Luckert, P.H. (1981a) Effect of indomethacin on intestinal tumors induced in rats by the acetate derivative of dimethylnitrosamine. *Science,* **214**, 558–559

Pollard, M. & Luckert, P.H. (1981b) Treatment of chemically-induced intestinal cancers with indomethacin. *Proc. Soc. exp. Biol. Med.,* **167**, 161–164

Pollard, M. & Luckert, P.H. (1983) Prolonged antitumor effect of indomethacin on autochthonous intestinal tumors in rats. *J. natl Cancer Inst.,* **70**, 1103–1105

Pollard, M. & Luckert, P.H. (1984) Effect of piroxicam on primary intestinal tumors induced by rats by *N*-methylnitrosourea. *Cancer Lett.,* **25**, 117–121

Pollard, M., Luckert, P.H. & Schmidt, M.A. (1983) The suppressive effect of piroxicam on autochthonous intestinal tumors in the rat. *Cancer Lett.,* **21**, 57–61

Powell, S.M., Zilz, N., Beazer-Barclay, Y., Bryan, T.M., Hamilton, S.R., Thibodeau, S.N., Vogelstein, B. & Kinzler, K.W. (1992) *APC* mutations occur early during colorectal tumorigenesis. *Nature,* **359**, 235–237

Prescott, S.M. & White, R.L. (1996) Self-promotion? Intimate connections between APC and prostaglandin H synthase-2. *Cell,* **87**, 783–786

Pretlow, T.P., O'Riordan, M.A., Pretlow, T.G. & Stellato, T.A. (1992) Aberrant crypts in human colonic mucosa: Putative preneoplastic lesions. *J. Cell Biochem.* **16G**, 55–62X

Rampton, D.S. (1987) Non-steroidal anti-inflammatory drugs and lower gastrointestinal tract? *Scand. J. Gastroenterol.*, **22**, 1–4

Ravi, S., Keat, A.C. & Keat, E.C.B. (1986) Colitis caused by non-steroidal anti-inflammatory drugs. *Postgrad. med. J.*, **62**, 773–776

Rao, C.V., Tokumo, K., Rigotty, J., Zang, E., Kelloff, G. & Reddy, B.S. (1991) Chemoprevention of colon carcinogenesis by dietary administration of piroxicam, α-difluoromethylornithine, 16α-fluoro-5-androsten-17-one, and ellagic acid individually and in combination. *Cancer Res.*, **51**, 4528–4534

Rao, C.V., Desai, D., Simi, B., Kulkarni, N., Amin, S. & Reddy, B.S. (1993) Inhibitory effect of caffeic acid esters on azoxymethane-induced biochemical changes and aberrant crypt foci formation in rat colon. *Cancer Res.*, **53**, 4182–4188

Reddy, B.S., Maruyama, H. & Kelloff, G. (1987) Dose-related inhibition of colon carcinogenesis by dietary piroxicam, a nonsteroidal antiinflammatory drug, during different stages of rat colon tumor development. *Cancer Res.*, **47**, 5340–5346

Reddy, B.S., Nayini, J., Tokumo, K., Rigotty, J., Zang, E. & Kelloff, G. (1990) Chemoprevention of colon carcinogenesis by concurrent administration of piroxicam, a nonsteroidal antiinflammatory drug with D,L-α-difluoromethylornithine, an ornithine decarboxylase inhibitor, in diet. *Cancer Res.*, **50**, 2562–2568

Reddy, B.S., Tokumo, K., Kulkarni, N., Aligia, C. & Kelloff, G. (1992) Inhibition of colon carcinogenesis by prostaglandin synthesis inhibitors and related compounds. *Carcinogenesis*, **13**, 1019–1023

Reddy, B.S., Rao, C.V. & Seibert, K. (1996) Evaluation of cyclooxygenase-2 inhibitor for potential chemopreventive properties in colon carcinogenesis. *Cancer Res.*, **56**, 4566–4569

Reed, G.A. (1988) Oxidation of environmental carcinogens by prostaglandin H synthase. *J. environ. Sci. Health*, C6, 223–259

Rice, J.R., Zenser, T.V. & Davis, B.B. (1985) Prostaglandin synthase-dependent cooxidation and aromatic amine carcinogenesis. *Prostaglandins Leukotrienes Cancer*, **2**, 125–129

Rigas, B., Goldman, I.S. & Levine, L. (1993) Altered eicosanoid levels in human colon cancer. *J. Lab. clin. Med.*, **122**, 518–523

Rioux, K.P. & Wallace, J.L. (1996) Mast cells do not contribute to nonsteroidal anti-inflammatory drug-induced gastric mucosal injury in rodents. *Aliment. pharmacol. Ther.*, **10**, 173–180

Rodenhuis, S. & Slebos, R.J. (1992) Clinical significance of *ras* oncogene activation in human lung cancer. *Cancer Res.*, **52**, 2665s–2669s

Rolland, P.H., Martin, P.M., Jacquemier, J., Rolland, A.M. & Toga, M. (1980) Prostaglandin in human breast cancer: Evidence suggesting that an elevated prostaglandin production is a marker of high metastatic potential for neoplastic cells. *J. natl Cancer Inst.*, **64**, 1061–1070

Said, S.A. & Foda, A.M. (1989) Influence of cimetidine on the pharmacokinetics of piroxicam in rat and man. *Arzneimittel.-forsch.*, **39**, 790–792

Salvemini, D., Misko, T.P., Masferrer, J.L., Seibert, K., Currie, M.G. & Needleman, P. (1993) Nitric oxide activates cyclooxygenase enzymes. *Proc. natl Acad. Sci. USA*, **90**, 7240–7244

Sandler, M., Karim, S.M. & Williams, E.D. (1968) Prostaglandins in amine-peptide-secreting tumours. *Lancet,* **ii**, 1053–1054

Sano, H., Kawahito, Y., Wilder, R.L., Hashiramoto, A., Mukai, S., Asai, K., Kimura, S., Kato, H., Kondo, M. & Hla, T. (1995) Expression of cyclooxygenase-1 and -2 in human colorectal cancer. *Cancer Res.*, **55**, 3785–3789

Santoro, M., Philpott, G.W. & Jaffe, B.M. (1976) Inhibition of tumour growth in vivo and in vitro by prostaglandin E. *Nature,* **263**, 777–779

Savage, R.L., Moller, P.W., Ballantyne, C.L. & Wells, J.E. (1993) Variation in the risk of peptic ulcer complications with nonsteroidal antiinflammatory drug therapy. *Arthr. Rheum.*, **36**, 84–90

Scheiman, J.M., Behler, E.M., Loeffler, K.M & Elta, G.H. (1994) Omeprazole ameliorates aspirin-induced gastroduodenal injury. *Dig. Dis. Sci.*, **39**, 97–103

Schlosser, M.J., Shurina, R.D. & Kalf, G.F. (1989) Metabolism of phenol and hydroquinone to reactive products by macrophage peroxidase or purified prostaglandin H synthase. *Environ. Health Perspect.*, **82**, 229–237

Schoon, I.M., Mellstrom, D., Oden, A. & Ytterberg, B.O. (1989) Incidence of peptic ulcer disease in Gothenburg, 1985 [published erratum appears in *Br. med. J.*, 1990, **301**, 906]. *Br. med. J.*, **299**, 1131–1134

Shimakura, S. & Boland, S.R. (1992) Eicosanoid production by the human gastric cancer cell line AGS and its relation to cell growth. *Cancer Res.*, **52**, 1744–1749

Shorr, R.I., Ray, W.A., Daugherty, J.R. & Griffin, M.R. (1993) Concurrent use of nonsteroidal anti-inflammatory drugs and oral anticoagulants places elderly persons at high risk for hemorrhagic peptic ulcer disease. *Intern. Med.*, **153**, 1665–1670

Silverstein, F.E., Graham, D.Y., Senior, J.Y., Davies, H.W., Struthers, B.J., Bittman, R.M. & Geis, G.S. (1995) Misoprostil reduces serious gastrointestinal complications in patients with rheumatoid arthritis receiving nonsteroidal anti-inflammatory drugs. A randomized, double-blind, placebo-controlled trial. *Ann. Intern. Med.*, **123**, 241–249

Smalley, W.E., Ray, W.A., Daugherty, J.R. & Griffin, M.R. (1995) Nonsteroidal anti-inflammatory drugs and the incidence of hospitalizations for peptic ulcer disease in elderly persons. *Am. J. Epidemiol.*, **141**, 539–545

Smalley, W.E., Griffin, M.R., Fought, R.L. & Ray, W.A. (1996) Excess costs for gastrointestinal disease among nonsteroidal anti-inflammatory drug users. *J. gen. intern. Med.*, **11**, 461–469

Smith, B.J., Curtis, J.F. & Eling, T.E. (1991) Bioactivation of xenobiotics by prostaglandin H synthase. *Chem.- biol. Interact.*, **79**, 245–264

Somerville, K., Faulkner, G. & Langman, M. (1986) Non-steroidal anti-inflammatory drugs and bleeding peptic ulcer. *Lancet,* **i**, 462–464

Spalding, J.W. (1988) Toxicology and carcinogenesis studies of malondialdchydc sodium salt (3-hydroxy-2-propenal, sodium salt) in F/344 N rats and B6C3F1 mice. *NTP tech. Rep.*, **331**, 5–13

Staton, G.W.J., Ingram, R.H., Dale, D.C. & Federman, D.D., eds (1996) *Asthma*, New York, Scientific American Inc., pp. 9–10

Steering Committee of the Physicians' Health Study Research Group (1989) Final report on the aspirin component of the ongoing Physicians' Health Study. *New Engl. J. Med.*, **321**, 129–135

Su, L.-K., Kinzler, K.W., Vogelstein, B., Preisinger, A.C., Moser, A.R., Luongo, C., Gould, K.A. & Dove, W.F. (1992) Multiple intestinal neoplasia caused by a mutation in the murine homolog of the APC gene. *Science*, **256**, 668–670

Suh, O., Mettlin, C. & Petrelli, N.J. (1993) Aspirin use, cancer and polyps of the large bowel. *Cancer*, **73**, 1171–1177

Szczeklik, A. (1994) Aspirin-induced asthma: An update and novel findings. *Adv. Prostaglandin Thromboxane Leukotriene Res.*, **22**, 185–198

Taha, A.S., Hudson, N.J., Hawkey, C.J., Swannell, A.J., Trye, P.N., Cottrell, J., Mann, S.G., Simon, T.J., Sturrock, B.R. & Russell, R.I. (1996) Famotidine for the prevention of gastric and duodenal ulcers caused by nonsteroidal anti-inflammatory drugs. *New Engl. J. Med.*, **334**, 1435–1439

Takeuchi, K., Takehara, K. & Ohuchi, T. (1996) Diethyldithiocarbamate, a superoxide dismutase inhibitor, reduces indomethacin induced gastric lesions in rats. *Digestion*, **57**, 201–209

Thun, M.J., Namboodiri, M.N., Calle, E.E., Flanders, W.D. & Heath, C.W. (1993) Aspirin use and risk of fatal cancer. *Cancer Res.*, **53**, 1322–1327

Tsujii, M. & DuBois, R.N. (1995) Alterations in cellular adhesion and apoptosis in epithelial cells overexpressing prostaglandin endoperoxide synthase 2. *Cell*, **83**, 493–501

Tutton, P.J. & Barkla, D.H. (1980) Influence of prostaglandin analogues on epithelial cell proliferation and xenograft growth. *Br J. Cancer*, **41**, 47–51

Van Der Ouderaa, F.J., Buytenhek, M., Nugteren, D.H. & Van Dorp, D.A. (1980) Acetylation of prostaglandin endoperoxide synthetase with acetylsalicylic acid. *Eur. J. Biochem.*, **109**, 1–8

Vane, J.R. (1971) Inhibition of prostaglandin synthesis as a mechanism of action for aspirin-like drugs. *Nature new Biol.*, **231**, 232–235

Vane, J.R., Flower, R.J. & Botting, R.M. (1990) History of aspirin and its mechanism of action. *Stroke*, **21**(Suppl. 4), 12–23

Verbeeck, R.K. (1990) Pharmacokinetic drug interactions with nonsteroidal anti-inflammatory drugs. *Clin. Pharmacokinet.*, **19**, 44–66

Vogelstein, B. & Kinzler, K.W. (1993) The multistep nature of cancer. *Trends Genet.*, **9**, 138–141

Vogelstein, B. & Kinzler, K.W. (1994) Colorectal cancer and the intersection between basic and clinical research. *Cold Spring Harbor Symp. Quant. Biol.*, **59**, 517–521

Wallace, J.L. (1997) Nonsteroidal anti-inflammatory drugs and gastroenteropathy. The second hundred years. *Gastroenterology*, **112**, 1000–1016

Wargovich, M.J., Chen, C.D., Harris, C., Yang, E. & Velasco, M. (1995) Inhibition of aberrant crypt growth by non-steroidal anti-inflammatory agents and differentiation agents in the rat colon. *Int. J. Cancer*, **60**, 515–519

Watson, S.A., Clifford, T., Sykes, R.E., Robinson, E. & Steele, R.J.C. (1995) Gastrin sensitivity of primary human colorectal cancer: The effect of gastrin receptor antagonism. *Eur. J. Cancer*, **31**A, 2086–2092

Williams, C.S. & DuBois, R.N. (1996) Prostaglandin endoperoxide synthase: Why two isoforms? *Am. J. Physiol.*, **270**, 393–400

Williams, E.D., Karim, S.M. & Sandler, M. (1968) Prostaglandin secretion by medullary carcinoma of the thyroid. A possible cause of the associated diarrhoea. *Lancet*, **i**, 22–23

Williams, C.W., Luongo, C., Radhika, A., Zhang, T., Lamps, L.W., Nanney, L.B., Beauchamp, R.D. & DuBois, R.N. (1996) Elevated cyclooxygenase-2 levels in Min mouse adenomas. *Gastroenterology*, **110**, 1134–1140

Wright, V. (1993). Historical overview of NSAIDs. *Eur. J. Rheum. Inflamm.*, **13**, 4–6

Yoshikawa, T., Naito, Y., Kishi, A., Tomii, T., Kaneko, T., Linuma, S., Ichikawa, H., Yasucda, M., Takahashi, S. & Kondo, M. (1993) Role of active oxygen, lipid peroxidation, and antioxidants in the pathogenesis of gastric mucosal injury induced by indomethacin in rats. *Gut*, **34**, 732–737

Zahavi, I., Fisher, S., Marcus, H., Heckelman, B., Kiro, A. & Dinari, G. (1995) Oxygen radical scavengers are protective against indomethacin-induced intestinal ulceration in the rat. *J. Pediatr. Gastroenterol. Nutr.*, **21**, 154–157

The Handbooks

Aspirin[1]

1. Chemical and Physical Characteristics

1.1 Name

Chemical Abstracts Services Registry Number
50-78-2

Chemical Abstracts Primary Name
Salicylic acid acetate

IUPAC Systematic Name
Benzoic acid, 2-acetyloxy

Synonyms
2-(Acetyloxy)benzoic acid; 2-acetoxybenzoic acid; o-acetylsalicylic acid; acidum acetylsalicylicum; acetylsalicylic acid

1.2 Structural and molecular formulae and relative molecular mass

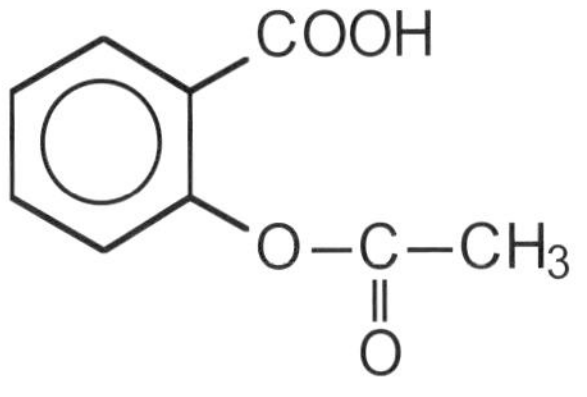

$C_9H_8O_4$ Relative molecular mass: 180.15

1.3 Physical and chemical properties

The data presented are taken from Budavari (1989) and Reynolds (1993), unless otherwise specified.

Description
Colourless or white needle-like crystals or white crystalline powder; odourless or almost odourless

Melting-point
135 °C

Solubility
One gram dissolves in 300 ml water at 25 °C, in 100 ml water at 37 °C, in 5 ml ethanol, 17 ml chloroform, 10–15 ml ethyl ether; less soluble in anhydrous ether

Spectroscopy
Ultraviolet, infrared, nuclear magnetic resonance and mass spectral data have been reported.

Stability
Stable in dry air but gradually hydrolyses in contact with moisture to acetic and salicylic acids. Decomposes in boiling water. Also unstable in solutions of alkali hydroxides and carbonates (pK_a 3.49 at 25 °C)

1.4 Technical products

Trade names
Aspirin is marketed throughout the world under many trade names, which include the following: AAS, Acentérine, Acesal, Acetard, Aceticyl, Acetilum Acidulatum, Acetophen, Acetosal, Acetosalic Acid, Acetyl, Acetylin, Acetylo, Acetylsal, Actispirine, Acylpyrin, Adiro, Albyl, Albyl-Selters, Angettes, Apernyl, Arthrisin, Artria, A.S.A., Asadrine, Asaferm, Asalite, Asatard, Aspalox, Aspegic, Aspergum, Aspinfantil, Aspirin, Aspirina, Aspirinetta, Aspirisucre, Aspisol, Aspro, Asrivo, ASS, Asteric, Astrix, Bamycor, Bamyl, Bamyl S, Bebesan, Bonakiddi, Bufferin, Calmantina, Calmo Yer Analgesico, Caprin, Cardiprin, Cartia, Casprium Retard, Catalgine, Cemirit, Chefarine-N, Claradin, Claragine, Codalgina Retard, Colfarit, Contradol, Contrheuma, Cosprin, Delgesic, Dispril, Disprin, Dolean pH 8, Doleron, Dolomega, Domupirina, Dreimal, Dulcipirina, Duramax, Easprin, ECM, Ecotrin, Empirin, Encaprin, Endydol, Enterosarin, Enterosarine, Entrophen, Extra Strength Tri-Buffered Bufferin, Flectadol, Gepan, Globentyl, Godamed, Halgon, Helicon, Helver Sal, Idotyl,

---

[1] Aspirin® is the Bayer trade mark for acetylsalicylic acid in more than 70 countries.

Istopirine, Ivépirine, Juvéprine, Kalcatyl, Kilios, Kynosina, Lafena, Levius, Licyl, Longasa, Magnecyl, Magnyl, Measurin, Mejoral Infantil, Melabon, Monobeltin 350, Neuronika, Novasen, Novid, Nu-Seals, Okal Infantil, Orravina, Platet, Premaspin, Primaspan, Primaspin, Protectin-OPT, Pyracyl, Rectosalyl, Resprin, Reumyl, Rhodine, Rhonal, Riane, Sal, Salacetin, Salcetogen, Saletin, Salicilina, Sanocapt, Santasal, Saspryl, Sinaspril, Solprin, Solpyron, Solusprin, Soparine, Spalt, SRA, Supasa, Superaspidin, Temagin ASS, Togal ASS, Trineral, Trombyl, Winsprin, Xaxa, ZORprin.

Aspirin is also marketed in many fixed combinations with other compounds, and especially with ascorbate, codeine and caffeine.

2. Occurrence, Production, Use, Analysis and Human Exposure

2.1 Occurrence

Aspirin is not known to occur as a natural product.

2.2 Production

Aspirin, the acetyl derivative of salicylic acid, is synthesized from the acid with acetic anhydride using sulfuric acid as catalyst (Roberts & Caserio, 1965). The basis of commercial production, which is approximately 40 000 t/year worldwide, was not known to the Working Group.

2.3 Use

Aspirin and its salicylate metabolite have analgesic, anti-inflammatory and antipyretic properties. Aspirin was first marketed in 1899 (Vane *et al.*, 1990). It is used for the relief of mild-to-moderate pain such as headache, dysmenorrhoea, myalgia and dental pain. It is also used in acute and chronic inflammatory disorders such as rheumatoid arthritis, juvenile rheumatoid arthritis and osteoarthritis. Aspirin inhibits platelet aggregation and is used in the prevention of arterial and venous thrombosis.

Aspirin is usually taken by mouth. Various dosage forms are available, including plain uncoated, buffered, dispersible, enteric-coated and modified-release tablets. Aspirin may be administered rectally or intravenously as a complex with lycin.

When aspirin is used as an analgesic and antipyretic, the conventional dose is 0.3–0.9 g, which may be repeated every 4–6 h according to clinical needs, up to a maximum of 4 g daily (Reynolds & Prasad, 1982). Generally, 4–8 g daily in divided doses are used for acute musculoskeletal and joint disorders such as rheumatoid arthritis and osteoarthritis.

Use of aspirin in children has been dramatically decreased after reports of a relationship between its use and the development of Reye syndrome, a very rare but possibly fatal combination of hepatic insufficiency and encephalopathy. One of the few indications in which aspirin therapy is still considered for children is juvenile rheumatoid arthritis. Suggested doses for this condition are 80 and 100 mg/kg bw daily in five or six divided doses, although up to 130 mg/kg daily are employed for some children.

Aspirin is used for the secondary prevention of myocardial infarct and stroke in patients with a history of such disorders. Large clinical studies have shown that doses of more than 300–325 mg daily are unnecessary, and some authorities recommend doses of about 75–100 mg daily.

2.4 Analysis

Accepted standard procedures for the assay of aspirin are given in the national pharmacopoeias of Argentina, Australia, Brazil, China, the Czech Republic, Egypt, France, Germany, Hungary, India, Italy, Japan, Mexico, the Netherlands, Poland, Portugal, Romania, the Russian Federation, Spain, Switzerland, Turkey, the United Kingdom and the United States, and in the European, Nordic and international pharmacopoeias.

Aspirin as its metabolite salicylic acid can be analysed in urine, plasma and saliva by colorimetry, thin-layer chromatography and high-performance liquid chromatography (Legaz *et al.*, 1992). In pharmaceutical preparations, it can be determined by high-performance liquid chromatography (Menouer *et al.*, 1982) gas-liquid chromatography (Galante *et al.*, 1981) and differential spectrophotometric analysis (Amer *et al.*, 1978) using proton magnetic resonance spectrometry (Vinson & Kozak, 1978; Al-Badr & Ibrahim, 1981).

2.5   Human exposure

Use of aspirin in the general population has been estimated from studies on use of non-steroidal anti-inflammatory drugs (NSAIDs) and cancer risk with data on the consumption of aspirin by study cohorts and by community control groups.

In a study by Kune *et al.* (1988) in Australia, of 727 community controls (average age, 65 years), 67 of the 398 men (17%) and 80 of the 329 women (24%) reported using aspirin. No data were provided on the frequency or duration of use. Paginini-Hill *et al.* (1989) reported aspirin use in a California retirement community (Table 1). The average age at the time of responding to the questionnaire was 73 years. Schreinemachers and Everson (1994) found that 59% of 12 668 subjects (age range, 25–74 years) had reported aspirin use within 30 days of interview in the US National Health and Examination Study.

In a study by Giovannucci *et al.* (1994), 47 900 US male health professionals aged 40–75 years were surveyed by questionnaire. Regular aspirin use was defined as more than twice weekly. A total of 33 806 (70%) did not use aspirin (average age, 56 years) and 14 094 (30%) did (average age, 59 years). The reasons for taking aspirin were surveyed in 185 men, who reported one or more of the following: cardiovascular disease, 25%; decrease in risk for cardiovascular disease, 58%; joint or musculoskeletal pain, 33%; headache, 25% and other reasons, 7.0%.

Giovannucci *et al.* (1995a) also questioned 121 701 female participants in the Nurses' Health Study (age range, 30–55 years) on four occasions over eight years; 15% reported regular aspirin use (defined as two or more tablets

Table 1. Aspirin use in a California retirement community

Aspirin use	Men (5051)		Women (8818)	
	No.	%	No.	%
None	3490	69	6021	68
Less than daily	685	14	1417	16
Daily	876	17	1380	16
Total use	1561	31	2797	32

From Paganini-Hill *et al.* (1989)

per week) in each questionnaire and 15% reported no aspirin use in any of the periods.

Greenberg *et al.* (1993) questioned 793 patients involved in a clinical trial of nutrient supplements on two occasions and categorized them as using aspirin not at all, intermittently or consistently, depending on whether they listed aspirin as one of their medications on zero, one or two questionnaires, respectively. The results are shown by age in Table 2.

Aspirin use increased by 4% among men with coronary heart disease or at high risk for coronary heart disease following publication of the results of trials on the cardiovascular prevention effects of aspirin. Nearly 50% of participants who reported a history of myocardial infarct, however, apparently did not take aspirin regularly (Shahar *et al.*, 1996).

Although the population-based data on aspirin use are limited, particularly with respect to dose, two general observations are warranted:
•   Aspirin consumption is high, in keeping with its ready availability, low cost and value in a wide range of conditions.
•   Because the incidence of musculoskeletal and cardiovascular disease increases with age, aspirin use rises concomitantly.

Table 2. Aspirin use in a clinical trial of nutrient supplements, by age

Age (years)	No use		Intermittent use		Consistent use	
	No.	%	No.	%	No.	%
< 50	54	82	8	12	4	6
50–59	170	79	26	12	19	9
60–69	277	72	51	13	59	15
≥ 70	92	74	13	10	20	16

From Greenberg *et al.* (1993)

3.   Metabolism, Kinetics and Genetic Variation

3.1   Human studies

3.1.1   Metabolism

The metabolism of acetylsalicylic acid (aspirin) is summarized in Figure 1.

Aspirin is rapidly hydrolysed to salicylic acid (2-hydroxybenzoic acid) in the intestinal wall (Spenney, 1978), liver (Ali & Kaur, 1983) and erythrocytes (Costello et al., 1984). Salicylic acid is further metabolized in the liver and kidneys into its glycine conjugate salicyluric acid and its glucuronic acid conjugates, salicyl phenolic glucuronide and salicyl acyl glucuronide. Ring hydroxylation products of salicylic acid are also formed, albeit in much smaller amounts; these include gentisic acid

Figure 1. Main metabolic pathways of aspirin

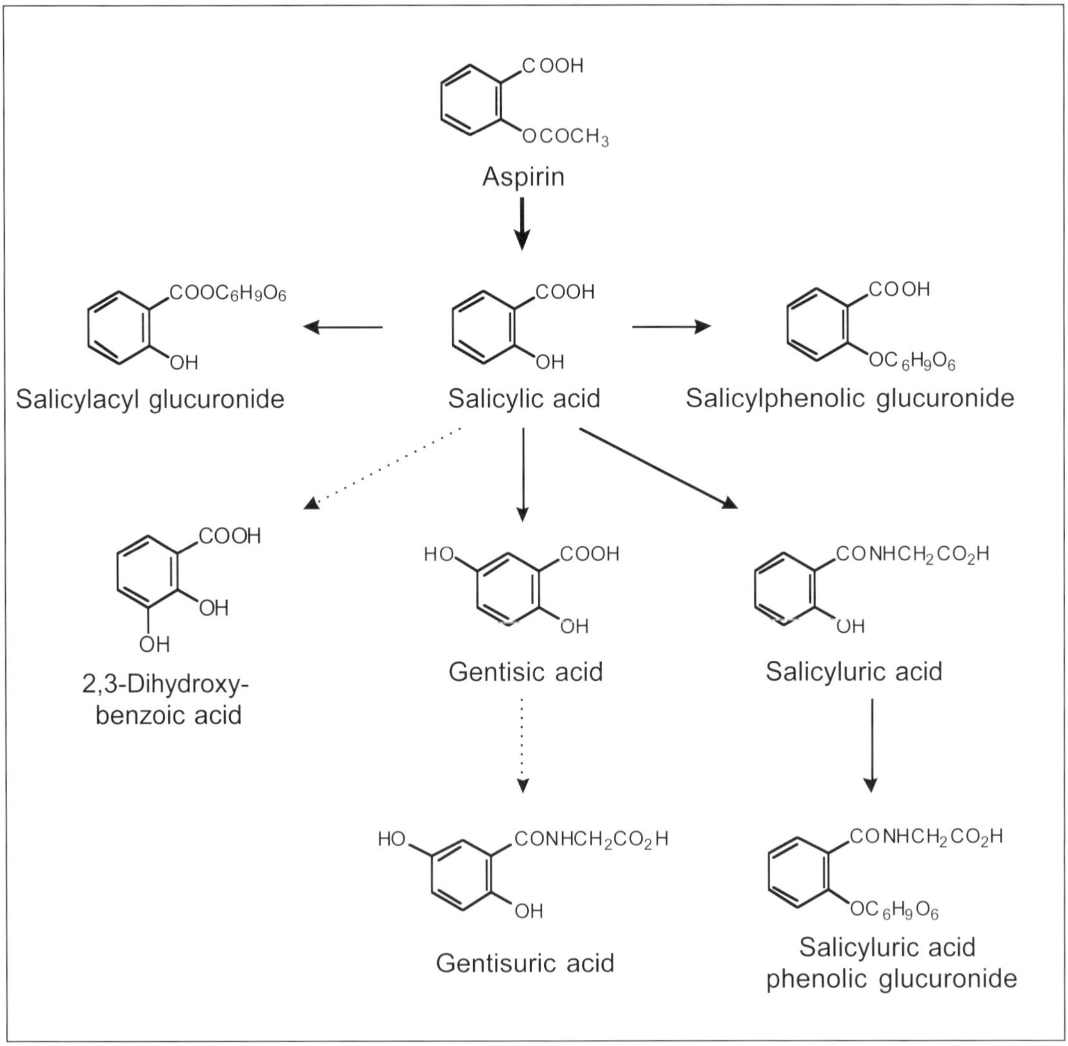

From Patel et al. (1990). Dotted lines indicate minor pathways

(2,5-hydroxybenzoic acid) and 2,3-dihydroxy-benzoic acid. Additional metabolites, also formed in minor amounts, include gentisuric acid and salicyluric acid phenolic glucuronide (Ali & Kaur, 1983; Costello *et al.*, 1984; Hutt *et al.*, 1986; Grooteveld & Halliwell, 1988). Small amounts of salicylic acid remain unchanged and are excreted.

The first step in the metabolism of aspirin, its hydrolysis to salicylic acid, is catalysed by a family of enzymes that are all serine esterases (Inoue *et al.*, 1979a,b, 1980; White & Hope, 1984). The esterases in the intestinal wall and liver perform most of the hydrolysis of aspirin (Rowland *et al.*, 1972); however, the erythrocyte esterases also contribute significantly to this process (Costello *et al.*, 1984). Thus, the haematocrit can be an important determinant of the half-life of aspirin. The rate of hydrolysis of aspirin to salicylic acid can vary considerably with age (Windorfer *et al.*, 1974), sex (Gupta & Gupta, 1977) and concomitant disease (Needs & Brooks, 1985).

After conversion of aspirin to salicylic acid, several fairly well characterized metabolic and elimination pathways affect the ultimate disposition of aspirin (Needs & Brooks, 1985). The major pathways for the metabolism of salicylic acid are conjugation with glycine to form salicyluric acid and conjugation with glucuronic acid to form salicyl phenolic glucuronide. Both follow Michaelis–Menten kinetics and are saturable. In contrast, the remaining pathways are minor and follow first-order kinetics (Levy & Tsuchiya, 1972).

Two properties of these pathways are critical to the metabolism and elimination of aspirin: the saturability of the 'primary' pathways and the self-induction of the metabolism. These phenomena are summarized below.

Salicylic acid, formed after a low, 325-mg, dose of aspirin, is metabolized by the pathways leading to salicyluric acid and salicyl phenolic glucuronide. As the amount of aspirin ingested is increased, these two pathways become saturated and the minor pathways are used to a greater extent, leading to increased amounts of their products. Thus, when increasing doses of aspirin saturate the two main metabolic pathways, the serum salicylate levels increase, the amounts of salicyluric acid and salicyl phenolic glucuronide do not increase further and larger amounts of gentisic acid, salicyl acyl glucuronide and other compounds are produced. As would be expected, the percentage of each metabolic product in the total pool of aspirin metabolites varies with dose (Patel *et al.*, 1990).

These findings, consistent with those of others (Levy *et al.*, 1969; Levy, 1979; Bochner *et al.*, 1981; Hutt *et al.*, 1986), demonstrate clearly the dose-dependent saturability of the primary pathways and the contribution of salicylic acid to the total elimination of salicylate after toxic doses, when the other major metabolic pathways are saturated.

Auto-induction of aspirin metabolism was suggested by observations in patients treated with aspirin for long periods. In these patients, the serum salicylate levels decreased with the length of treatment (Furst *et al.*, 1977; Muller *et al.*, 1977; Rumble *et al.*, 1980). The amount of salicyluric acid in urine was increased, indicating self-induction of aspirin metabolism.

3.1.2 *Pharmacokinetics*
The pharmacokinetic properties of aspirin have been reviewed by Needs and Brooks (1985).

(a) Absorption
After oral administration, aspirin is rapidly and extensively absorbed from the stomach but mostly from the upper small intestine (Flower *et al.*, 1985). Absorption occurs rapidly, by passive diffusion of the non-ionized lipophilic molecules; for example, the absorption half-life of aqueous aspirin ranges from 4.5 to 16 min (Rowland *et al.*, 1972). In this study, 68% of the dose reached the systemic circulation unhydrolysed.

Many factors affect the rate of absorption of aspirin, including the pH at the mucosal surfaces, the rate of gastric emptying, conditions that affect intestinal transit time and, if tablets are given, their dissolution rate. Of these factors, the most important is the last. Liquid preparations are absorbed most rapidly: Serum levels peak 15–20 min after intake of liquid formulations, 2–4 h after ingestion of regular tablets, and 4–6 h or more after intake of enteric–coated aspirin. The latter, which resists dissolution in the acidic stomach, dissolves mainly after passing into the alkaline environment of the small intestine (Liberman & Wood, 1964; Briggs *et al.*, 1977; Ross-Lee *et al.*, 1982).

It is of interest that, in patients on long-term treatment, the bioavailability of enteric-coated aspirin is similar to that of regular preparations, as the two formulations provide comparable steady-state concentrations of salicylate (Orozco-Alcala & Baum, 1979). When absorption is delayed by prolonged gastric emptying, metaclopramide can accelerate it (Ross-Lee *et al.*, 1983).

The effect of pH is of particular interest (reviewed by Gugler & Allgayer, 1990; Brouwers & De Smet, 1994). Aspirin, with a pK_a of 3.5, is a weak acid and is 99% non-ionized at pH 1; it can therefore diffuse through lipid membranes. If the pH of the stomach is increased, more aspirin is ionized, and this decreases its rate of absorption (Flower *et al.*, 1985). In the case of tablets, however, a rise in pH increases the solubility and thus tablet dissolution; the overall effect is to enhance absorption. High doses of antacids increase urinary pH, thus increasing urinary excretion of salicylic acid, leading to decreased plasma levels (Clissold, 1986).

In patients prescribed long-term aspirin use, the rate of absorption is not very important: accumulation is controlled entirely by oral bioavailability and the rate of plasma clearance (Verbeeck, 1990). A high absorption rate reduces the lag time between drug intake and the pharmacological effect, such as pain relief. This type of effect is useful in the treatment of acute conditions such as dysmenorrhoea and headaches (Chan, 1983; Diamond & Freitag, 1989).

(b)   Distribution
After absorption, aspirin is distributed throughout the body tissues and fluids, mainly by pH-dependent passive processes, and binds to plasma proteins, especially albumin. The apparent volume of distribution of salicylate ranges from 9.6 to 13 litres in adults (Graham *et al.*, 1977) and children (Wilson *et al.*, 1982).

Aspirin has unusual accumulation characteristics. The plateau level of salicylate in the body attained by repetitive administration of fixed doses of aspirin at constant intervals increases more than proportionally with increasing doses. The time required to attain the plateau also increases with dose. It was observed clinically that a 50% increase in the daily dose of aspirin produced about a 300% rise in the concentration of salicylate in the serum (Paulus *et al.*, 1971). This rise was attributed to the fact that the saturable processes (formation of salicyluric acid and salicyl phenolic glucoronide) contribute less to the elimination of salicylate from the body as the amount of salicylate in the body increases. These observations account for the pronounced effects that relatively small changes in the maintenance dosage of aspirin have on salicylate concentrations in body fluids and the pharmacological effects of aspirin.

A compartmental model has been used to evaluate the absorption, metabolism and excretion of aspirin and salicylic acid given in low (30 and 100 mg) or moderate (400 mg) doses (Dubovska *et al.*, 1995). The model confirmed the linearity of the kinetics of aspirin, showed that the apparent volume of distribution and clearance of aspirin are independent of dose and showed that the metabolic kinetics of salicylic acid at 400 mg are dose-dependent.

Both aspirin and salicylic acid are partially bound to proteins, especially albumin; 80–95% of salicylic acid is bound to plasma albumin (Murray & Brater, 1993). The binding of salicylic acid is reversible, but aspirin acetylates human serum albumin (Hawkins *et al.*, 1968; Pinckard *et al.*, 1968). Salicylic acid reaches: (i) synovial fluid, where its concentration is lower than that in plasma (Rabinowitz *et al.*, 1982); (ii) cerebrospinal fluid, where both aspirin and salicylic acid diffuse slowly because of the high degree of ionization at plasma pH (Flower *et al.*, 1985); (iii) saliva, where its concentration is proportional to that in plasma (Roberts *et al.*, 1978) and (iv) breast milk (Findlay *et al.*, 1981).

Salicylates administered to the mother are transferred readily to the fetus (Schoenfeld *et al.*, 1992). As aspirin has a short half-life, only a small amount of unmetabolized compound reaches the fetus. The fetus binds less salicylates in plasma than adults and has reduced metabolic activity, in particular glucuronidation, and less effective elimination. Therefore, fetuses and newborns whose mothers took salicylates before delivery may have plasma concentrations up to four times higher than those of their mothers.

(c)   Elimination

After oral intake, the plasma levels of aspirin rise sharply, reaching a maximum at 15–20 min. They then decline rapidly, and only small amounts remain after 2 h (Rowland et al., 1972). Although the half-life in the declining phase is short, it is always longer than the half-life of aspirin administered intravenously, due to continued absorption of aspirin during the declining phase. The salicylic acid levels rise rapidly and eventually exceed those of aspirin, because of slower elimination rather than differences in distribution (Rowland et al., 1967).

Hydrolysis of aspirin to salicylic acid in the plasma is rapid, with a half-life of 15–20 min (Rowland et al., 1972). Salicylic acid is removed from the body by parallel, competing pathways of renal elimination and formation of metabolites. Renal excretion of salicylic acid is saturable (Dubovska et al., 1995), occurs by first-order kinetics and is extremely sensitive to urinary pH, urinary organic acids and urinary flow rate.

No differences in pharmacokinetics have been demonstrated between old and young adults (Roberts et al., 1983; Silagy, 1993). Diseases in which the serum albumin concentration is altered are characterized by changes in the free salicylate fraction. For example, hypoalbuminaemic cirrhotic patients had increased unbound salicylic acid concentrations, although the kinetics of aspirin and salicyclic acid were not altered (Roberts et al., 1983). Zapadnyuk et al. (1987) reported, however, that the pharmacokinetics of aspirin were not the same in people aged 20–30, 60–74 and 75–89 years after a single oral administration of 14 mg/kg body weight (bw). The constants of absorption and elimination and the total clearance value decreased with age; and the half-life declined from 4 to 12 h across the age range. In the older patients, the area under the concentration–time curve increased.

The pharmacokinetics of a low dose of aspirin (60 mg/day) were studied during the second and third trimesters in pregnant women at high risk for placental insufficiency (Asymbekova et al., 1995). In the 16 women with uncomplicated pregnancies, the changes in the kinetics of aspirin were a lower concentration–time index, higher total clearance and a larger distribution volume. Similar changes were found in the four women with advanced placental insufficiency.

(d)   Drug interactions

The pharmacokinetic interactions of aspirin and various salicylates have been reviewed extensively (Miners, 1989; Verbeeck, 1990). Metabolic drug interactions involving aspirin are theoretically possible, but no studies have shown conclusively that hydrolysis of aspirin is altered by co-administered drugs. A number of treatments, however, affect the rate or extent of absorption of aspirin, including activated charcoal, antacids, cholestyramine and metoclopramide. Caffeine and metoprolol have been reported to increase the peak salicylic acid concentration after administration of aspirin, and co-administration of dipyridamole and aspirin results in higher plasma aspirin concentrations. The mechanism(s) responsible for the latter observation remains unknown.

Many of the drug interactions involve displacement of the co-administered drug from plasma protein, as, for example, in the case of interactions with diclofenac, flurbiprofen, ibuprofen, isoxicam, ketoprofen, naproxen, phenytoin and tolmetin. After displacement of these agents, the clearance of total drug increases and, consequently, the plasma concentration of total drug decreases. Although generally not measured, the unbound concentration of the interacting drug should not be markedly altered. Salicylic acid also increases the total plasma clearance of fenoprofen, but, unlike the interactions with other propionic acid non-steroidal compounds, plasma protein binding displacement does not appear to be involved.

There is no firm evidence that salicylic acid induces the metabolism of co-administered drugs; however, it can inhibit their metabolism. Such an effect has been reported for salicylamide, valproic acid and zomepirac. Certain co-administered drugs may alter the metabolism of salicylic acid; its metabolism is inhibited after treatment with benzoic acid, salicylamide, zomepirac and possibly cimetidine. Salicylic acid elimination is enhanced by oral contraceptives and by corticosteroids.

3.2 Experimental models

The pharmacokinetics of aspirin have been studied in many species, including rats and dogs (Sechserova *et al.*, 1979; Aonuma *et al.*, 1982; Rabinowitz *et al.*, 1982; Laznicek & Laznickova, 1994). The fate of aspirin has been followed by using radiolabelled salicylate or by simply measuring its plasma concentrations or those of its metabolites (Iwamoto *et al.*, 1982; Hatori *et al.*, 1984).

After intravenous or oral administration of aspirin at 10 mg/kg bw to male Wistar rats, 88 and 86% of the dose, respectively, was excreted in urine, mostly as salicylic acid and its conjugated forms. This finding suggests that the gastrointestinal absorption of aspirin in rats is essentially complete. Orally administered aspirin is subject to first-pass metabolism in both the gut and liver of rats (Iwamoto *et al.*, 1982).

The kinetics of sodium salicylate are dose-dependent, and its plasma concentration declines by a first-order process (Yue & Varma, 1982). The metabolism of orally administered ^{14}C-aspirin in rats over a 10-fold dose range (10–100 mg/kg bw) resulted in excretion of 81–91% of the dose in urine during the first 24 h; salicylic acid was the major urinary metabolite (43–51%) (Patel *et al.*, 1990). The excretion of salicyluric acid decreased with increasing dose, whereas that of gentisic acid and salicyl phenolic and acyl glucuronides increased. The profile of aspirin metabolites was qualitatively similar in humans and rats, but there were quantitative differences. A limited capacity to form salicyluric acid was observed in both species. In rats, the dependence on this pathway was low and was compensated by increased use of other routes. In contrast, in humans, the dependence on salicy-

luric acid formation was high and, in cases of overdose, compensation by other routes was incomplete.

In another study in rats, the concentration in major tissues and organs of aspirin labelled with ^{14}C on both the acetyl and carboxyl groups was determined by measuring the distribution of ^{14}C tracers in tissue sections (Hatori *et al.*, 1984). During the first 10–30 min after oral administration, the degradation to salicylate was 38% in the stomach wall, 64% in the liver and 86% in the lung.

The age-dependence of aspirin metabolism was demonstrated in a study in calves (Sechserova *et al.*, 1979). The older the animals, the lower were the total salicylate and salicylic acid levels and the higher the salicyluric acid level.

Two serine esterases involved in the hydrolysis of aspirin to salicylic acid have been purified to homogeneity from rat liver (Kim *et al.*, 1990). Both have a low K_m for aspirin and a wide substrate spectrum. At present, these enzymes are categorized as arylesterases (EC 3.1.12) and carboxyesterases (EC 3.1.1.1).

3.3 Genetic variation

No data were available to the Working Group.

4. Cancer-preventive Effects

4.1 Human studies
4.1.1 Studies of colorectal cancer

(a)   Methodological considerations

Most of the data on aspirin and colorectal cancer or adenomas come from epidemiological (observational) studies of sporadic disease in the general population. It was not possible in these studies to completely separate use of aspirin from that of other NSAIDs; however, as use of non-aspirin NSAIDs became widespread relatively recently, long-term use in studies of the general population involved predominately aspirin.

Intervention studies are generally considered to be more reliable than observational studies in the investigation of causal relationships. This may not be the case, however, if long-term use is a necessary parameter, and clinical trials may be limited by the fact that the randomized treatment is too brief. In such instances, observational studies may be informative because individuals who report longer use can be identified and studied.

Several potential problems should be considered in interpreting the epidemiological studies: (i) bleeding and other aspirin-induced symptoms can prompt closer medical surveillance earlier than would otherwise occur; (ii) changes in aspirin use may be precipitated by the early symptoms of neoplasia; and (iii) other behaviour that affects colorectal cancer risk may be associated with use of aspirin. An overall perspective of these issues is presented on p. 63.

Throughout this section, the term 'relative risk' is used in a generic sense to refer to measures of association such as odds ratios, risk ratios and 'rate ratios'.

(b)   Cohort studies

Nine published cohort studies provide information on aspirin-containing drugs and the risk for colorectal cancer. The studies are discussed chronologically; those completed before 1991 address NSAIDs as a side issue, whereas later studies focus directly on aspirin and other NSAIDs. The relevant studies are summarized in Table 3.

Studies of cancer occurrence in patients with rheumatoid arthritis have been conducted in Finland and Sweden. Such studies were considered to be relevant by the Working Group because of the prolonged, intense use of aspirin and to a lesser extent NSAIDs by such patients; however, it was recognized that the effects of aspirin could not be separated from those of other drugs used to treat rheumatoid arthritis or from those of the disease itself.

Isomäki et al. (1978) identified 46 101 patients (11 483 men, 34 618 women) in Finland who were reimbursed for treatment of rheumatoid arthritis by the national health insurance between 1967 and 1973. Using computer linkage with the national cancer registry for that period, the authors found approximately the same numbers of newly diagnosed cases as expected among the arthritis patients for cancers of the oesophagus (males: 5 observed, 7.5 expected; females: 21/20), and colon (11/9.9 and 33/39, respectively) and for

cancers of the stomach (51/54) and rectum (7/11) in males. Women had fewer than expected cancers of the stomach (80/100) and rectum (20/35); the reductions were statistically significant ($p < 0.05$).

Laakso et al. (1986) conducted a much smaller study of 500 men and 500 women treated for rheumatoid arthritis at a National Rheumatism Foundation hospital in Finland between 1970 and 1980. The cohort largely overlapped with that of Isomäki et al. (1978) and is omitted from Table 3. The numbers of deaths from cancer were: one from oesophageal cancer (2 expected), three from stomach cancer (11 expected), none from colon cancer (3 expected) and one from rectal cancer (none expected). None of these differences was significant.

A larger study in Sweden by Gridley et al. (1993) comprised 11 683 men and women with a diagnosis of rheumatoid arthritis recorded in a population-based registry between 1965 and 1983. These patients were followed from the date of discharge from hospital through 1984 in the national cancer and mortality registries. For men and women combined, the numbers of cases observed and expected, the standardized incidence ratio (SIR) and the 95% confidence intervals (CIs) for cancers of the digestive tract were as follows: oesophagus, 11/8.3, SIR=1.32, 0.7–2.4; stomach, 39/62, SIR=0.63, 0.5–0.9; colon, 44/70, SIR=0.63, 0.5–0.9; rectum, 28/39, SIR=0.72, 0.5–1.1.

[The Working Group noted the potential for confounding by underlying disease in these studies.]

Stemmermann et al. (1989) wrote a brief description of the Japan–Hawaii Cancer Study conducted in 1971–75 on 137 Japanese men residing in Hawaii who reported use of aspirin, an aspirin and caffeine combination, or dextropropoxyphene for at least one week during the previous month. Among analgesic users, three colorectal cancers were observed, with 4.3 expected on the basis of the incidence among 652 non-users in the study.

Paganini-Hill et al. (1989) identified newly diagnosed cases of various chronic diseases from hospital records for 13 987 residents of a California retirement community between

Table 3. Cohort studies of use of non-steroidal anti-inflammatory drugs and the risk for colorectal cancer in the general population

Reference	Population	Study size	End-point	Drug	Frequency	Results (RR)[a]	Comments
Isomäki et al. (1978)	Rheumatoid arthritis, Finland; 34 618 women and 11 483 men, 1967–73	**Women** 33 cases 20 cases **Men** 11 cases 7 cases	Colon cancer Rectal cancer Colon cancer Rectal cancer (incidence)	Therapy for arthritis	Heavy use	0.84 (NS) 0.58 (p < 0.05) 1.1 (NS) 0.64 (NS)	Risk for stomach cancer also reduced
Gridley et al. (1993)	Rheumatoid arthritis, Sweden: 7933 women and 3750 men, 1965–84	44 cases 28 cases	Colon cancer Rectal cancer (incidence)	Therapy for arthritis	Heavy use	0.63 (0.5–0.9) 0.72 (0.5–1.1)	
Paganini-Hill et al. (1989, 1991); Paganini-Hill (1995)	US retirement community; 13 987 elderly men, and women, 1981–87	181 cases	Colon cancer (incidence)	Aspirin	Daily	1.5 (1.1–2.2)	Median age. 73 No data on aspirin after baseline
Thun et al. (1991, 1992, 1993)	American Cancer Society, 662 424 US adults, 1982–88	950 deaths 138 deaths	Colon cancer (fatal) Rectal cancer (fatal)	Aspirin Aspirin	≥16 times/ month	0.58 (0.45–0.74) 0.66 (0.37–1.2)	Multivariate estimates No data on aspirin after baseline Decreased risk mostly confined to users of ≥10 years
Schreinemachers & Everson (1994)	12 688 US adults, 1971–87	169 cases	Colorectal cancer (incidence)	Aspirin	Last 30 days	0.74 (0.49–1.1)	RR reduced under age 65
Giovannucci et al. (1994)	Harvard Health Professionals: 47 900 US men, 1986–91	251 cases	Colorectal cancer (incidence)	Aspirin	≥ 2 tablets/ week	0.68 (0.52–0.92)	All cancers and metastatic or fatal cancers
Giovannucci et al. (1995)	US Nurses Health Study, 89 446 women, 1984–92	297 cases	Colorectal cancer (incidence)	Aspirin	≥ 2 tablets /week ≥ 20 years	0.56 (0.36–0.90)	Risk decreased with duration but not with dose > 2–4 months

RR, relative risk; NS, not significant
[a] In parentheses, 95% confidence interval

1981 and 1987. The median age of the participants at the time of enrolment was 73 years. The study population consisted mostly of white, moderately affluent, well-educated people, about two-thirds of whom were women. People who reported on a mailed questionnaire in 1989 that they used aspirin at least daily had a 50% higher incidence of colon cancer than did those who used aspirin less than monthly (40 cases; RR, 1.5; 95% CI, 1.1–2.2). Two subsequent reports on the same study reported follow-up of the cohort through May 1991 (Paganini-Hill et al., 1991; Paganini-Hill, 1995). A statistically nonsignificant 38% higher incidence of colon cancer was found in men but not women. This study differs from those that show an inverse relation between aspirin use and the risk for colorectal cancer: the participants were older, no data were available on the duration of aspirin use, and the participants lived in a single retirement community. The finding that ischaemic heart disease was significantly more common in daily aspirin users than in non-users (men: RR, 1.9; 95% CI, 1.1–3.1; women: RR, 1.7; 95% CI, 1.1–2.7) raises the possibility that patients with coronary symptoms or risk factors for vascular disease may have begun taking aspirin shortly before enrolment in the study because of local medical practices. [The Working Group noted that changing local medical practices disproportionately affect small regional studies, increasing misclassification of long-term exposures.]

Thun et al. (1991, 1992, 1993) measured death rates from colonic and other cancers according to aspirin use at enrolment in the American Cancer Society study of 662 424 US adults, who were followed from 1982 to 1988. People who reported using aspirin or an aspirin–caffeine combination 16 or more times per month for at least one year had 40% lower death rates from colon cancer than those who reported no aspirin use (men: RR, 0.60; CI, 0.40–0.89; women: RR, 0.58, CI, 0.37–0.90). Adjustment in the analysis for obesity, dietary vegetable and fat consumption and physical activity did not attenuate the reduction in risk. The results were also not changed by exclusion from the analysis of people whose underlying disease might have affected both aspirin use

and colon cancer risk; the diseases included prevalent cancer, heart disease, stroke or reporting being 'sick' at the time of enrolment. Use of acetaminophen was not associated with a lower risk for colon cancer (Thun et al., 1991).

The trend of decreasing colorectal cancer risk with more frequent aspirin use was stronger among people who had used aspirin for ≥ 10 years than in those with a shorter duration of use. Specifically, the RR for fatal colon cancer among people who reported using aspirin 16 or more times per month for ≥ 10 years was 0.36 in comparison with people who reported no aspirin use, whereas the RR for the group who reported this level of use for 1–9 years was 0.71. For both men and women, aspirin use 16 or more times per month for at least one year reduced the risk for fatal colon cancer (RR, 0.58; CI, 0.45–0.74) and fatal rectal cancer (RR, 0.66, CI, 0.37–1.2) (Thun et al., 1993).

Because of its size, prospective design, dose–response trends and internal consistency, the American Cancer Society study gave support to the NSAID hypothesis. Its limitations are the use of a single, brief, self-administered questionnaire, the lack of data on dose (as opposed to frequency or duration) and on use of NSAIDs other than aspirin and the reliance on death from cancer rather than incidence to define the presence of disease.

Schreinemachers and Everson (1994) reported on 12 668 people aged 25–74 who provided information on aspirin use when enrolled in the First National Health and Nutrition Examination Survey between 1971 and 1987. Over the average follow-up of 12 years (through 1987), the incidence of colorectal cancer was 26% lower among participants who had used any aspirin in the 30 days before interview than among those who had used no aspirin (RR, 0.74; CI, 0.49–1.1). The analyses controlled for obesity but not for physical activity or diet. The question on aspirin did not differentiate continuing use from brief or occasional use.

Giovannucci et al. (1994) assessed the incidence of colorectal adenoma and carcinoma among 47 900 men aged 40–75 in the Harvard Health Professionals study. Regular users of aspirin (two or more tablets per week in 1986) had a lower risk for colorectal cancer at all stages (RR, 0.68; CI, 0.52–0.92) and at advanced (metastatic or fatal) stages (RR, 0.51; CI, 0.32–0.84) than non-users. Age, history of polyps or previous endoscopy, parental history of colorectal cancer, smoking, body mass, leisure time physical activity and intakes of red meat, vitamin E and alcohol were controlled for in the analyses. The inverse association became progressively stronger with more consistent use of aspirin, i.e. regular use reported on more than one questionnaire. Colorectal adenomas were less common in aspirin users than in non-users whether or not the patients had been found to have occult blood in the faeces, suggesting that bleeding and early diagnosis of polyps did not account for the lower cancer risk in aspirin users. The inverse association was strongest with metastatic or fatal colorectal cancer.

Giovannucci et al. (1995) reported the incidence of colorectal cancer in relation to the dose and duration of use of aspirin among 89 446 US female nurses from 1984 through 1992. Data on aspirin use were obtained by questionnaire in 1980, 1982, 1984 and 1988,

and deaths and newly diagnosed cases of colorectal cancer were ascertained over eight years. The duration of aspirin use correlated most strongly with the reduced risk for colorectal cancer. The RR for colorectal cancer decreased progressively with years of use (Figure 2; *p* for trend = 0.008). Nurses who reported taking two or more aspirin tablets weekly for 20 or more years had a significantly lower risk than non-users (RR, 0.56; CI, 0.36–0.90). Although the RR appeared to be decreasing after five years of regular use, the decrement did not become statistically significant until more prolonged use. Controlling for several dietary factors, physical activity, alcohol and smoking did not alter these results. [The Working Group noted that one strength of this study is the repeated measures of aspirin use, which allow more detailed analysis of dose and duration than is possible in other studies.]

(c)   *Case–control studies*
Six published case–control studies examined the risk for colorectal cancer in relation to use of aspirin-containing drugs (Table 4). A further two studies addressed the risk for colorectal

Figure 2. Age-adjusted relative risks for colorectal cancer and 95% confidence intervals according to the number of consecutive years of regular use of aspirin as compared with non-users of aspirin

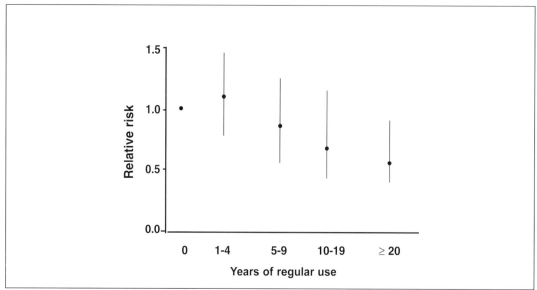

From Giovannucci *et al.* (1995). Regular aspirin use defined as consumption of two or more tablets per week

cancer in relation to medical conditions that served as a proxy for aspirin use.

Kune et al. (1988) assessed whether the risk for newly diagnosed colorectal cancer was associated with illnesses, operations and medications, using a population-based tumour registry in Melbourne, Australia. Personal interviews were conducted to determine whether 715 histologically confirmed cases and 727 randomly selected controls had used any of eight medications, two of which were aspirin-containing drugs or other NSAIDs. People who responded 'yes'; were asked to characterize their use as 'daily', 'weekly' or 'don't know'. Those who used aspirin [exact usage unspecified] had a 40% lower incidence of colorectal cancer than persons who reported no aspirin use (RR, 0.60; CI, 0.0.82). Persons who used other NSAIDs had a 23% lower incidence of colorectal cancer (RR, 0.77; CI, 0.60-1.0). Having chronic arthritis was also inversely associated with the risk for colorectal cancer (RR, 0.66, CI, 0.53–0.83). The association with aspirin use was similar in 392 cases of colon cancer and in 323 cases of rectal cancer, and the inverse association remained after adjustment in the analysis for diet and vitamin supplementation. Information on how long people in the study had used NSAIDs was collected but not presented. [The Working Group noted that controls were not selected contemporaneously and that the analyses of use of non-aspirin NSAIDs did not adjust for simultaneous use of aspirin.]

Rosenberg et al. (1991) examined the relationship between use of NSAIDs and newly diagnosed colorectal cancers in a large, hospital-based, case–control study in four northeastern US cities. Nurses interviewed 1326 patients with colorectal cancer, aged 30–69, and 4891 hospitalized controls (1011 with other cancers, 3880 with trauma or acute infection) about the use of salicylates (aspirin), indoles (indomethacin), fenamates (mefanamic acid), pyrazolones (phenylbutazone) and oxicams (piroxicam). Regular use was defined as use on at least four days a week for at least three months. Virtually all of the NSAID use was of aspirin. Regular NSAID users had a 50% lower risk for colorectal cancer than those who had never used NSAIDs (RR, 0.5; CI, 0.4–0.8). The risk

decreased with duration of use and increased after cessation of NSAID use, although neither trend was statistically significant. The hospital-based design of the study did not allow complete exclusion of bias from the selection of controls or confounding by diet or physical activity, which were not measured.

Suh et al. (1993) compared aspirin use among 830 patients hospitalized for colorectal cancer (490 colon, 340 rectum) at the Roswell Park Memorial Institute, USA, with that in two control groups: 1138 healthy visitors from a screening clinic and 524 hospital patients who had neither cancer nor digestive diseases. The cases were all diagnosed in 1982–91. Patients who took at least one aspirin daily had a lower risk for colorectal cancer than did non-users in analyses including the screening clinic controls (RR in men, 0.24; CI, 0.12–0.50; RR in women, 0.54; CI, 0.26–1.13). Similar estimates with wider confidence intervals were seen in analyses that included the hospitalized controls. No clear gradient of increasing risk was seen with the frequency of aspirin use, nor were analyses by duration of aspirin use presented.

Peleg et al. (1994) compared hospital pharmacy records for 97 newly diagnosed cases of colorectal cancer and 388 controls, who were followed for at least four years at a municipal hospital in Atlanta, Georgia, USA. Medications were supplied free or at low cost to poor patients, thus providing monthly records of the issuance of prescription and non-prescription aspirin, non-aspirin NSAIDs and acetaminophen. The risk for colorectal cancer decreased with the use of both aspirin and non-aspirin NSAIDs but not with acetaminophen. As shown in Table 4, The inverse trend was more strongly associated with duration of use (estimated as the number of days for which NSAIDs were dispensed during the four-year risk period) than with the dose of NSAIDs. Diet and physical activity could not be controlled for. In a second report, Peleg et al. (1996) described 93 cases of colorectal cancer that were included in the above study. The paper is discussed separately in relation only to sporadic adenomatous polyps (Table 5).

Muscat et al. (1994), at the American Health Foundation, interviewed 511 patients with

Table 4. Case–control studies of non-steroidal anti-inflammatory drugs (NSAIDs) and the risk for colorectal cancer in the general population

Reference	Population	Study size	End-point	Drug	Frequency	Results (RR)[a]	Comments
Kune et al. (1988)	Population-based, Melbourne, Australia, 1980–81	715 cases 727 controls	Colorectal cancer (incidence)	Aspirin NSAIDs	Daily (?) Daily (?)	0.60 (0.44–0.82) 0.77 (0.60–1.01)	Adjusted for diet Unadjusted for aspirin use
Rosenberg et al. (1991)	Hospital-based, four cities in eastern USA, 1977–88	1326 cases 4891 controls	Colorectal cancer (incidence)	Mostly aspirin	≥ 4 days/week ≥ 3 months	0.5 (0.4–0.8)	Trend with duration NS; risk increased after cessation
Suh et al. (1993)	Hospital-based, Roswell Park, USA, 1982–91	830 cases 1138 clinic controls 524 hospital controls	Colorectal cancer (incidence)	Aspirin	≥ 1 per day in 4 years before study	0.24 (0.12–0.50) 0.54 (0.26–1.1)	Men Women
Peleg et al. (1994)	Hospital-based, Atlanta, USA, 1988–90	97 cases 388 controls	Colorectal cancer (incidence)	Aspirin and non-aspirin	Used aspirin > 624 days in 4 years before study Used NSAIDs > 313 days in 4 years before study	0.08 (0.01–0.59) 0.25 (0.09–0.73)	Urban poor
Muscat et al. (1994)	Hospital-based, American Health Foundation, 1989–92	511 cases 500 controls	Colorectal cancer (incidence)	NSAIDs	≥ 3 times/week for ≥ 1 year	0.64 (0.42–0.97) 0.32 (0.18–0.57)	Men Women
Müller et al. (1994)	Hospital-based, US veterans, 1988–92	12 304 cases 49 216 controls	Colon cancer (incidence)	NSAIDs Other anticoagulants	Not stated	0.52–0.91 1.2–1.3	For 6 diseases treated with NSAIDs For diseases treated with other anticoagulants
Reeves et al. (1996)	Population-based, women in Wisconsin, 1991–92	184 cases 293 controls	Colorectal cancer (incidence)	Aspirin and non-aspirin	≥ 1 tablet at least twice weekly for ≥ 1 uear	0.65 (0.40-1.0)	Non-aspirin NSAIDs more strongly associated than aspirin
Bansal & Sonnenberg (1996)	Hospital-based, US veterans, 1981–93	371 cases among 11 446 veterans with and 52 243 without inflammatory bowel disease	Colorectal cancer (incidence)	NSAIDs	Not stated	0.68 (0.65–0.72)	

RR, relative risk; NS, not significant
[a] In parentheses, 95% confidence interval

colorectal cancer and 500 hospitalized controls about use of NSAIDs and acetaminophen. Use was defined as consumption at least three times a week for at least one year before hospitalization of the patient. By this definition, NSAID use was associated with a significantly lower risk for colorectal cancer in both men (RR, 0.64; CI, 0.42–0.97) and women (RR, 0.32; CI, 0.18–0.57). There were too few cancers for a reliable assessment of the trend in risk with duration of NSAID use or of differences among subgroups of people taking NSAIDs for different indications. Acetaminophen was not associated with a lower risk for colorectal cancer.

Müller *et al.* (1994) tested whether gastrointestinal bleeding induced by aspirin might lead to colonoscopy, early diagnosis and surgical removal of adenomatous polyps, rather than aspirin truly inhibiting tumorigenesis. By comparing 12 304 patients first treated for colon cancer at a Veterans Administration hospital in the USA between 1988 and 1992 with 49 216 controls matched to the cases for age, sex and race, the researchers assessed whether the incidence of colon cancer was increased or decreased among veterans with conditions treated by aspirin or NSAIDs (such as ischaemic heart disease, peripheral vascular disease, arterial embolism and thrombosis, osteoarthrosis and spondylosis), in comparison with patients with conditions treated with non-aspirin anticoagulants (atrial fibrillation, phlebitis and thrombophlebitis). The incidence of colon cancer was significantly lower in veterans with the six conditions generally treated with aspirin (RR, 0.52–0.91) and was significantly higher in those with the diseases treated with non-aspirin anticoagulants (1.2–1.3).

Reeves *et al.* (1996) conducted a population-based study of 184 women in Wisconsin, USA, whose invasive colorectal cancer was first reported to the State tumour registry between 1991 and 1992, and 293 population-based controls. All of the women were aged 40–74 years. NSAID use was ascertained by telephone interview; regular use was defined as taking at least one tablet at least twice weekly for at least one month. Regular use was associated significantly with a lower incidence of colorectal cancer (RR, 0.65; CI, 0.40–1.0) in analyses in which

adjustment was made for age, previous sigmoidoscopy, family history and body mass index. A statistically significant trend of decreasing risk was seen with increasing duration but not with the frequency of NSAID use. Non-aspirin NSAIDs were associated with a stronger reduction in colorectal cancer risk (RR, 0.43; CI, 0.20–0.89) than aspirin (RR, 0.79; CI, 0.46–1.4).

Bansal and Sonnenberg (1996) examined whether diseases potentially associated with use of NSAIDs were associated with the risk for colorectal cancer among 11 446 veterans hospitalized for inflammatory bowel disease at Veterans Administration hospitals between 1981 and 1993. In a comparison of 371 patients with both colorectal cancer and bowel disease and 52 243 with colorectal cancers only, the researchers found a lower risk for death from colorectal cancer in patients with other conditions usually associated with use of NSAIDs than in patients not likely to take these drugs (RR, 0.68; CI, 0.65-0.72). [The Working Group noted that the cases of colon cancer first diagnosed between 1988 and 1992 at a Veterans Administration hospital would overlap with those in the study of Müller *et al.* (1994); however, the designs of the two studies are sufficiently different to be reported separately.]

(d)   *Randomized clinical trial of colorectal cancer and adenomatous polyps*

One randomized clinical trial provides some information on aspirin use in relation to colorectal cancer. The US Physicians' Health Study (Gann *et al.*, 1993) was a double-blind, placebo-controlled trial of 22 071 male physicians, which was designed to evaluate the effects of alternate daily doses of aspirin (325 mg) and β-carotene on the risks for cardiovascular disease and cancer. The men taking aspirin were removed from the trial after a mean follow-up of five years because of a significant reduction in the incidence of non-fatal myocardial infarct. In a subsequent analysis of the 33 cases of colorectal cancer, an end-point that the trial had not been designed to evaluate, it was found that the RR for invasive cancer associated with use of aspirin compared with the placebo was 1.2 (95% CI, 0.80–1.7) over the five years of treatment. An additional analysis of colorectal cancer incidence by year of treatment showed RRs of 2.0 (0.75–5.3) for year 1, 1.2 (0.53–2.7) for year 2, 1.3 (0.58–2.8) for year 3, 1.0 (0.48–2.1) for year 4 and 0.77 (0.34–1.8) for year 5 or later, which may be compatible with an emerging protective effect of aspirin with increasing duration of treatment.

In a subsequent analysis of 13 years of follow-up, after most of the patients on placebo had begun taking aspirin, the findings for colorectal cancer were re-examined in two ways: by classifying participants according to their initial randomization [RR, 1.1; CI, 0.85–1.3 (Sturmer et al., 1996)] and by actual aspirin use (RR, 0.88; 0.59–1.3). [The Working Group noted that, even with the longer follow-up, use of aspirin could not have exceeded 13 years and the study still had limited statistical power for addressing the risk for colorectal cancer.]

4.1.2 Studies of sporadic adenomatous polyps in the colon

The relationship between the presence of adenomatous polyps and subsequent development of colorectal cancer is discussed in the General Remarks. The studies described below are summarized in Table 5.

(a)   Cohort studies

Greenberg et al. (1993) assessed whether self-reported use of aspirin modified the recurrence of adenomatous polyps among 793 patients participating in a randomized trial of nutrient supplements and antioxidants. All participants had a histologically confirmed colorectal adenoma removed within three months before enrolment in the study, leaving no known polyps in the colon. Participants reported their use of medications at six and 12 months after enrolment, and had a second colonoscopy after one year. 'Consistent' aspirin users (people who reported taking aspirin on both questionnaires) had a lower recurrence of adenomatous polyps than did non-users (25% vs 34%, RR, 0.52; CI, 0.31–0.89). Similar results were found after four years of observation (RR, 0.58; CI, 0.36–0.91) (Tosteson et al., 1995). An important strength of this study, despite the self-reported non-randomized aspirin use, was

that all participants underwent full colonoscopy at predefined intervals, minimizing the possibility that bleeding induced by aspirin might bias detection of polyps.

Giovannucci et al. (1994) examined colorectal adenomas as well as carcinomas in the Harvard Health Professionals study. The analysis was based on 472 distal adenomas among 10 521 men who reported having had a colonoscopy or sigmoidoscopy between 1982 and 1986 for reasons other than bleeding. The diagnosis of adenoma was verified from medical records. The RR, adjusted for other measured risk factors for the occurrence of adenomas of the descending and sigmoid colon and rectum, in men who reported aspirin use in 1986 was 0.65 (CI, 0.42–1.0) in comparison with non-users. Adenomas were less common among aspirin users than non-users whether or not the patients had faecal occult blood.

Giovannucci et al. (1995) also assessed colorectal adenoma incidence in relation to aspirin use among 89 446 US nurses from 1980 through 1990. The analyses included 564 cases of adenomatous polyps of the descending and sigmoid colon (371) or rectum (193), confirmed by a histopathological report. Having had an endoscopy between 1980 and 1990 was reported slightly more often by women who took 14 or more aspirin tablets per week in 1980 than in non-users (21.5% vs. 17.6%); however, large adenomas (> 1 cm in diameter) were no more common in women who used aspirin at this level (0.38%) than in non-users (0.40%). [The Working Group noted that these findings could be compatible either with inhibition of the growth by aspirin or early detection and removal of smaller adenomas in nurses taking aspirin.]

(b)   Case–control studies

Logan et al. (1993) examined the risk for colorectal adenomas in relation to aspirin use among subjects in a randomized trial of faecal occult blood screening in Nottingham, United Kingdom. A total of 147 patients who had faecal occult blood and an adenomatous polyp were compared with two control groups: 176 with blood in the faeces but no adenoma or carcinoma detected by colonoscopy, sigmoidoscopy or barium enema and 153 people with

Table 5. Studies of non-steroidal anti-inflammatory drugs (NSAIDs) and risk for sporadic adenomatous polyps

Reference	Population	Study size	Drug	Frequency	Results (RR)[a]	Comments
Cohort studies						
Greenberg et al. (1993)	US polyp prevention trial; 793 adults with previous adenomas	259 recurrent polyps	Aspirin	Any use at start and end of 1 year	0.52 (0.31–0.89)	Colonoscopy minimized detection bias
Giovannucci et al. (1994b)	Harvard Health Professionals: 10 521 US men, 1986–91	472 distal adenomas	Aspirin	≥ 2 tablets/week	0.65 (0.42–1.0)	Inverse association stronger with regular use reported on more than one questionnaire
Giovannucci et al. (1995)	Harvard Health Professionals, 89 446 US female nurses, 1980–90	564 distal adenomas	Aspirin	≥ 14 tablets	Not given	No effect on incidence of adenomas > 1 cm
Case–control studies						
Logan et al. (1993)	Within randomized trial of FOB testing; Nottingham, United Kingdom	147 cases Controls: 176 negative FOB 153 positive FOB	NSAIDs	Any use	0.49 (0.3–0.8) 0.66 (0.4–1.1)	vs. controls with no FOB vs. controls with FOB
Suh et al. (1993)	Hospital-based, Roswell Park, USA	212 cases Controls: 1138 screening clinic 524 hospital	Aspirin	≥ 2 times/day	0.61 (0.26–1.4) 0.53 (0.19–1.5)	vs. screening clinic controls vs. hospital controls
Martinez et al. (1995)	Endoscopy patients at gastrointestinal clinics, Texas, USA	157 cases 480 controls	NSAIDs	≥ 1 daily ≥ weekly	0.36 (0.20–0.63) 0.77 (0.39–1.6)	
Peleg et al. (1996)	Hospital-based, Atlanta, USA, 1990–93	113 cases with adenoma 226 controls	NSAIDs (aspirin and non-aspirin)	< 320 CCDs 320–700 CCDs ≥ 700 CCDs	0.59 (0.23–1.5) 0.56 (0.20–1.5) 0.31 (0.11–0.84)	CCD ≥ 700 equals 'standard dose' of NSAIDs on 42% of days of observation

RR, relative risk; FOB, faecal occult blood; CCD, calculated cumulative dose

[a] In parentheses, 95% confidence interval

no blood in the faeces and who were not examined further. When the latter were used as the referent, the RR for colorectal adenoma in persons ever having used aspirin was 0.49 (CI, 0.3–0.8). This inverse association was also present, but weaker, when the cases were compared with the controls who had faecal occult blood (RR, 0.66; CI, 0.4–1.1). There were no clear trends with frequency of use, but use for longer than five years resulted in a lower risk than use for shorter periods. NSAIDs other than aspirin, but not acetaminophen, were also associated with a lower risk for adenomas.

Suh *et al.* (1993), at the Roswell Park Memorial Institute, compared aspirin use among 212 hospitalized patients found to have adenomatous polyps of the colon or rectum with that of two control groups: 1138 healthy visitors from a screening clinic and 524 hospital patients who had neither cancer nor digestive diseases. All of the cases were diagnosed between 1982 and 1991. Patients who took aspirin two or more times daily had a lower risk for colorectal cancer than did non-users. The RR for adenomas in comparison with the screening clinic controls was 0.61 (CI, 0.26–1.4) and that in comparison with the hospital controls was 0.53 (0.19–1.5).

Martinez *et al.* (1995) conducted a retrospective, clinic-based study of 157 patients with adenomatous polyps and 480 controls, all of whom had undergone endoscopy at collaborating gastroenterology clinics in Houston, Texas, USA. The RR for adenomatous polyps among persons who took aspirin or other NSAIDs at least daily when compared with those who never used NSAIDs was 0.36 (CI, 0.20–0.63); the estimate for use one to six times per week was 0.77 (CI, 0.39–1.6). An advantage of this study was that all of the patients underwent endoscopy, reducing the potential for screening bias.

Peleg *et al.* (1996) compared the hospital pharmacy records for 113 cases of colorectal adenoma diagnosed between 1 August 1990 and 1 March 1993 with those of 226 controls from the same municipal hospital in Atlanta, Georgia, USA. Using these records, the researchers computed calculated cumulative doses of all NSAIDs over the 55-month study: This corresponds roughly to the number of

days a patient was prescribed a 'standard daily dose' of any NSAID during the study. Patients prescribed a cumulative dose of ≥ 700 (equivalent to receiving a 'standard dose' of NSAIDs for 400 days during the two-year-and-seven-month study), had a significantly reduced risk for adenoma than controls (RR, 0.31; CI, 0.11–0.84). Data for cumulative doses of < 320 and 320–700 are given in Table 5. [The Working Group noted that the 'standard daily dose' defined in this study is intermediate between an anti-inflammatory dose and an analgesic dose and approximately one-half of the anti-inflammatory level. The researchers did not define their interpretation of a 'standard dose' of aspirin.]

(c)   Randomized clinical trial
The efficacy of aspirin in inhibiting sporadic adenomatous polyps was examined in one randomized trial (Gann *et al.*, 1993). In the US Physicians' Health Study, men randomized to 325 mg aspirin every other day for five years had a slightly lower risk for cancer *in situ* or self-reported polyps than did men receiving the placebo (122 vs. 142 cases; RR, 0.86; CI, 0.68–1.1). [The Working Group noted that it was impossible to exclude the possibility that polyps existed at the time of enrolment. This would have tended to dilute any beneficial effect of aspirin on colorectal cancer incidence. It was also impossible to distinguish between adenomatous and hyperplastic polyps.]

4.1.3 Studies of oesophageal and gastric cancers
These studies are summarized in Table 6.

Isomäki *et al.* (1978) found five incident cases of cancer of the oesophagus (7.4 expected) and 51 cases of cancer of the stomach (54 expected) in patients with rheumatoid arthritis in Finland in 1967–73. The number of cases expected was calculated from general population rates. Gridley *et al.* (1993) likewise found fewer cases of gastric cancer than expected (observed/expected, 39/62; RR, 0.63; CI, 0.5–0.9) but not of oesophageal cancer (11/8.3; RR, 1.3; CI, 0.7–2.4) among patients with rheumatoid arthritis in Sweden. In neither of these studies were covariates other than age, sex and time period controlled for.

Table 6. Cohort studies of use of non-steroidal anti-inflammatory drugs and risks for oesophageal and gastric cancers

Reference	Population	Study size	End-point	Drug	Frequency	Results (RR)[a]	Comments
Isomäki et al. (1978)	Rheumatoid arthritis, Finland; 34 618 women and 11 483 men, 1967–73	5 cases	Oesophageal cancer	Therapy for arthritis	Heavy use	0.67 (NS)	
		51 cases	Gastric cancer (incidence)			1.1 (NS)	
Gridley et al. (1993)	Rheumatoid arthritis, Sweden; 8787 women and 3750 men, 1965–84	11 cases	Oesophageal cancer	Therapy for arthritis	Heavy use	1.3 (0.7–2.4)	
		39 cases	Gastric cancer (incidence)			0.63 (0.5–0.9)	
Thun et al. (1993)	American Cancer Society, 635 031 US adults, 1982–88	176 deaths	Oesophageal cancer (fatal)	Aspirin	≥ 16 times/month	0.78 (0.42–1.4)	Multivariate estimates
		308 deaths	Gastric cancer (fatal)	Aspirin		0.49 (0.22–1.12)	No data on aspirin after baseline Decreased risk mostly confined to users of ≥ 10 years
Schreinemachers & Everson (1994)	12 688 US adults, 1971–87	20 cases	Gastric cancer (incidence)	Aspirin	Last 30 days	0.93 (0.49–1.7)	
Funkhouser & Sharp (1995)	12 688 US adults, 1971–87	15 cases	Oesophageal cancer	Aspirin	Last 30 days	0.10 (0.01–0.76)	Multivariate estimate, also for alcohol use and smoking

RR, relative risk; NS, not significant

[a] In parentheses, 95% confidence interval

Thun *et al.* (1993), in a study described on p. 52, found lower death rates from cancers of the oesophagus and stomach among regular aspirin users (16 or more times per month in the past year) than in people who had never used aspirin. The trend of decreasing risk with more frequent aspirin use was statistically significant for gastric cancer (*p* for trend = 0.002) and of borderline significance for oesophageal cancer (*p* = 0.054). Smoking, alcohol consumption, dietary consumption of fat and fruit, vegetables and grains and obesity were adjusted for in the analysis.

Schreinemachers and Everson (1994) found no difference in the number of newly diagnosed cases of gastric cancer among participants in the National Health and Nutrition Examination Survey who were followed from 1971 to 1987 (RR, 0.93; CI, 0.49–1.7; 30 cases). These authors did not consider oesophageal cancer, but in another report of the same study, Funkhouser and Sharp (1995) found significantly fewer oesophageal cancers among people who used aspirin occasionally than in non-users (RR, 0.10; CI, 0.01–0.76), although this is based on only 15 cases. No cases of oesophageal cancer were observed among regular aspirin users.

Garidou *et al.* (1996) conducted a small, hospital-based case–control study in Greece. They found that chronic intake of any analgesic was non-significantly inversely associated with both squamous-cell carcinoma (five cases; RR, 0.6; CI, 0.2–1.9) and adenocarcinoma (four cases; RR, 0.5; CI, 0.2–1.6) of the oesophagus. [The Working Group noted that chronic analgesic use was not defined. Some controls may have used analgesics for long periods because of chronic or recurrent injuries.]

4.1.4 Studies of cancers other than in the digestive tract

Aspirin was included in a hypothesis-generating cohort study designed to screen 215 drugs for possible carcinogenicity, which covered more than 140 000 subscribers enrolled between July 1969 and August 1973 in a prepaid medical care programme in northern California (USA). Computer records of persons to whom at least one drug prescription was dispensed were linked to cancer records from hospitals and the local cancer registry. The observed numbers of cancers were compared with the expected numbers, standardized for age and sex, derived from the entire cohort. Three publications have summarized the screening findings for follow-up periods of up to seven years (Friedman & Ury, 1980), nine years (Friedman & Ury, 1983) and 15 years (Selby *et al.*, 1989). Among 2393 persons who received aspirin–phenacetin–caffeine–butalbital in combination, there was a significant (*p* < 0.01) deficit of breast cancer (two observed, 9.6 expected) in the seven-year follow-up. No negative or positive association with use of this combination was reported in the 15-year follow-up.

The incidences of cancers of the lung, bladder, prostate and breast were similar among daily aspirin users and non-users in the study of Paganini-Hill *et al.* (1989).

In the previously described study of the incidence of cancer among Swedish patients with rheumatoid arthritis (Gridley *et al.*, 1993), women with this condition, who probably had prolonged exposure to NSAIDs, had reduced rates of breast cancer (SIR, 0.79; CI, 0.6–1.0). There was no evidence of protection from cancers other than of the breast, colon and rectum and oesophagus.

Thun *et al.* (1993) found no consistent differences in the death rates of aspirin users and non-users from cancers outside the digestive tract among over 600 000 US adults in the American Cancer Society study. The death rates were either not statistically significantly different or were seen in one sex only, with no dose–response trend. Cancer sites that were examined included buccal cavity and pharynx, respiratory system, breast (female), genital system, urinary system, lymphatic and haematopoietic systems and other or unspecified. The RR for breast cancer among women who reported taking aspirin 16 or more times monthly was 0.88 (CI, 0.62–1.2) in comparison with non-users.

Schreinemachers and Everson (1994) reported significantly lower incidences among users of aspirin than non-users for cancers of the trachea, bronchus and lung (RR, 0.68; CI,

0.49-0.94; 72 cases in aspirin users, 91 cases in non-users) and breast cancer in women (RR, 0.70; CI, 0.50–0.96; 79 cases in aspirin users, and 68 cases in non-users).

In a large, international, population–based, case–control study, salicylates were not associated with renal-cell cancer (McCredie *et al.*, 1995). No dose–response relationship was found. Moreover, the lack of association was not altered by restricting analgesic use to that five or 10 years before the year of diagnosis.

Egan *et al.* (1996) found no association between regular aspirin use and the incidence of breast cancer in a cohort study of 89 528 registered US nurses in 1990. The analyses were based on 2414 cases identified over 12 years of follow-up (RR, 1.0; CI,. 0.95–1.1). Rosenberg *et al.* (1991) reported no associations between regular use of aspirin and cancers of the breast, lung, endometrium, ovary, testis or urinary bladder or leukaemia, lymphoma or malignant melanoma in preliminary analyses of a case–control study of drug use in Boston, USA.

Harris *et al.* (1996) described a case–control study of breast cancer and NSAID use in the USA. They interviewed 511 women with newly diagnosed breast cancer at one centre and 1534 women who had undergone screening mammography. Use of any NSAID three or more times weekly for at least one year was associated with a reduced risk for breast cancer (RR, 0.66; CI, 0.52–0.83). The risks were similar for users of aspirin alone, ibuprofen alone and all NSAIDs combined. The most heavily exposed women, with regard to dose and duration, had the lowest risk. [The Working Group noted the incomplete descriptions of the study population, the participation rates and exposure categories. An earlier report (Harris *et al.*, 1995) probably covered a subset of this study and was therefore not considered separately.]

4.1.5   Issues in interpreting the evidence for prevention of colorectal cancer

In considering the epidemiological data on use of aspirin and risk for colorectal cancer, the Working Group carefully considered the following sources of potential bias and confounding because of their concern about the implications for colorectal cancer prevention in the general population.

Publication bias. The Working Group was not aware (and did not think it plausible) that informative studies have been excluded from the literature.

Screening/detection. It is possible that bleeding induced by NSAIDs including aspirin may lead to endoscopy and earlier detection and removal of colorectal adenomas, resulting in a lower incidence of and death rates from colorectal cancer. Earlier detection of invasive cancer might also reduce mortality. This hypothesis cannot, however, explain the lower prevalence and incidence of colorectal adenoma among aspirin users observed in several studies, which contradicts the hypothesis of screening bias.

Indications for usage. It is possible that the reasons why aspirin users take aspirin influence the risk for colorectal cancer. In many of the studies, the reasons for aspirin use are not well characterized. This uncertainty is particularly apparent for long-term users, among whom the putative protective effect appears to be most marked. Nevertheless, two considerations reduce this concern. First, the association is observed in a variety of populations with different underlying morbidities. Second, the association is not observed with acetaminophen.

Life-style factors potentially associated with aspirin use and colorectal cancer. The Working Group considered possible confounding by physical activity, diet, obesity and other life-style factors that potentially affect the risk for colorectal cancer. In studies in which these factors were addressed, no diminution of the association was found, and no other known risk factor is sufficiently strong to account for the association with aspirin. It is possible but implausible that unknown risk factors could be associated strongly enough with both aspirin use and the risk for colorectal cancer to account for the findings.

Factors associated with aspirin intolerance. The possibility that genetic or life-style factors associated with intolerance to aspirin use could also be associated with risk for colorectal cancer was considered. The Working Group was unaware of any evidence to support this hypothesis.

Also, the small proportion of the general population who are intolerant to aspirin makes this implausible.

Exposure measurement. Information on the effects of prolonged use of aspirin is available in only a few studies; this is an important limitation of the aggregated epidemiological data. In most studies, measurement of aspirin use was based on self-reports relating to use a few years before the onset of the studied end-point (adenomas or cancers). This is likely to be a misclassified surrogate for long-term aspirin use; however, non-differential misclassification would have the effect of minimizing any true effect of aspirin. Differential misclassification leading to a spurious association is conceivable only in the case–control studies, but the Working Group concluded that this was unlikely to explain the observed findings. The Group also considered the biological plausibility of an association between aspirin use and colorectal cancer, given the short interval between reported exposure and outcome. Two interpretations are compatible with a causal association: recent aspirin use is a good surrogate for long-term use, and/or aspirin has a fairly rapid effect on cancer prevention. In view of the evidence that duration of exposure is important — and that a reduced risk for colorectal cancer may indeed be achieved, at least in part, through prevention of adenomas — the Working Group recognized that the interpretation of a causal association depends on the assumption that reported recent aspirin use is a good surrogate for long-term use. There was no independent evidence to support or refute this assumption.

4.2 Experimental models[1]
4.2.1 Experimental animals

(a) Colon
Short-term studies. Aspirin was evaluated for its ability to reduce the incidence and growth of aberrant crypt foci in the rat colon (Mereto *et al.*, 1994). Forty-eight male Sprague-Dawley rats were treated with either aspirin (10 mg/kg bw per day) by intragastric administration for 12 consecutive days, then given saline or 1,2-dimethylhydrazine (25 mg/kg bw) on days 4 and 9 or were treated with 1,2-dimethylhydrazine only. About half of the animals in all groups were killed four weeks after the first administration of 1,2-dimethylhydrazine; the rest were killed after eight weeks, and colonic aberrant crypt foci were quantified after methylene blue staining. When given both four and eight weeks after the beginning of treatment with 1,2-dimethylhydrazine, aspirin caused a significant (60%) decrease in the number of foci ($p < 0.01$–0.001). In addition, the numbers of larger foci (with three or more aberrant crypts per focus) were significantly lower (70% reduction; $p < 0.01$) at both times in aspirin-treated rats.

Groups of 14 seven-week-old male Fischer 344 rats were given subcutaneous injections of aspirin at doses of 0.2 and 0.4 mg/kg diet [200 and 400 ppm] for 35 days. Azoxymethane in saline (15 mg/kg bw) was given on days 7 and 14 of the experiment. Control rats were injected with saline only. All rats were killed on day 35, and aberrant crypt foci were quantified after methylene blue staining. At the doses used, aspirin did not inhibit either the number of aberrant crypt foci or the number of crypts per focus (Pereira *et al.*, 1994).

In a similar experiment, 20 adult male Fischer 344 rats received subcutaneous injections of azoxymethane at a dose of 15 mg/kg bw once per week for two weeks. Rats were then randomized to diets containing 0, 0.2 or 0.4 g/kg [200 or 400 ppm] aspirin; these doses represented 40 and 80% of the maximum tolerated dose (MTD; see General Remarks) of aspirin determined in the same laboratory. Azoxymethane had induced about 170 aberrant crypt foci by eight weeks. Aspirin at either dose suppressed the formation and progression of foci to foci of multiple aberrant crypts ($p < 0.05$), although the degree of inhibition was greater at 400 than 200 ppm (Wargovich *et al.*, 1995).

Long-term studies. These studies are summarized in Table 7.

---

[1] In this section, the concentrations of aspirin in the diet are given in the units used by the authors of the study and in square brackets as ppm, to allow ready comparison of studies.

Table 7. Results of experiments on the chemopreventive activity of aspirin on colon carcinogenesis in male rats

Strain	Carcinogen, dose and route of administration	Aspirin, dose, route and duration of administration	Tumour incidence (% animals with tumours)		Tumour multiplicity (tumours/tumour-bearing animal)		Reference
			Control	Aspirin	Control	Aspirin	
Sprague-Dawley	DMH, 30 mg/kg bw intragastrically, once	10 mg/kg bw per day, subcutaneously, − 1 and + 1 week	50	17	1.0	1.0	Craven & DeRubertis (1992)
	DMH, 30 mg/kg bw intragastrically, once	10 mg/kg bw per day, subcutaneously, 2 + 36 weeks	42	42	1.2	1.0	
Wistar	DMH 30 mg/kg bw, subcutaneously 18 times, weekly	5 mg/kg bw per day 30 mg/kg bw per day 60 mg/kg bw per day intragastrically, 18 weeks	100 100 100	100 50 25	NR	NR	Davis & Patterson (1994)
Fischer 344	AOM, 15 mg/kg bw, subcutaneously, twice, weekly	200 ppm 400 ppm − 2 to + 50 weeks in the diet	78 78	53 47	1.7 1.7	0.80 0.70	Reddy et al. (1993)

DMH, 1,2-dimethylhydrazine; AOM, azoxymethane; NR, not reported

Groups of 12–20 male Sprague-Dawley rats, 21 days of age, were given subcutaneous injections of aspirin at 10 mg/kg bw per day one week before and one week after a single dose of 1,2-dimethylhydrazine at 30 mg/kg bw by intragastric administration or were given aspirin four weeks after administration of 1,2-dimethylhydrazine up to the end of the experiment at 36 weeks. A 66% reduction in the incidence of 1,2-dimethylhydrazine-induced adenocarcinomas was seen in rats receiving aspirin for one week before and after the carcinogen, but aspirin had no effect on the tumour response when given four weeks after the carcinogen (Craven & DeRubertis, 1992). [The Working Group noted the small numbers of animals per group.]

In a similar study, groups of 16 male Wistar rats, two months old, received daily doses of aspirin at 0, 5, 30 or 60 mg/kg bw by intragastric administration for 18 weeks. One-half of each group also received weekly injections of 30 mg/kg bw 1,2-dimethylhydrazine for 18 weeks. Aspirin at all doses progressively reduced the number of tumours ($p < 0.03$) and the percentage of tumours ≥ 5 mm in diameter ($p < 0.03$). At the two higher doses, aspirin significantly reduced the incidence of tumours ($p < 0.03$–0.01) (Davis & Patterson, 1994). [The Working Group noted the small number of animals per group.]

In a further study, groups of 48 male Fischer 344 rats, five weeks old, were fed diets containing 0, 200 ppm (40% MTD) or 400 ppm (80% MTD) aspirin. Two weeks later, 36 rats per group were given subcutaneous injections of 15 mg/kg bw azoxymethane once weekly for two weeks; the other 12 rats per group were treated with the vehicle only. After 52 weeks on their respective dietary regimens, all rats were necropsied, and all tumours were subjected to histopathological examination. At both dietary concentrations, aspirin reduced the incidence, multiplicity and size of azoxymethane-induced colon adenocarcinomas ($p < 0.5$–0.01) (Reddy et al., 1993).

(b)   Liver

The chemopreventive effect of aspirin on hepatocarcinogenesis induced by a choline-deficient semisynthetic diet containing 1.75 g/kg methionine, 0 mg/kg choline and 0.11 mmol/kg phosphatidylcholine, was examined in male Fischer 344 rats. The levels of aspirin in the diet were 0.1, 0.2, 0.4 or 0.8% [1000, 2000, 4000 or 8000 ppm]. The duration of the study was 30 weeks. Administration of aspirin at the two higher concentrations reduced the development of preneoplastic and neoplastic nodules in the liver ($p < 0.05$–0.001). In the group fed 0.4% aspirin the number of γ-glutamyl transpeptidase-positive nodules per square centimetre was reduced from 1.7 in the group on control diet to 0.20, and the size of the nodules was decreased from 4.82 to 0.39 mm². No nodules were seen in the group given the diet containing 0.8% aspirin (Denda et al., 1994).

Male Fischer 344 rats, six to eight weeks of age, were fed a commercial diet and hepatocellular carcinomas were induced in all animals by initiation with an intraperitoneal injection of 200 mg/kg bw N-nitrosodiethylamine and selection by feeding 0.002% 2-acetylaminofluorene for two weeks and giving a single intragastric intubation of 1 mg/kg bw carbon tetrachloride. Aspirin, mixed in the diet and administered at a concentration of 0.75% [7500 ppm] one week later, decreased the multiplicity of hepatocellular carcinomas from 4.08 to 2.21 ($p < 0.01$). No significant differences in incidence were observed (Tang et al., 1993).

In an initiation–promotion model of hepatocarcinogenesis, nine male Fischer 344 rats were given a single intraperitoneal injection of 200 mg/kg bw N-nitrosodiethylamine; after two weeks of recovery, the animals received the basal diet supplemented with 0.05% phenobarbital for 10 weeks and were then killed. Another group also received aspirin in the diet at a concentration of 0.75 or 1.0% [7500 or 10 000 ppm]. Aspirin treatment significantly retarded the body-weight gain and reduced the average food intake throughout the experiment; it also reduced the number and percent of areas of the liver occupied by γ-glutamyl transpeptidase-positive foci in a dose-dependent manner ($p < 0.01$) but did not appreciably influence the average size of foci (Denda et al., 1989).

Groups of 14–16 male Fischer 344 rats received a choline-deficient, L-amino acid-defined diet or the same diet containing 0.1 or 0.2% [1000 or 2000 ppm] aspirin for 12 and 30 weeks, at which time the surviving animals were killed. By 12 weeks, the number and areas of the liver staining for γ-glutamyl transferase- positive foci were decreased in a dose-dependent manner by aspirin ($p < 0.05–0.01$), and by 30 weeks, the numbers and percent area of the liver occupied by nodules staining for glutathione S-transferase placental form were also decreased dose-dependently ($p < 0.05–0.01$) (Endoh et al., 1996).

(c) Urinary bladder
In a study in B6D2F$_1$ mice, the MTD for aspirin was first determined in a preliminary experiment for dose selection and dietary tolerance and found to be 1000 mg/kg diet [1000 ppm]. Groups of 75 male mice, five to six weeks of age, then received weekly oral doses of 7.5 mg N-nitrosobutyl(4-hydroxybutyl)amine in ethanol:water (ratio not given) or vehicle only for eight weeks (total dose, 60 mg/mouse). Aspirin was administered in the diet at doses of 400 and 800 ppm (representing 40 and 80% of the MTD) beginning one week before the first dose of nitrosamine and continuing until termination of the study at 24 weeks. The terminal body weights and survival were not reduced by inclusion of aspirin in the diet. The incidence of transitional-cell carcinomas in the urinary bladders of nitrosamine-treated mice (22/75) was similar to that in mice treated with the carcinogen plus aspirin (22/73) (Rao et al., 1996).

Groups of 32 Fischer 344 rats received 2% N-[4-(5-nitro-2-furyl)-2-thiazolyl]formamide in the diet with 0.5% aspirin [5000 ppm] for 12 weeks; aspirin was continued for one week, and then the animals were given control diet for 56 weeks. Aspirin significantly reduced the incidence of urinary bladder carcinomas: in only 10 of 27 (37%) rats treated with aspirin but in 18 of 21 (87%) rats treated with the carcinogen only. Forestomach tumours, however, were not seen in rats fed the carcinogen alone but developed in 7 of 27 rats fed carcinogen plus aspirin (Murasaki et al., 1984).

Groups of 32 five-week-old male Wistar rats received basal diet for 32 weeks; basal diet for 32 weeks with water containing 0.05%

N-nitrosobutyl(4-hydroxybutyl)amine in weeks 2–10; a diet containing aspirin at 1 g/kg [1000 ppm] in weeks 1–20 and water *ad libitum* for 32 weeks; or a diet containing aspirin at 1 g/kg [1000 ppm] in weeks 1–20, drinking-water containing the nitrosamine at 0.05% during weeks 2–10 and then basal diet and water for the remainder of the 32 weeks. Aspirin significantly reduced ($p < 0.05$) the incidence of carcinogen-induced urinary bladder tumours: 8 of 32 rats treated with the nitrosamine developed bladder tumours, whereas only 1 of 32 rats treated with carcinogen plus aspirin developed a bladder tumour (Klän et al., 1993).

(d) Pancreas
Groups of 20 outbred female Syrian golden hamsters, five weeks old, received five weekly doses of 10 mg/kg bw N-nitrosobis(2-oxopropyl)amine by subcutaneous injection; one group of 19 hamsters was also given aspirin (purity, 99.5%) from weeks 6 to 32 (time of terminal kill). A control group of 30 hamsters was given tap-water. Aspirin treatment had no effect on body-weight gain. Neither the reduction in the incidence of pancreatic tumours, from 20/28 to 10/19, nor the reduction in the multiplicity of pancreatic adenocarcinomas, from 1.3 to 0.84, was significant (Takahashi et al., 1990).

4.2.2 In-vitro models
No data were available to the Working Group.

4.3 Mechanisms of chemoprevention
Most research into the mechanisms of the chemopreventive action of aspirin has been centred around four areas that are thought to be related to the development of colorectal cancer: (i) activation of carcinogens, (ii) cell proliferation, (iii) apoptosis and (iv) immune surveillance. These hypotheses are summarized in Figure 3.

4.3.1 Inhibition of carcinogen activation
Cyclooxygenases (COX-1 and COX-2)[1] may be involved in the initiation of carcinogenesis in three general ways: activation of carcinogens to DNA-binding forms, production of malondialdehyde and formation of peroxyl radicals.

[1] Used as synonyms for prostaglandin endoperoxide synthases (PGH synthases)

Figure 3. Proposed mechanisms of prevention of colon cancer by aspirin

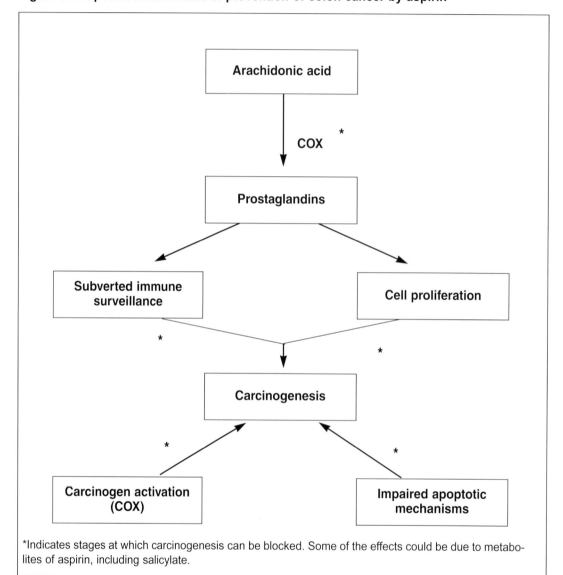

*Indicates stages at which carcinogenesis can be blocked. Some of the effects could be due to metabolites of aspirin, including salicylate.

Activation of carcinogens by COX is well documented (reviewed by Eling *et al.*, 1990), and it has also been demonstrated that aspirin can inhbit such processes (Krauss & Eling, 1985; Levy & Weber, 1992; Liu *et al.*, 1995). An illustrative example is the conversion of 2-aminofluorene to a DNA-binding product by both COX isozymes. This conversion is inhibited by aspirin.

Malondialdehyde is produced by the enzymic and nonenzymic breakdown of prostaglandin H and during lipid peroxidation (reviewed by Marnett, 1992). It is a directly acting mutagen in bacterial and mammalian systems and it is also carcinogenic in rats. Aspirin and other NSAIDs inhibit the formation of malondialdehyde only *via* the breakdown of prostaglandin H_2.

Minchin *et al.* (1992) demonstrated in an enzyme-free system *in vitro* that aspirin directly activates several *N*-hydroxyarylamines by *O*-acetylation.

4.3.2 *Inhibition of cell proliferation*

An indirect pathway by which aspirin could inhibit the proliferation of colonocytes is inhibition of the proliferative effect of prostaglandins. This effect, which requires acetylation of COX by aspirin, has been documented only in cultured colon cancer cells. The plausibility of this idea rests on the already mentioned observations that colon tumours produce increased amounts of prostaglandin E_2, colon adenomas and carcinomas overexpress COX and mice lacking both the *Apc* and *Cox-2* genes have 90% fewer intestinal tumours than those lacking only *Apc*.

Aspirin induced a concentration-dependent reduction in the proliferation rate of HT-29 human colon cancer cells. This effect was accompanied by distinctive morphological changes in these cells. Of greater interest, aspirin altered the distribution of HT-29 cells in the various phases of the cell cycle in a non-liear, concentration-dependent fashion at concentrations starting at 1 mmol/litre (Shiff *et al.*, 1996).

Salicyclic acid, the metabolite of aspirin, also inhibited the growth of human colorectal tumour cell lines at concentrations of 1–5 mmol/litre (Elder *et al.*, 1996). The inhibitory effect was greater against carcinoma and adenoma cell lines transformed *in vitro* than against adenoma cell lines. Accumulation of many cells in the G_0/G_1 cell cycle phase and apoptosis were also noted. It is doubtful that the inhibition of cell proliferation in these studies was due to a reduction in prostaglandin production (Hanif *et al.*, 1996). [The Working Group noted that as the typical concentrations in humans *in vivo* would be less than 1 μmol/litre, the physiological significance of these in-vitro observations remains in doubt.]

4.3.3 *Apoptosis*

Most NSAIDs can induce apoptosis in colon cancer cell lines *in vitro*, but conflicting findings are reported for aspirin. Shiff *et al.* (1996) found that although indomethacin, naproxen and piroxicam induced apoptosis in HT-29 cells, aspirin at 1500 μmol/litre did not. Three methods were used to detect apoptosis: DNA laddering on agarose gel electrophoresis, fluorescent-activated cell sorting to detect sub-diploid peaks based on DNA content and acridine orange staining to highlight cellular morphological changes such as DNA condensation. Elder *et al.* (1996), however, demonstrated a convincing, dose-dependent apoptotic response of HT-29 colon cancer cells to salicylate and a similar response in transformed adenoma cells but not in all adenoma cell lines. Acridine orange staining of floating cells was used to quantify apoptosis. Elder *et al.* used concentrations up to 5 mmol/litre but did detect an effect at 1500 μmol/litre, equivalent to the concentration used by Shiff *et al.*. The latter group tested aspirin, whereas Elder *et al.* tested salicylate, which is more appropriate, since it is the predominant pharmacological metabolite in patients on long-term aspirin treatment.

4.3.4 *Immune surveillance*

The role of aspirin in immune surveillance is uncertain, as is the central idea that immune surveillance is important in carcinogenesis. The role of aspirin in immune surveillance has been addressed both directly and indirectly in cell culture systems. The finding that colon cancers contain elevated levels of prostaglandin E_2 (Rigas *et al.*, 1993) prompted studies of the role of this compound in regulation of the expression of classes I and II HLA antigens in SW1116 colon cancer cells. Prostaglandin E_2 down-regulated the expression of the class II antigen HLA-DR in SW1116 cells in a concentration- and time-dependent manner. The effect of aspirin at 100–200 μmol/litre was reversible and specific (Arvind *et al.*, 1995). Other eicosanoids such as prostaglandin F_{2a} and leukotriene B_4 had no such effect. The reduction of HLA-DR by prostaglandin E_2 was accompanied by reduced mRNA levels of *HLA-DRa* and reduced transcription of the corresponding gene. (*HLA-DRa* is one of the two genes that code for the heterodimeric HLA-DR protein). In contrast, the expression of HLA class I genes was not affected. An additional study by the same group confirmed that prostaglandin, E_2, prostaglandin $F_{2\alpha}$ and leukotriene B_4 did not affect the expression of MHC class I antigens in SW1116 and HT-29 human colon adenocarcinoma cells. Furthermore, 16,16-dimethyl prostaglandin E_2, a stable analogue of prostaglandin E_2, did not affect their expression in mice, even when treated with a colon carcinogen (Feng *et al.*, 1996).

The effect of aspirin on the expression of class II antigens was also assessed from a different viewpoint (Arvind *et al.*, 1996). Aspirin induced a several-fold increase in the expression of HLA-DR in HT-29 human colon adenocarcinoma cells, which do not normally express these antigens. These effect was accompanied by increased steady-state mRNA levels of *HLA-DRa* and an increased transcription rate of the gene. The study clearly established a transcriptional effect of aspirin on an HLA class II gene, suggesting a potentially important immunological effect of this versatile compound. This finding is consistent with results showing up-regulation of MHC expression in rats after treatment with piroxicam (Rigas *et al.*, 1994).

Several studies (reviewed by Rumore *et al.*, 1987) have demonstrated that aspirin induces interferon, decreases the antibody response, inhibits antigen–antibody interactions, alters T-lymphocyte functions and alters leukocyte migration.

Nitric oxide synthesized by inducible nitric oxide synthase has been implicated as a mediator of inflammation. Aspirin and salicylate at millimolar concentrations have been reported to inhibit induction of inducible nitric oxide synthase in murine macrophages activated by lipopolysaccharide (Amin *et al.*, 1995; Brouet & Ohshima, 1995) and in neonatal rat cardiac fibroblasts treated with interferon-γ and tumour necrosis factor-α (Farivar & Brecher, 1996).

5. Other Beneficial Effects

5.1 Antiplatelet effects

5.1.1 Background

Aspirin is widely used to prevent myocardial infarct, thrombotic stroke and death from vascular events in populations at high risk for vascular conditions. Randomized trials have confirmed the efficacy of aspirin in secondary prevention in patients with documented coronary, cerebral or peripheral vascular disease. The absolute benefits are smaller for healthy people, however, and the net improvement less certain. This section covers the mechanism whereby aspirin inhibits platelet aggregation, how aspirin differs mechanistically from other NSAIDs and from non-NSAID antiplatelet drugs and what is known currently about the lowest effective dose.

5.1.2 Mechanism

Aspirin inhibits platelet aggregation and thrombosis by permanently inactivating COX-1 in platelets (Moncada & Vane, 1979). Irreversible acetylation of the hydroxyl group of a single serine residue essentially stops platelet thromboxane A_2 production for the 7–10-day life of the platelet. Unlike nucleated cells, platelets cannot resynthesize COX-1. Aspirin is a more potent inhibitor of platelet thromboxane production than other NSAIDs because it binds covalently, rather than reversibly, to COX-1 (Patrono, 1994). The mechanism by which aspirin inhibits platelet aggregation and prevents clot propagation differs fundamentally from that of various recently developed antiplatelet drugs, which block the binding of fibrinogen to receptors on the platelet membrane but do not inhibit COX or the production of platelet thromboxane (CAPRIE Steering Committee, 1996; Cohen, 1996).

5.1.3 Secondary prevention in populations at high risk for cardiovascular events

Prophylactic aspirin therapy is known to reduce the risk for vascular thrombosis in high-risk populations (Antiplatelet Trialists' Collaboration, 1988, 1994a,b). A comprehensive overview of 145 randomized trials, 50 involving aspirin alone, found aspirin to be beneficial in high-risk settings: patients with acute myocardial infarct, those with a past history of myocardial infarct or clinical cerebrovascular disease, those with a past history of stroke or transient ischaemic attack and those with various other vascular problems (including unstable angina, stable angina, a history of vascular surgery, angioplasty, atrial fibrillation, valvular disease and peripheral vascular disease). Most of the trials involved daily doses of 75–325 mg aspirin (Antiplatelet Trialists' Collaboration, 1994b).

In absolute terms, the benefit of aspirin is greatest in patients with acute myocardial infarct, among whom 38 vascular events were prevented per 1000 patients treated for only about one month. Similar benefits were seen for patients with prior myocardial infarct, prior stroke, transient ischaemic atack or other 'high risk' cardiovascular conditions, although longer treatment (16–33 months) was required to obtain them. Much smaller benefits were observed in primary prevention trials, with four vascular events prevented in 1000 patients over an average of 62 months of therapy (Antiplatelet Trialists' Collaboration, 1994; Hirsh et al., 1995).

5.1.4 Primary prevention in populations at average risk for cardiovascular events

Among men in the general population, prophylactic aspirin administration reduces the incidence of non-fatal myocardial infarct but has not yet been demonstrated to reduce overall mortality from cardiovascular disease (Hirsh et al., 1995).

5.1.5 Lowest effective dose for prevention of cardiovascular events in high-risk populations

The optimal dose of aspirin for long-term prophylactic cardiovascular therapy is unknown. In the randomized trials reviewed by the Antiplatelet Trialists' Collaboration (1994b), daily doses of 75–150 mg seemed to be as effective as higher doses in preventing vascular events, although the statistical power to examine this issue was limited. Several well-designed

randomized trials of secondary prevention have shown aspirin to be effective in preventing thrombosis at doses of 75 mg/day (RISC Group, 1990; SALT Collaborative Group, 1991; Juul-Moller et al., 1992; Lindblad et al., 1993). One study indicated that a dose as low as 30 mg/day may be protective (Dutch TIA Trial Study Group, 1991). The theory that very low doses of aspirin might be as effective and less toxic than higher doses is biologically plausible because aspirin inhibits platelet thromboxane A2 production almost completely (Patrono, 1994). The efficacy of doses lower than 325 mg every other day has not yet been tested in randomized trials in the context of primary prevention.

5.2 Alzheimer disease

McGeer et al. (1996) recently reviewed 17 epidemiological studies of the use of NSAIDs and steroids as possible protective factors against Alzheimer disease. Five of six case–control studies in which 'arthritis' was used as a surrogate for use of NSAIDs or steroids and one of two in which rheumatoid arthritis was examined reported a reduced risk for Alzheimer disease associated with those diagnoses (combined data for arthritis, RR, 0.56; CI, 0.44–0.70). In three other studies of patients with rheumatoid arthritis, Alzheimer disease was noted to be uncommon. The summary measure of risk in three additional case–control studies of the use of NSAIDs and risk for Alzheimer disease was 0.50 (0.34–0.72) as a group; similarly, steroids were associated with a summary odds ratio of 0.66 (0.43–0.99) in four case–control studies.

In nearly all of the reviewed studies, the diagnosis of Alzheimer disease was made clinically, usually by a neurologist, so that attempts were made to exclude vascular and other dementias. In all of these studies, information on use of aspirin was obtained retrospectively, so that recall bias or change in use of aspirin precipitated by the disease itself could not be reliably excluded.

5.3 Reproductive outcomes

Combined analyses of all randomized trials of antiplatelet therapy in the possible prevention of pregnancy-induced hypertension have been published (CLASP Collaborative Group, 1994; ECPPA Collaborative Group, 1996). Most of the trials were of aspirin (50–150 mg/day), but a few were of aspirin with dipyridamole. When the results of all the trials were taken together, antiplatelet therapy was associated with a reduction of 23% in the incidence of pre-eclampsia (ECPPA Collaborative Group, 1996). The results are heterogeneous, however, and when the small trials (including fewer than 200 women) are excluded, the apparent reduction is 17%. All of the trials that found strong effects of antiplatelet therapy on the prevention of pre-eclampsia were very small, and at least as many women are known to have been randomized in other small but unpublished trials (CLASP Collaborative Group, 1994). If some small trials with unpromising results were not published, the available results from the small trials would give a biased estimate of the effects of antiplatelet therapy, but the large trials would not. The findings of the analysis of the data from the large trials are consistent with this assumption.

In five of the larger trials included in these combined analyses, information on pre-term delivery was presented (Hauth *et al.*, 1993; Italian Study of Aspirin in Pregnancy, 1993; Sibai *et al.*, 1993; CLASP Collaborative Group, 1994; ECPPA Collaborative Group, 1996). No noteworthy effect of aspirin (50 or 60 mg/day) on preterm delivery was observed; however, in the large trial of the CLASP Collaborative Group (1994), the absolute risks of preterm delivery differed substantially between the categories of women studied. Among about 8000 women entered for prophylactic reasons, only one-fifth of the placebo group had pre-term delivery, and the absolute benefit appeared to be about two fewer preterm deliveries per 100 women allocated aspirin. Among just over 1000 women entered for therapeutic reasons, two-fifths of the placebo group had preterm delivery, and the absolute benefit appeared to be about 5 per 100.

In some of the trials of the use of low doses of aspirin in the prevention of pregnancy-induced hypertension or pre-eclampsia, data on intrauterine growth retardation were presented (Uzan *et al.*, 1991; Hauth *et al.*, 1993; Italian Study of Aspirin in Pregnancy, 1993;

Sibai *et al.*, 1993; Viinikka *et al.*, 1993; CLASP Collaborative Group, 1994; ECPPA Collaborative Group, 1996). The RRs associated with use of aspirin were in the range 0.5–1.0. A significant effect was found only in the relatively small trial of Uzan *et al.* (1991).

A combined analysis of antiplatelet therapy in the prevention of perinatal mortality was presented by the CLASP Collaborative Group (1994) and was subsequently updated by the ECPPA Collaborative Group (1996). This analysis suggested a 1% (standard deviation, 10) reduction in the incidence of perinatal mortality associated with antiplatelet therapy. Data from the trials in which at least 200 women were enrolled suggested a 1% (standard deviation, 10) increase in perinatal mortality associated with antiplatelet therapy.

Shapiro *et al.* (1976) examined the relationship between perinatal mortality and reported aspirin use at any time during pregnancy in a multicentre cohort study of 41 337 women whose pregnancies lasted at least seven months. Data on drug use were recorded at each antenatal visit and were confirmed for most women by the attending physician or by review of the hospital or clinical record. The women were divided into 1515 who were heavily exposed, 24 866 with intermediate exposure and 14 956 who were not exposed. Heavy exposure was defined as use for at least eight days per month for at least six lunar months. There were 371 (2.5%) perinatal deaths in the unexposed group, 548 (2.2%) in the group with intermediate exposure and 38 (2.5%) in the group with heavy exposure. Thus, there was no association between perinatal mortality and level of exposure to aspirin.

6. Carcinogenicity

6.1 Humans
6.1.1 Renal cancer
Paganini-Hill *et al.* (1989) reported significantly more hospitalizations from renal cancer among men who used aspirin daily than among non-users in a cohort in a retirement community followed up from 1981 through 1987 (RR, 6.3; CI, 2.2–17; nine exposed cases, six unexposed). Only three cases of renal

cancer were observed among exposed women (RR, 2.1; 0.53–8.5) in the initial report. After 3.5 additional years of follow-up, the statistically significant excess remained in male but not female aspirin users (Paganini-Hill, 1995). No information was available in this study on the duration of aspirin use, past use of phenacetin or current exposure to other analgesics.

Aspirin use was not associated with cancers of the urinary system in the large American Cancer Society cohort (Thun *et al.*, 1993) nor with renal cancer in the two largest trials of aspirin in the primary prevention of heart disease (Hennekens *et al.*, 1990). Steineck *et al.* (1995) found an increased risk for transitional-cell urothelial cancer among people who reported acetaminophen use (1.6, 1.1–2.3) but not aspirin use (0.7; 0.5–1.0) in a population-based case–control study of 325 cases and 393 controls.

[The Working Group noted that a major limitation of the studies that show aspirin to be associated with urinary tract cancers is the inability to control for past use of phenacetin. A number of the studies did not distinguish between renal-cell and renal pelvic cancer.]

Ross *et al.* (1989) also found aspirin use to be associated with cancer of the renal pelvis and ureter in a population-based case–control study of 187 cases from the Los Angeles Tumor Registry and 187 neighbourhood controls (RR among nonsmokers, 5.0, 1.7–14); the association with renal pelvis cancer was confined to women. In a large-scale study in Minnesota, USA, no relationship was found between renal-cell carcinoma and regular use or duration of use of aspirin (Chow *et al.*, 1994).

6.1.2 Haematopoietic malignancies

In the studies of rheumatoid arthritis patients in Finland and Sweden (see p. 51), the incidence of haematopoietic malignancies was about twice that of the general population (Isomäki *et al.*, 1978; Gridley *et al.*, 1993). In the study of Gridley *et al.* (1993), described on p. 51, there was an increased risk for lymphomas (SIR, 2.0; CI, 1.5–2.6). [The Working Group noted that the underlying rheumatoid arthritis and other treatment could account for differences in lymphoma risk in this study.]

6.1.3 Childhood cancer

In some case–control studies of childhood cancer, data on recalled aspirin use during pregnancy was obtained by interviewing the mothers. In a study of 188 cases of leukaemia and 93 controls with other cancers and a second control group of people hospitalized for reasons other than cancer (Manning & Carroll, 1957), the RR for leukaemia associated with reported use of aspirin was 1.5 (CI, 0.87–2.5), in comparison with controls with other cancers and 2.3 (CI, 1.1–.4.8) in comparison with the other control group.

In single studies, no significant association was found between reported aspirin use during pregnancy and brain tumours (Preston-Martin *et al.*, 1982), neuroblastoma (Schwartzbaum, 1992) or rhabdomyosarcoma (Grufferman *et al.*, 1982) in the offspring.

6.2 Experimental animals

No data were available to the Working Group.

7. Other Toxic Effects

7.1 Adverse effects
7.1.1 Humans

(a) Upper gastrointestinal tract toxicity

All NSAIDs, including aspirin, cause a dose-dependent increase in the incidence of upper gastrointestinal toxic effects, ranging in severity from dyspepsia to gastrointestinal haemorrhage, ulceration and perforation. The severity and frequency of these complications vary greatly with the dose and duration of use. Aspirin is the only NSAID for which substantial data exist on the toxicity of both prolonged use of low doses and exposure to anti-inflammatory doses.

Toxicity of high doses. At high anti-inflammatory doses of aspirin (> 2400 mg daily), gastrointestinal bleeding and ulceration become important individual and public health problems. In several randomized trials of cardiovascular disease and aspirin use, patients receiving 1 g of aspirin per day had an incidence of six episodes of haematemesis per 10 000 person-months of treatment (Aspirin

Myocardial Infarction Study Research Group, 1980). The incidence during the three-year treatment period was two times higher than that of untreated patients. The incidence of upper gastrointestinal tract ulcers (per 10 000 patient-months of treatment) was 9.7 in patients treated with 972–1500 mg aspirin daily (Coronary Drug Project Research Group, 1976; Britton *et al.*, 1987; Ehresmann *et al.*, 1977; Hess *et al.*, 1985; Fields *et al.*, 1978; Lemak *et al.*, 1986) and 2.1 in the group receiving placebo in the US Physicians' Health Study (Steering Committee of the Physicians' Health Study Research Group, 1989). The absolute rates in these trials may not be generalizable to the general population because people with ulcers were excluded from the study, but they indicate that gastric toxicity due to anti-inflammatory doses of aspirin is a serious problem. Gastric toxicity due to use of NSAIDs, including aspirin, by rheumatoid arthritis patients has been estimated to cause 240 000 hospitalizations and 2600 deaths per year in the USA (Fries *et al.*, 1991).

Toxicity of low doses. Among men in the US Physicians' Health Study who received either placebo or 325 mg aspirin every other day for five years, the incidence of haematemesis or melaena was approximately 1.5 times higher than that in the controls. This corresponds to about 19 episodes of major gastrointestinal bleeding attributable to 100 000 person-months of aspirin treatment. In a trial in the United Kingdom in which some 2400 persons were randomized to receive 300 or 1200 mg of aspirin daily or placebo, the RR for upper gastrointestinal tract haemorrhage in people at 300 mg daily was 3.3 (1.2–9.0) in comparison with those on placebo (Slattery *et al.*, 1995).

(b)   Non-gastrointestinal bleeding, including haemorrhagic stroke

A dose-dependent increase in the risk for serious blood loss requiring transfusion was observed in the combined data from 34 randomized trials (Antiplatelet Trialists' Collaboration, 1994b, Appendix 1; Table 8). Aspirin at doses of 75 mg daily increases the risk for non-fatal extracerebral bleeding requiring transfusion.

Aspirin may also increase the risk for haemorrhagic stroke (Hirsh *et al.*, 1995). In both the British doctors study (Peto *et al.*, 1988) and the US Physicians' Health Study (Steering Committee of the Physicians' Health Study Research Group, 1989), statistically insignificant increases in total stroke incidence were reported in healthy men treated with aspirin. Ten stroke deaths were observed in the US Physicians Study among people treated with aspirin, versus seven in the placebo group (RR, 1.4; CI, 0.54–3.9). The incidence of non-fatal disabling stroke was higher among British doctors treated with aspirin (19 per 10 000 man-years) than in the placebo group (7.4 per 10 000; $p < 0.05$). The total stroke incidence was not increased in an observational study of aspirin use among healthy US nurses (Manson *et al.*, 1991). The net effect of aspirin prophylaxis is consistently beneficial in populations at high risk for ischaemic stroke who have already experienced a cerebrovascular event or symptoms (Antiplatelet Trialists' Collaboration, 1994b). Ishaemic and haemorrhagic strokes cannot be reliably separated in many of the trials of aspirin in secondary prevention.

(c)   Blood pressure

In a meta-analysis of 50 randomized, placebo-controlled trials, short-term treatment with aspirin appeared to have no demonstrable effect on blood pressure, in contrast to many other NSAIDs (Johnson *et al.*, 1994).

(d)   Reye syndrome

Reye syndrome is an acute condition characterized by non-inflammatory encephalopathy and liver injury. This extremely rare syndrome has been reported primarily, although not exclusively, in children (Sullivan-Bolyai & Corey, 1981). A review of six case–control studies from the USA — four published before 1981 and two subsequent studies — designed specifically to address methodological flaws in the earlier studies, supported the role of use of aspirin during a period of antecedent illness (Hurwitz, 1989). A seventh case–control study from the United Kingdom further supports this association (Hall, 1990).

Table 8. Incidence of non-fatal extracerebral bleeding requiring transfusion according to aspirin dose in 34 randomized clinical trials

Aspirin dose[a] (mg/day)	Person-years of treatment	No. of people	Per 100 000 treatment years	
			Incidence	95% CI
Placebo	95 591	75	0.54	0.42–0.67
75–170	62 863	63	0.81	0.63–1.0
300–500	26 134	41	1.1	0.75–1.4
1200–1500	6 590	20	2.2	1.2–3.0

From Antiplatelet Trialists' Collaboration (1994b)

[a] Reflects actual dose used in trials; therefore, scale not continuous

Since 1980, publicity and advice has been followed by a marked decline (at least 50%) in aspirin use among children in the USA. This decline was accompanied by a drastic reduction in the reported number of cases of Reye syndrome in children, notably those over five years old. At these ages, the problems in the differential diagnosis of metabolic disorders and Reye syndrome that may occur with younger children are unlikely (Hurwitz, 1989). Therefore, the consistent positive association between Reye syndrome and aspirin use observed in case–control studies is supported by a temporal association between the use of aspirin in children and the occurrence of the syndrome.

Controlled studies of aspirin use and Reye syndrome are confined to the USA and the United Kingdom. Few children with Reye syndrome who were exposed to aspirin have been reported from other countries. Among 20 children with Reye syndrome reported over a 10-year period in Australia when paediatric aspirin use of aspirin was low, prior exposure to aspirin was found in only one child (Orlowski et al., 1987). In a series of 15 children with Reye syndrome in Germany, three had been exposed to aspirin (Gladtke & Schausiel, 1987). It remains unknown whether aspirin-associated Reye syndrome has occurred outside the USA and the United Kingdom.

(e)   Asthma

Approximately 10% of adults with asthma develop acute, idiosyncratic bronchoconstriction after ingesting aspirin or other NSAIDs (Fischer et al., 1994; Staton & Ingram, 1996). Often called 'aspirin-sensitive' asthma, this condition can be precipitated by any currently available NSAID. Symptoms begin within 15 min to 4 h (usually 1 h) after ingestion, and may include rhinorrhoea, conjunctival irritation, scarlet flushing of the head and neck and severe, even life-threatening asthma. The respiratory symptoms can continue beyond discontinuation of NSAID use (Szczeklik, 1994).

(f)   Nephrotoxicity

The relationship between chronic use of analgesics, most notably phenacetin, and chronic renal failure has been recognized for over 30 years. Although epidemiological studies have consistently found an increased risk for chronic renal failure associated with phenacetin use and prolonged use of mixtures of analgesics, the findings with regard to aspirin have been inconsistent. Two large case–control studies of end-stage renal disease (Pernerger et al., 1994) and early chronic renal failure (Sandler et al., 1989) and one cohort study with a 20-year follow-up (Dubach et al., 1991) reported no excess risk for chronic renal failure in association with aspirin use. In another large case–control study (Pommer et al., 1989), an increased risk for chronic renal disease was associated with aspirin used in combination with other analgesics, but not when used as a single agent. In a further large case-control study, the RR was 2.5 (CI, 1.2–5.2) for chronic renal failure associated with regular aspirin use alone (Morlans et al., 1990); however, in this study, the probability that the association was confounded by prior use of phenacetin-containing compounds could not be excluded completely. At doses of 1–2 g/day, aspirin may decrease urate excretion, increase plasma urate concentrations and potentially precipitate clinical gout. At higher doses, aspirin either does not affect urate excretion or lowers it (Goodman Gilman *et al.*, 1990). As aspirin inhibits the effects of uricosuric agents, its use in patients treated with these agents is not advised (Editions du Vidal, 1995).

(g)   Reproductive and developmental effects

Abruptio placentae. In a randomized controlled trial, Sibai *et al.* (1993) found an increased incidence of abruptio placentae among women who received 60 mg of aspirin per day over that of women who received placebo (Table 9). This was not a primary outcome of the trial, nor indeed of any other trial (Hauth *et al.*, 1995), as no evidence of an increase in the incidence of abruptio placentae was found in randomized trials in which at least 200 women were enrolled. The increased risk found by Sibai *et al.* (1993) may be a chance observation or due to a low incidence of the disorder in the placebo group in that trial (Hauth *et al.*, 1995).

Maternal bleeding around the time of delivery. Hertz-Picciotto *et al.* (1990) reviewed studies of the association between taking aspirin late in pregnancy and maternal haemostatic abnormalities. Clinically observable effects on maternal haemostasis were seen at an average dose of 1500 mg/day or more. Platelet dysfunction was observed at lower doses, such as 60 mg/day. In a randomzed trial of the use of 60 mg of aspirin per day, no noteworthy difference in the incidence of antepartum haemorrhage, other than abruptio placentae or post-partum bleeding of 500 ml or more, was observed in comparison with women given placebo (CLASP Collaborative Group, 1994). A significantly higher percentage (4%) of women allocated to aspirin received blood transfusions after delivery than women allocated placebo (3.2%), independently of differences in the occurrence or degree of post-partum haemorrhage. No effect of aspirin on maternal bleeding complications was observed in other large trials (Italian Study of Aspirin in Pregnancy, 1993; Sibai *et al.*, 1993; Viinikka *et al.*, 1993; ECPPA Collaborative Group, 1996).

Table 9. Use of low doses of aspirin and abruptio placentae: data from randomized trials in which at least 200 women were enrolled

Dose of aspirin (mg per day)	No. of women		Abruptio placentae				RR	95% CI[a]	Reference
	Aspirin	Placebo	Aspirin		Placebo				
			No.	%	No.	%			
60	1485	1500	11	0.7	2	0.1	5.6	1.2–25	Sibai *et al.* (1993)
150	156[b]	74	7[b]	4.5	6	8.1	0.6	0.2–1.6	Uzan *et al.* (1991)
60	302	302	3[c]	1.0	2[c]	0.7	1.5	0.3–8.9	Hauth *et al.* (1993)
50	561	471[d]	7[c]	1.2	9[c]	1.9	0.7	0.2–1.7	Italian Study of Aspirin in Pregnancy (1993)
50	97	100	0[c]		0[c]		Undefined		Viinikka *et al.* (1993)
60	4659	4650	86	1.8	71	1.5	1.2	0.9–1.7	CLASP Collaborative Group (1994)
60	476	494	5	1.1	7	1.4	0.7	0.2–2.3	ECPPA Collaborative Group (1996)

[a] Calculated by the Working Group
[b] Some women received 225 mg/day diprimadole
[c] Data from Hauth *et al.* (1995)
[d] No treatment

Neonatal haemostatic abnormalities. There is a consistent association between bleeding in the newborn and maternal exposure to aspirin at analgesic or antipyretic doses late in pregnancy (Hertz-Picciotto *et al.*, 1990). Such abnormalities may include intracranial haemorrhage, particularly in preterm babies and those with a low birth weight.

In a large randomized trial of 60 mg/day aspirin or placebo, fewer intraventricular haemorrhages were reported among babies born to women allocated aspirin (0.7%) than among those in the placebo group (0.9%); this difference was not statistically significant (CLASP Collaborative Group, 1994). No significant differences in fetal or neonatal deaths attributed to haemorrhage or in the incidence of other neonatal haemorrhages were seen, and no differences in the incidence of fetal bleeding complications were observed in other large trials of low doses of aspirin (Italian Study of Aspirin in Pregnancy, 1993; Sibai *et al.*, 1993; Viinikka *et al.*, 1993; ECPPA Collaborative Group, 1996).

Preterm constriction of the ductus arteriosus. During fetal life, the patency of the ductus arteriosus is maintained by prostaglandins, while COX inhibitors constrict it. As aspirin inhibits COX, it has been postulated that maternal use of aspirin late in pregnancy may lead to preterm constriction of the ductus arteriosus, leading to abnormalities in pulmonary vasculature that would promote pulmonary hypertension in the newborn. Few data are available, however, as abnormalities of pulmonary vasculature are not easy to diagnose, even at routine autopsy (Hertz-Picciotto *et al.*, 1990).

Congenital anomalies. Studies of the association between maternal aspirin use in the first trimester and congenital anomalies are summarized in Table 10. The studies are difficult to compare because of differences in the definition and characterization of anomalies. The only statistically significant increases associated with reported aspirin use were for congenital heart defects (Rothman *et al.*, 1979; Zierler & Rothman, 1985) and for orofacial clefts (Saxén, 1975).

Congenital abnormalities were not found to be associated with aspirin use during the first 14 days of pregnancy (Nelson & Forfar, 1971) or during the first trimester (Weatherall & Greenberg, 1979).

In a comparison of prescriptions for 764 mothers whose children had a defect of the central nervous system with those of an equal number of mothers of control babies, aspirin use for the three months before the last menstrual period and for the first trimester of pregnancy was not associated with increased risk (Winship *et al.*, 1984). This finding was corroborated for all congenital defects in a similar study of prescribed analgesics (Hill *et al.*, 1988), and by McDonald (1994) for use of any analgesic during the first trimester.

The study of Rothman *et al.* (1979) was designed to investigate the relationship between exposure to exogenous sex hormones and congenital heart disease. A total of 460 cases was ascertained among infants born in Massachusetts, USA, during the period 1973–75. Most of the cases were ascertained from a programme designed to provide special care to infants born in New England with serious congenital heart disease, the diagnosis being determined by cardiac catheterization, surgery or, ultimately, autopsy. The remaining cases were ascertained from death certificates. The control series comprised 1500 births selected randomly from all births in Massachusetts during the study period. At the end of each year, questionnaires were sent to the mothers of control infants, and cases were identified from the specialized care programme. Mothers of cases identified from death certificates were interviewed by telephone. Data were obtained on 390 cases (85% of those eligible) and 1254 controls (89%). The RR associated with aspirin consumption at about the time the pregnancy began was 1.3 (one-tailed $p = 0.02$). The authors noted that information about use of non-hormonal drugs was obtained from an open-ended questionnaire and therefore may have been subject to some recall bias. For the cases in which a specific diagnosis was known, reported medication was compared for the major diagnostic

Table 10. Association between maternal aspirin use in the first trimester and congenital malformations

Area and period of study	Cases Type[a]	Cases No.	Controls or cohort Type	Controls No.	Aspirin Source	Method of assessing use[b]	Prevalence of use in controls	Contrast	RR	95% CI	Reference
UK, South Wales, 1964–66	CNS	279	Population	279	Any	IR, MR	17	Any versus none	1.6[c]	1.1–2.4	Richards (1969)
	CVS	100		100			15		0.8[c]	0.4–1.9	
	Ali	173		173			13		2.2[c]	1.3–3.9	
	MSK	152		152			14		1.8[c]	1.0–3.3	
	All	833		833			14		1.7[c]	1.3–2.2	
UK, Scotland (3 maternity units over 2 years)	Major	175	Hospital	916	Any	Q, Pres	3	Any versus none	1.2	0.6–2.5	Nelson & Forfar (1971)
	Minor	283					2		1.7	1.0–2.9	
	All	458					5		1.5	0.9–2.4	
Finland, 1967–71	ICP	232	Population	226	Any (salicylates)	IA, IR	6	Any versus none	1.9	0.9–3.8	Saxén (1975)
	ICL(P)	232		230			5		4.5	2.3–8.6	
	CLP	599		590			6		2.5	1.6–3.7	
USA, multicentre, 1959–65	CNS	266	Cohort	50 282	Any	IA	30[d]	Heavy[e] versus none	0.8[f]		Slone et al. (1976)
	CVS	404							0.9[f]		
	MSK	395							1.0[f]		
	RT	218							1.0[f]		
	GI	301							1.2[f]		
	Major	1393							0.9[f]	0.8–1.1	
USA, Massachusetts, 1973–75	CVS	390	Population	1254	Any	Q	16[g]	Any versus none	1.3	1.0–1.8	Rothman et al. (1979)
UK, England and Wales	Serious[h]	836	General population	836	Prescribed	MR	1.3	Any versus none	1.7	0.7–4.2	Weatherall & Greenberg (1979)
UK, England and Wales, 1971	CNS	764	General population	764	Prescribed	MR	0.4	Any versus none	2.7	0.6–16	Winship et al. (1984)

Table 10 (contd)

Area and period of study	Cases		Controls or cohort		Aspirin		Prevalence of use in controls	Association with aspirin			Reference
	Type[a]	No.	Type	No.	Source	Method of assessing use[b]		Contrast	RR	95% CI	
USA, Massachusetts, 1980–83	CVS	298	Population	738	Any	IR, MR	9	Any versus none	1.4	1.0–2.0	Zierler & Rothman (1985)
UK, England and Wales, 1983–84	CLP	676	Population	676	Prescribed analgesics	MR	4	Any versus none	1.3	0.8–2.1	Hill et al. (1988)
	LRD	115		115			4		0.6	0.1–2.5	
USA and Canada, multicentre, 1976–86	CVS	1381	Other[i]	6966	Any	IR	27	Any versus none	0.9	0.8–1.1	Werler et al. (1989)
Canada, Montreal, 1987–94	Major	787	Hospital	787	Any analgesic	IR	17	Any versus none	1.1		McDonald (1994)
	Minor	2386		2386					1.3		

[a] CNS, central nervous system; CVS, cardiovascular system; Ali, alimentary system (including orofacial clefts); MSK, musculoskeletal system; ICP, cleft palate without other anomaly; ICL(P), cleft lip ≥ palate without other anomaly; CLP, all orofacial clefts, with or without anomalies of other systems; RT, respiratory tract (including orofacial clefts); LRD, limb reduction defects

[b] IR, maternal interview after delivery of index child; MR, review of medical records; Q, questionnaire; Pres, prescription information; IA, maternal interview at antenatal clinic visit

[c] Crude unmatched analysis of matched data

[d] Drug use: prevalence of heavy use, 10%

[e] Defined as taken for at least eight days during at least one of the first four lunar months

[f] Adjusted for range of potentially confounding variables

[g] In periconceptional period

[h] 23% had neural tube defects, 7% limb malformations, 49% oral clefts and 21% other serious malformations

[i] 90% confidence interval

categories. The RR for transposition of the great arteries associated with use of aspirin was 3.3 (90% CI, 1.7–6.6, based on 12 exposed cases).

Zierler and Rothman (1985) carried out a further study of severe congenital heart disease and maternal use of medications in early pregnancy in Massachusetts during the period 1980–83. Congenital heart disease was considered to be severe if the diagnostic and therapeutic procedures included cardiac catheterization or surgery during the first year of life, or if death occurred before the first birthday. Controls were randomly selected from birth certificates filed in Massachusetts. Maternal interviews were completed for 298 cases (68% of those potentially eligible) and 738 controls (79% of those eligible). A positive association was found with reported aspirin use during the first trimester (RR, 1.4; 90% CI, 0.95–2.0). The most frequently reported indications for aspirin use were fever, cold and flu symptoms. The mothers of affected children reported use of aspirin for controlling fever more often than mothers of controls. Confounding by maternal illness did not account for the relationship with aspirin. Because of concern about potential recall bias, the authors also considered information on exposure from obstetric records. The RR associated with use of aspirin was 2.4 (95% CI, 0.6–10). [The Working Group noted that information on aspirin obtained over the counter would be unlikely to be recorded in obstetric records, and that no information was given on the numbers of cases and controls exposed according to these records.] When the data on specific types of cardiac anomalies among the cases were analysed, the RR, adjusted for use of other drugs, reported symptoms and laboratory reports of infection, were 2.4 (90% CI, 0.9–6.4) for aortic stenosis; 3.1 (1.2–8.0) for coarctation of the aorta; 3.2 (1.3–7.5) for hypoplastic left ventricle and 1.7 (0.9–3.7) for transposition of the great arteries.

Werler et al. (1989) analysed data from an on-going surveillance case–control study of birth defects in relation to exposure to drugs and other environmental factors in centres in Greater Boston and Philadelphia, USA, and south-eastern Ontario, Canada, during the period 1976–86 and in five counties in Iowa, USA, in 1983–85. Data on medications taken for various indications were obtained by maternal interview. Cases with identified syndromes that included cardiac abnormalities such as Down syndrome and Holt-Oram syndrome, were excluded. More than 80% of cases and 80% of controls (mothers of infants with non-cardiac malformations) participated. No association was seen between reported aspirin use during the first trimester and total cardiac defects. In addition, no association was apparent for specific defects, comprising aortic stenosis, coarctation of the aorta, hypoplastic left ventricle, transposition of the great arteries or conotruncal defects.

No association between use of aspirin and anomalies of the cardiovascular system was found in a case–control study in South Wales, United Kingdom (Richards, 1969), or in a multicentre cohort study in the USA (Slone et al., 1976). The latter study is the only one in which information relevant to the investigation of a possible dose–response relationship was available. Another analysis of the data collected in the latter study related to specific types of congenital anomaly (Heinonen et al., 1977). The RRs, adjusted for hospital of delivery, were 2.4 (eight exposed cases) for aortic stenosis, 1.5 (seven exposed cases) for transposition of the great arteries, 2.1 (17 exposed cases) for coarctation of the aorta and 3.0 (eight exposed cases) for the tetralogy of Fallot.

A case–control study of orofacial clefts in Finland during the period 1967–71, in which information on exposure was obtained prospectively from prenatal clinic records and retrospectively by interview by the midwife during the mother's first visit to the maternity welfare centre after delivery, suggested a positive association with maternal exposure to salicylates (Saxén, 1975). This was largely accounted for by exposure during the first trimester. [The Working Group noted that, as positive associations were also seen with use of other antipyretic analgesics, opiates (mainly codeine) and penicillins, confounding by pyrexia may have occurred.]

No association between the prevalence of orofacial clefts and aspirin use during the first trimester was found in the multicentre cohort study in the USA (Heinonen *et al.*, 1977). RRs greater than 3 were associated with any exposure to aspirin during the first trimester and the prevalence of rachischisis or cranioschisis, situs inversus or dextrocardia, other adrenal syndromes, abnormal hands and fingers and miscellaneous foot abnormalities. Multivariate analyses were not carried out for specific defects, and these observations may be chance findings. No elevation in risk was found for the broader categories of anomalies considered in the analysis of aspirin categorized by degree of exposure (Slone *et al.*, 1976; Heinonen *et al.*, 1977).

In two of the randomized trials of use of low doses of aspirin during pregnancy, information on follow-up of the offspring was reported (Parazzini *et al.*, 1994; CLASP Collaborative Group, 1995). No difference in the frequency of congenital anomalies was found.

Morbidity later in childhood. In two cohort studies, the relationship between use of aspirin during pregnancy and the IQ of the offspring was investigated (Hertz-Picciotto *et al.*, 1990). In one of these, use of aspirin at least seven times per week was associated with a 10-point lower mean IQ for girls and 1.3-point lower mean IQ for boys at the age of four. Use of aspirin was also related to attention decrement. The credibility of these findings may be strengthened by the lack of association between use of acetaminophen (paracetamol) and either IQ or attention decrement (Streissguth *et al.*, 1987). No association between aspirin use and IQ at the age of four was observed in a multicentre cohort study in the USA (Klebanoff & Berendes, 1988).

An 18-month follow-up of children born to women participating in the Italian Study of Aspirin and Pregnancy (1993) was undertaken by postal questionnaire. Information was obtained on 427 children (72%) of the women given aspirin and 361 (73%) of those who received no treatment. No difference between the groups was apparent in height, weight, respiratory, hearing or vision problems or other disorders. In addition, there was no difference between the groups in terms of the gross or fine motor and language development of the child (Parazzini *et al.*, 1994).

Follow–up of children born to women in the trial of the CLASP Collaborative Group (1994) was restricted initially to children in the United Kingdom and Canada (CLASP Collaborative Group, 1995). Thus, 4168 children in the United Kingdom were assessed at 12 months from information provided by general practitioners and 4365 children in the United Kingdom and Canada were assessed at 18 months from responses to a questionnaire by their parents. The response rate at 12 months was 89% and that at 18 months, 86%. There were no differences between the groups in the frequency of hospital visits during the first 18 months of life for motor deficits, developmental delay, respiratory problems or bleeding. In addition, there were no differences in the proportion of children whose height or weight was below the third centile, in the frequency of abnormal gross motor, fine motor or language development or in the prevalence of abnormal sleep patterns, and there were no differences in feeding problems, mood, behaviour, hearing, vision or respiratory symptoms.

7.1.2 Experimental animals

(a) Gastrointestinal tract toxicity

It has been shown in animal models that aspirin is harmful to the gastric mucosa and is associated with irritation, ulceration and bleeding of the stomach (Kauffman, 1989). These studies have indicated two broad mechanisms by which aspirin causes gastric mucosal damage: one related to inhibition of COX activity and the other independent of the effect of aspirin on COX.

Gastric toxicity due to COX inhibition. Aspirin makes the gastric mucosa more susceptible to injury, inhibits mucus and bicarbonate secretion, alters the physiochemical nature of mucus, stimulates fundic but not antral ^{3}H-thymidine incorporation and makes the epithelial surface less hydrophobic (reviewed by Kauffman, 1989).

Aspirin given intravenously or intragastrically at 60 mg/kg bw per h to rats inhibited COX activity and caused macroscopic mucosal injury; these two effects were well correlated (Konturek *et al.*, 1981). Exogenous prostaglandin E_2 and I_2 completely prevented this mucosal injury. In addition, dose–response studies with lower doses of aspirin showed a significant correlation between COX inhibition and mean ulcer area. Further support for the hypothesis that reduction of endogenous prostaglandins predisposes the mucosa to injury comes from studies in which rabbits were immunized with prostaglandin E_2–thyro-globulin conjugate (Olson *et al.*, 1985; Redfern *et al.*, 1987), which resulted in the production of circulating prostaglandin E_2 antibodies. Gastrointestinal ulcers occurred as early as six weeks after the beginning of immunization. These observations support the notion that endogenous prostaglandins are important for the maintenance of mucosal defence and that their inhibition is an important mechanisms of aspirin-induced mucosal injury.

Gastric toxicity independent of COX inhibition. In most of the studies described below, the similarity of the effects of aspirin and salicylic acid was used to deduce that the mechanism of action of aspirin is not via COX inhibition, since salicylic acid is a less efficient COX inhibitor (Mitchell *et al.*, 1994). As aspirin is rapidly deacetylated to salicylic acid in cells, the half-life of aspirin in interstitial fluid and serum after oral administration is short. Salicylic acid is, however, toxic to cells and affects epithelial function. Salicylates are associated with mucosal barrier injury, resulting in large net cation fluxes, hydrogen back-diffusion and a fall in the transmucosal difference in potential. The mucosal content of ATP is reduced by salicylic acid, affecting ion transport and increasing proton dissipation from surface epithelial cells (reviewed by Kauffman, 1989).

The effects of single and repeated doses of aspirin have been examined by light and electron microscopy. The gastric mucosa of dogs showed dose-dependent epithelial damage and haemorrhage into the lamina propria within 4 h after intraluminal administration of aspirin

(Lev *et al.*, 1972). The damage was more pronounced after one than four weeks, suggesting adaptation to repeated administration of aspirin. Electron microscopic evaluation of the gastric mucosa of mice exposed to 20 mmol/litre aspirin in 1, 10 or 100 mmol/litre HCl for 8 min showed many lysed and exfoliated surface epithelial cells and swelling and disruption of all cells, with enlarged nuclei and clumped nuclear chromatin (Fromm, 1976). Davenport (1967) demonstrated that the gastric mucosal barrier of rats is lost after exposure to either aspirin or salicylic acid. Both drugs increase the proton flux into the mucosa and cause a drop in potential difference, a sensitive measure of epithelial integrity. The back-diffusion of protons leads to cellular acidification and altered cellular metabolism. Studies in rats (Rowe *et al.*, 1987) and rabbits (Fromm & Kolis, 1982) suggest, however, that aspirin and salicylic acid damage the mucosa equally, but only after the gastric luminal pH has been lowered to 1.0. Guinea-pig gastric mucosa perfused with 2 mmol/litre aspirin at pH 4 showed a fall in transmucosal potential, a reduction in ATP content and acid secretion and an increase in proton back-diffusion (Ohe *et al.*, 1980). These observations suggest that one action of aspirin is to damage the energy metabolism of mucosal cells, causing cell death with resultant back-diffusion of protons.

Membrane transport mechanisms are also affected by salicylates. Observations on rabbit antral mucosa exposed to aspirin or salicylic acid at low pH (Fromm, 1976; Kuo & Shanbour, 1976) suggest that salicylates inhibit active ion transport in the gastric mucosa, possibly through decreased ATP production as a result of either enzyme inhibition or their uncoupling effect.

(b)   Nephrotoxicity
Aspirin causes a wide spectrum of renal damage including nephrotic syndrome, acute interstitial nephritis, acute tubular necrosis, acute glomerulonephritis and nonspecific renal failure (Clive & Stoff, 1984; Carmichael & Shankel, 1985).

Chronic administration of aspirin at 120–500 mg/kg per day to rats over 18–68 weeks caused renal papillary necrosis and decreased urinary concentrating ability (Burrell *et al.*, 1991; D'Agati, 1996); however, some investigators have been unable to induce renal papillary necrosis in other species or in rats at lower divided doses, as used in humans (Owen & Heywood, 1986). In a variety of rat strains, administration of aspirin as a single high dose intravenously or by gavage produced acute necrosis of the proximal tubules, rarely accompanied by renal papillary necrosis in susceptible strains like homozygous Gunn rats (Axelsen, 1980; Mittman *et al.*, 1985). This strain of rat, which has an inactivating mutation in one glucuronyl transferase relevant to aspirin, develops renal papillary necrosis after a single oral dose of aspirin (Axelsen, 1976).

A study of administration of 500 mg/kg ^{14}C-aspirin to 3- and 12-month-old male rats showed an age-dependent effect of aspirin on the kidneys (Kyle & Kocsis, 1985). Aspirin induced proximal tubular necrosis in the older animals but only mild, nonspecific cellular changes in the younger group. In addition, the mitochondrial pathway for salicylurate synthesis was significantly inhibited in the older animals. These findings suggest that mitochondrial injury plays an important role in the development of salicylate-induced proximal tubular necrosis.

(c) Hepatotoxicity

Aspirin-induced liver injury probably has an immunological basis, but neither the detailed mechanism nor the precise incidence rates are known. Studies in mice (Cai *et al.*, 1994, 1995) have demonstrated that long-term treatment with aspirin leads to increased proliferation of hepatic peroxisomes. According to the oxidative stress hypothesis (Reddy & Lalwani, 1983), peroxisome proliferation results in excess formation of hydrogen peroxide, which induces lipid peroxidation. In fact, treatment of mice (Cai *et al.*, 1995) and rats (Goel *et al.*, 1986) with aspirin induced a 1.3-fold increase in basal hydrogen peroxide levels in liver homogenates. It is possible that products of lipid peroxidation interact with DNA, leading to adducts, DNA strand breaks and DNA–protein cross-linking (Vaca *et al.*, 1988).

Long-term treatment of rats with peroxisome proliferators like aspirin decreases the cellular antioxidant defenses (Glauert *et al.*, 1992).

Thus, aspirin may initiate or promote neoplastic change by installing a long-term imbalance between cellular oxidative stress and antioxidant defence.

(d) Ototoxicity

Aspirin causes mild to moderate, temporary hearing loss in laboratory animals. The deficit is detected behaviourally or electrophysiologically (Boettcher & Salvi, 1991). There appear to be some species differences in susceptibility to salicylate ototoxicity, presumably due in part to differences in the pharmacokinetics of salicylates among species (Myers & Bernstein, 1965; Gold & Wilpizeski, 1966; Eddy *et al.*, 1976). The hearing loss caused by aspirin is accompanied by supra-threshold changes in hearing, including a decrease in temporal integration, poorer frequency selectivity and poorer temporal resolution. The supra-threshold changes are not severe and appear to be quite variable among subjects. Animals exposed to both noise and aspirin have greater hearing loss and cochlear damage than those exposed to noise alone (Eddy *et al.*, 1976; Carson *et al.*, 1989).

(e) Reproductive and developmental effects
Reproductive effects. Administration of aspirin to adult male rats at a dose of one-tenth of the LD_{50} value for six weeks was accompanied by a decrease in the functional activity of spermatozoids. Repeated inhalation of a concentration of 25 mg/m^3 for four months produced morphological changes in the spermatogenic epithelium and abnormal antenatal development of the progeny (Vasilenko *et al.*, 1979).

Developmental toxicity. Congenital malformations were induced in rats by salicylate poisoning of the mother while the embryos were in early stages of development (Warkany & Takacs, 1959). Among the defects produced were craniorachischisis with well-preserved cerebral and spinal nervous tissues. Other malformations encountered were anencephaly, hydrocephaly, facial clefts, gastroschisis and irregularities of the vertebrae and ribs.

The doses of aspirin most commonly used in animal models are 250–1000 mg/kg of maternal weight. In all species, these doses usually cause malformations in the surviving fetuses, 25–80% of which are affected. The malformations include cleft lip and palate, hydrocephaly, gastroschisis and skeletal dysplasias (Lubawy & Burriss Garrett, 1977). In mice, aspirin at high doses (500 mg/kg) over a 24-h period on days 8 and 9 or 9 and 10 of gestation induces cleft lip (Trasler, 1965).

When rat embryos were cultured with 100–300 mg/ml salicylic acid, decreases in crown–rump length, somite number and yolk sac diameter are observed (Joschko et al., 1993). A significant increase in the prevalence of malformations is seen, including anomalies of the eye, branchial arch and heart and an absence of forelimb buds. The neural tube is especially vulnerable and frequently fails to close. Cellular and ultrastructural examination reveals extensive cell death in the neuroepithelium, with a lesser effect on mesenchymal cells. It is likely that the extensive cell necrosis and blebbing in the developing neuroepi-thelium at the site of neural tube fusion are involved in failed neurulation, while necrosis at other sites in the cranial neuro-epithelium is linked with intellectual and behavioural abnormalities.

Salicylic acid, the product of aspirin hydrolysis, is considered to be the causative agent in teratogenicity associated with aspirin (Kimmel et al., 1971; Koshakji & Schulert, 1973). Early studies (Goldman & Yakovac, 1963) showed that the teratogenic action of salicylate compounds occurs through maternally mediated metabolic factors; however, more recent studies with fluorimetric techniques (Kimmel et al., 1971) and culture in vitro (McGarrity et al., 1981) demonstrated that aspirin has a direct effect in the rat embryo in the absence of any maternal influence.

The teratogenicity of aspirin may be mediated via its obvious target, COX, and altered prostaglandin synthesis (Vane, 1971), interference with oxidative phosphorylation (Bostrom et al., 1964) or altered biosynthesis of nucleic acids and proteins (Janakidevi & Smith, 1970). Alternative explanations include a direct effect of salicylic acid on cell membranes, particularly those close to the mesenchyme (Joschko et al., 1993).

Doses of 250–1000 mg/kg of maternal weight cause a high rate of embryo deaths and stillbirths in all animal species, and fetuses of rats given 125 or 250 mg/kg bw per day of aspirin were shorter and weighed less than those from control rats (Lubawy & Burriss Garrett, 1977).

When aspirin was co-administered with ethanol, as in a study in TO mice (Padmanabhan et al., 1994), it significantly reduced the rate of prenatal ethanol-induced mortality. Pre-administration of a low dose (150 mg/kg bw) of aspirin reduced the ethanol-induced exencephaly, while a higher dose (200 mg/kg bw) increased the incidence of this malformation.

7.2 Genetic and related effects
7.2.1 Humans
No data were available to the Working Group.

7.2.2 Experimental models
The results of tests for genetic and related effects in model systems are summarized in Table 11 and Figure 4. The genetic and related effects of aspirin have been reviewed (Giri, 1993). Aspirin induced DNA damage in *Bacillus subtilis* (Kawachi et al., 1980; Kuboyama & Fujii, 1992) but not in *Escherichia coli* (King et al., 1979) or in *Salmonella typimurium* tester strains (Bruce & Heddle, 1979; King et al., 1979; Bartsch et al., 1980; Kawachi et al., 1980; Oldhham et al., 1986; Jasiewicz & Richardson, 1987; Kuboyama & Fujii, 1992). It did not induce sex-linked recessive lethal mutation in *Drosophila melanogaster* or mutations in a host-mediated assay (King et al., 1979), and it did not induce mutation, cell transformation (Patierno et al., 1989), aneuploidy (Watanabe, 1982; Ishidate, 1988) or micronucleus formation (Dunn et al., 1987) in mammalian cells in vitro. Mixed results were reported for chromosomal aberrations in mammalian cells in vitro (Meisner & Inhorn, 1972; Kawachi et al., 1980; Watanabe, 1982; Ishidate, 1988; Muller et al., 1991). It induced chromosomal aberrations (Kawachi et al., 1980) but not micronuclei (Bruce & Heddle, 1979; King et al., 1979) in bone-marrow cells of rodents treated in vivo. It did not induce sperm abnormalities in mice in vivo (Bruce & Heddle, 1979).

Table 11. Genetic and related effects of aspirin

End-point	Test-code	Test system	Results[a] −	Results[a] +	Dose[b] (LED or HID)	Reference
D	BSD	*B. subtilis rec*, differential toxicity	+	0	0.00	Kawachi *et al.* (1980)
D	BSD	*B. subtilis rec*, differential toxicity	(+)	0	5000	Kuboyama & Fujii (1992)
G	SA5	*S. typhimurium* TA1535, reverse mutation	−	−	250	Jasiewicz & Richardson (1987)
G	SA5	*S. typhimurium* TA1535, reverse mutation	−	−	1800	King *et al.* (1979)
G	SA5	*S. typhimurium* TA1535, reverse mutation	−	−	250	Oldham et al. (1986)
G	SA7	*S. typhimurium* TA1537, reverse mutation	−	−	250	Bruce & Heddle (1979)
G	SA7	*S. typhimurium* TA1537, reverse mutation	−	−	250	Jasiewicz & Richardson (1987)
G	SA7	*S. typhimurium* TA1537, reverse mutation	−	−	1800	King *et al.* (1979)
G	SA7	*S. typhimurium* TA1537, reverse mutation	−	−	250	Oldham *et al.* (1986)
G	SA8	*S. typhimurium* TA1538, reverse mutation	−	−	250	Jasiewicz & Richardson (1987)
G	SA8	*S. typhimurium* TA1538, reverse mutation	−	−	1800	King *et al.* (1979)
G	SA8	*S. typhimurium* TA1538, reverse mutation	−	−	250	Oldham *et al.* (1986)
G	SA9	*S. typhimurium* TA98, reverse mutation	−	−	250	Bruce & Heddle (1979)
G	SA9	*S. typhimurium* TA98, reverse mutation	−	−	250	Jasiewicz & Richardson (1987)
G	SA9	*S. typhimurium* TA98, reverse mutation	−	−	0	Kawachi *et al.* (1980)
G	SA9	*S. typhimurium* TA98, reverse mutation	−	−	1800	King *et al.* (1979)
G`	SA9	*S. typhimurium* TA98, reverse mutation	−	−	27	Kuboyama & Fujii (1992)
G	SA9	*S. typhimurium* TA98, reverse mutation	−	−	250	Oldham *et al.* (1986)
G	SA0	*S. typhimurium* TA100, reverse mutation	−	−	180	Bartsch *et al.* (1980)
G	SA0	*S. typhimurium* TA100, reverse mutation	−	−	250	Bruce & Heddle (1979)
G	SA0	*S. typhimurium* TA100, reverse mutation	−	−	250	Jasiewicz & Richardson (1987)
G	SA0	*S. typhimurium* TA100, reverse mutation	−	−	0	Kawachi *et al.* (1980)
G	SA0	*S. typhimurium* TA100, reverse mutation	−	−	1800	King *et al.* (1979)
G	SA0	*S. typhimurium* TA100, reverse mutation	−	−	27	Kuboyama & Fujii (1992)
G	SA0	*S. typhimurium* TA100, reverse mutation	−	−	250	Oldham *et al.* (1986)
G	ECK	*E. coli* K12, forward or reverse mutation	−	−	1800	King *et al.* (1979)
G	DMX	*D. melanogaster*, sex-linked recessive lethal mutation	−	0	1800	King *et al.* (1979)
G	GIA	Mutation, other animal cells *in vitro*	−	0	3000	Patierno *et al.* (1989)
M	MIA	Micronucleus test, animal cells *in vitro*	−	0	3600	Dunn *et al.* (1987)
C	CIC	Chromosomal aberration, Chinese hamster cells *in vitro*	+	0	0.00	Ishidate (1988)
C	CIC	Chromosomal aberration, Chinese hamster cells *in vitro*	+	0	15.6	Ishidate (1988)
C	CIC	Chromosomal aberration, Chinese hamster cells *in vitro*	−	+	0.00	Kawachi *et al.* (1980)
C	CIC	Chromosomal aberration, Chinese hamster cells *in vitro*	−	0	1800	Muller *et al.* (1991)
A	AIA	Aneuploidy, animal cells *in vitro*	−	−	1500	Ishidate (1988)
T	TCM	Cell transformation, C3H10T1/2 cells *in vitro*	−	0	3000	Patierno *et al.* (1989)
C	CHF	Chromosomal aberration, human fibroblasts *in vitro*	−	0	250	Meisner & Inhorn (1972)
C	CHL	Chromosomal aberration, human lymphocytes *in vitro*	+	0	75	Watanabe (1982)
A	AIH	Aneuploidy, human cells *in vitro*	−	0	300	Watanabe (1982)
H	HMM	Host-mediated assay, microbial cells	−	0	180	King *et al.* (1979)
M	MVM	Micronucleus formation, mice *in vivo*	−	0	1000	Bruce & Heddle (1979)
M	MVM	Micronucleus formation, mice *in vivo*	−	0	360	King *et al.* (1979)
C	CBA	Chromosomal aberration, animal bone marrow *in vivo*	+	0	0.00	Kawachi *et al.* (1980)
P	SPM	Sperm morphology, mice *in vivo*	−	0	1000	Bruce & Heddle (1979)

Definitions of the abbreviations and terms used are given in Appendix 1.

[a] In the absence (−) and presence (+) of an exogenous metabolic activation system; +, positive; (+), weakly positive; −, negative; 0, not done

[b] Lowest effective dose (LED) or highest ineffective dose (HID), expressed as μg/ml for *in-vitro* studies and as mg/kg body weight per day for *in-vivo* studies

Figure 4. Profile of genetic and related effects of aspirin

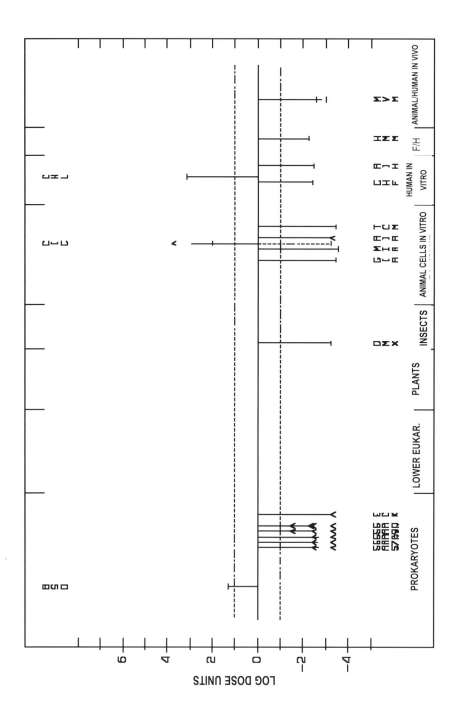

8. Summary of Data

8.1 Chemistry, occurrence and human exposure

Aspirin has been used for nearly a century as an analgesic, anti-inflammatory and antipyretic agent. It is used in the treatment of rheumatism, fever and related conditions; it is also used in the prevention of arterial and venous thrombosis. The doses of aspirin usually used vary according to the therapeutic indication. Low doses (75–300 mg/day) are conventionally used in the prophylaxis of cardiovascular disease; daily doses up to 5 g are used in the treatment of pain and fever. Doses up to 8 g three or four times daily are used in the management of rheumatic complaints. In view of its ready availability, low cost and efficacy in a wide range of conditions, aspirin consumption is common and widespread.

8.2 Metabolism and kinetics

Aspirin is rapidly hydrolysed to salicylic acid in the intestinal wall, liver and erythrocytes. Aspirin is absorbed rapidly after oral administration. Both aspirin and salicylate are partially bound to proteins, especially albumin. Salicylate reaches the synovial fluid, the cerebrospinal fluid, saliva, breast milk and the fetus. Hydrolysis of aspirin to salicylate in the plasma occurs with a half-life of 15–20 min. Salicylate is removed by renal elimination and formation of metabolites. The hydrolysis of aspirin is not altered by concurrent administration of other drugs.

8.3 Cancer-preventive effects
8.3.1 Humans

(a) Colorectal cancer

Most of the data on aspirin and colorectal cancer come from epidemiological studies of the disease in the general population. In several studies, use of aspirin was not separated from use of other non-steroidal anti-inflammatory drugs. Relevant data are also available with respect to adenomatous colorectal polyps, which are thought to be precursor lesions for colorectal cancer. In a few studies, adenomatous and hyperplastic polyps were not distinguished.

Overall, the observational epidemiological studies cover more than 18 000 cases of colorectal cancer and more than 2000 cases of adenomatous polyps. The studies differ in design, location, population and motivating hypothesis. In 12 studies (four cohort and eight case–control) out of 13 that assessed the risk for colorectal cancer, there was a reduced risk associated with sustained aspirin use. In nine of these 12 studies, the reduction in risk was statistically significant, with relative risks of 0.4–0.6 in regular users in comparison with non-users. In all six studies on adenomatous colorectal polyps (two cohort and four case–control), there was a reduction in risk with aspirin use, which was statistically significant in four of them. In addition, two studies on patients with rheumatoid arthritis showed a significant reduction in colorectal cancer incidence in comparison with general population rates.

While information on the duration of treatment and dose of aspirin that are necessary for prevention is limited, the prophylactic effect appears to increase with increasing duration of use.

The observational studies are sufficiently large, taken together, and consistent, despite their diversity, that chance alone cannot explain their results. The Working Group considered several possible problems in the interpretation of the evidence, including publication bias, detection bias, bias due to indications for use of aspirin, genetic predisposition, other confounding factors and problems in the measurement of aspirin use. There is no obvious bias or confounding that could explain the findings. Collectively, the published observational studies provide consistent evidence that aspirin may inhibit one or more stages in the development of colorectal cancer.

The negative findings in the randomized US Physicians' Health Study neither support nor convincingly refute the aspirin–colorectal cancer prevention hypothesis. Factors that could obscure protection by aspirin against colorectal polyps or cancer in this trial include its short duration (randomized aspirin treatment being stopped after a mean of five years) and the small number of cases of cancer expected.

(b) Gastric cancer

Two population-based cohort studies addressed use of aspirin and gastric cancer. In the larger of these, a statistically significant inverse trend for gastric cancer was found with aspirin use. In one of two other population-based cohort studies of similar size and design, in which a diagnosis of rheumatoid arthritis was used as a proxy for exposure to non-steroidal anti-inflammatory drugs, rheumatoid arthritis was associated with a significantly lower risk for gastric cancer. In the other study, no such relationship was found.

(c) Oesophageal cancer

Three studies addressed the relationship between aspirin use and oesophageal cancer. One of these studies demonstrated a statistically significant inverse relationship.

(d) Breast cancer

No consistent association has been observed between use of aspirin and the occurrence of cancer of the breast in women. The larger studies generally found no association, but a reduced risk was reported in two of six cohort studies and in one of two case–control studies.

(e) Cancers at other sites

No reduction in the risks for cancers of the lung, bladder, prostate, buccal cavity, pharynx or genital system or melanoma was found to be associated with aspirin use in the few studies in which results were reported for cancers at these sites.

8.3.2 Experimental animals

Aspirin had chemopreventive activity in two of three studies in rat models in which colonic aberrant crypt foci were used as the end-point. In three studies with rat models of colon cancer, administration of aspirin significantly reduced the incidence and (in one case) the size of colon tumours. Aspirin inhibited hepatocarcinogenesis in four studies in rat models. In a single study in mice, aspirin was ineffective in inhibiting carcinogenesis in a urinary bladder model, but it inhibited bladder carcinogenesis in rats.

8.3.3 Mechanism of action

Aspirin can irreversibly inhibit cyclooxygenases, which may be involved in the initiation of carcinogenesis in three general ways: activation of carcinogens to DNA-binding forms, production of malondialdehyde and formation of peroxyl radicals.

Aspirin at high concentrations reduces the proliferation rate of cultured human colon cancer cells, alters their distribution in the various phases of the cell cycle, increasing the proportion of cells in G_0 or G_1 phase, and can induce apoptosis.

Non-cyclooxygenase-dependent mechanisms have been described that could play a role in its chemopreventive effects.

8.4. Other beneficial effects

Prophylactic aspirin therapy has been proven in large, reliable, randomized trials to reduce by about 25% the risk for myocardial infarct, stroke and vascular death in people with pre-existing cardiovascular conditions. The absolute benefits are greatest for patients with acute myocardial infarct and are smaller in patients with conditions posing a less acute risk. Two randomized trials of healthy people did not show any benefit of aspirin in preventing deaths from circulatory disease.

Although studies of clinically diagnosed Alzheimer disease and non-steroidal anti-inflammatory drugs consistently suggest a 50% reduction in risk, the temporal relationship between such exposure and disease development or progression has not been convincingly demonstrated.

8.5 Carcinogenicity
8.5.1 Humans

Many large-scale epidemiological studies have been conducted of aspirin use and cancer. There is no consistent evidence of an increased risk for cancer at any specific site.

8.5.2 Experimental animals

No data were available to the Working Group.

8.6 Toxic effects
8.6.1 Humans

Aspirin causes a dose-dependent increase, with no known lower threshold, in the incidence of upper gastrointestinal toxicity, including dyspepsia, gastrointestinal haemorrhage, oesophageal and gastric erosion, perforation and death. Low doses (40 mg) of aspirin inhibit platelet aggregation and can increase the risk for non-fatal bleeding requiring transfusion. The risk for haemorrhagic stroke may also be increased by relatively low doses. A positive association has been observed between use of aspirin in children and Reye syndrome. Aspirin can precipitate or aggravate asthma. Maternal exposure to high but not low doses of aspirin prior to delivery has consistently been associated with bleeding in the mother and the newborn.

8.6.2 *Experimental animals*

Aspirin is harmful to the gastric mucosa and can result in irritation, ulceration and bleeding in the stomach. Aspirin induces a wide spectrum of renal damage. In rats, it causes papillary necrosis and decreased urinary concentrating ability or acute necrosis of the proximal tubules. Susceptibility to the nephrotoxicity of aspirin appears to be age-dependent. In mice, long-term treatment with aspirin is associated with proliferation of hepatic peroxisomes. High doses of aspirin cause mild to moderate temporary hearing loss, accompanied by changes in suprathreshold hearing, including a decrease in temporal integration, poorer frequency selectivity and poorer temporal resolution.

Congenital malformations can be induced in rats after administration of aspirin at high doses to dams while the embryos are in early stages of development, leading to a variety of anomalies. There is a clear correlation between ingestion of aspirin and congenital malformations, but these adverse effects occur at doses far in excess of those likely to be encountered in the therapeutic setting.

Aspirin induced chromosomal aberrations in Chinese hamster cells and in human lymphocytes *in vitro* in one study. It induced chromosomal aberrations in the bone marrow of rats treated *in vivo* in one study.

9. Recommendations for Research

Definitive evidence for chemopreventive activity nominally requires data from appropriately designed randomized trials. In practice, the duration that is necessary for aspirin to exert the sought-after effect may, for practical purposes, preclude the execution of the necessary randomized trials. Rather, it may be necessary to rely upon observational studies. Such studies can be performed using existing databases, and this possibility merits high priority.

Adenomatous polyps may be perceived as biomarkers for the probable development of colorectal cancer; however, confidence in this perception is progressively increased as the relationship between these lesions and the later stages of colorectal cancer is more fully understood. It is important, therefore, that studies of these biomarkers include, where possible, monitoring of subsequent disease development.

Cohort studies on sporadic cancer are needed, with prospective evaluation of aspirin use over long periods of time — 10 or more years. In addition, the Group identified the need for clinical trials of aspirin use for the prevention of recurrent or primary sproadic adenomas, of colorectal adenomas in patients with familial predisposition and of recurrent colorectal cancer after surgical treatment of a first case.

The Working Group was aware that certain trials are in progress, apart from published data cited in this volume. Obviously, the results of such trials will influence current evaluations of NSAIDs as cancer-preventive agents. The knowledge that trials are in progress mitigates against specific recommendations for future trial design; however, one matter that necessitates attention is determination of the lowest dose of aspirin necessary for effective chemopreventive activity. This parameter should be a specific concern in the design of future trials and/or observational studies.

10. Evaluation[1]

10.1 Cancer-preventive activity

10.1.1 Humans

There is *limited evidence* in humans that aspirin reduces the risk for colorectal cancer, based on the finding of a consistent moderate reduction in risk in observational studies. Individually, none of the potential sources of bias or confounding provides a reasonable explanation for the reduction in risk for colorectal cancer that has been reported; however, the possible cumulative effect of these issues, although not quantifiable, cannot be excluded. Therefore, the Working Group concluded that bias and confounding could not be ruled out with reasonable confidence.

10.1.2 Experimental animals

There is *sufficient evidence* for the cancer-preventive activity of aspirin in experimental animals. This evaluation is based on models of cancers of the colon and liver.

10.2 Overall evaluation

Epidemiological studies in humans provide *limited evidence* for the cancer-preventive activity of aspirin, based on over 20 observational studies (both cohort and case–control), which show a moderately reduced risk for colorectal cancer in people using aspirin regularly, and an indication of greater reduction in risk with prolonged use. In experimental animal models, there is *sufficient evidence* for the prevention of colon cancer by aspirin. Aspirin is toxic, especially at high doses, but beneficial effects for humans have been demonstrated at relatively low doses, especially a reduction in the risk for myocardial infarct and thrombotic stroke in populations with pre-existing disease. These findings indicate the need for more detailed research on cancer prevention, including controlled trials with different regimens of aspirin, including dose, route of administration, frequency and duration, and different cohorts, in an endeavour to determine whether aspirin can be shown to be of greater benefit in reducing cancer in human populations than its possible off-setting toxicity. Detailed consideration of the total benefits in the prevention of cancer and other diseases in contrast to toxicity will be required before use of aspirin for the prevention of cancer in humans, particularly in asymptomatic populations, can be recommended.

11. References

Al-Badr, A.A. & Ibrahim, S.E. (1981) Simultaneous quantitative analysis of aspirin, phenacetin and caffeine in pharmaceutical preparations by proton magnetic resonance spectrometry. *Zbl. Pharm. Pharmakother. Laboratoriumsdiagn.*, 120, 1251–1254

Ali, B. & Kaur, S. (1983) Mammalian tissue acetylsalicylic acid esterases. Identification, distribution and discrimination from other esterases. *J. Pharmacol. exp. Ther.*, 226, 589–594

Amer, M.M., Wanbi, A.M. & Aboul-Eialah, M.K. (1978) Differential spectrophotometric analysis of aspirin in some pharmaceutical preparations. *Bull. Fac. Pharm. Cairo Univ.*, 15, 311–323

Amin, A.R., Vyas, P., Attur, M., Leszczynska-Piziak, J., Patel, I.R., Weissmann, G. & Abramson, S.B. (1995) The mode of action of aspirin-like drugs: Effect on inducible nitric oxide synthase. *Proc. natl Acad. Sci. USA*, 92, 7926–7930

Antiplatelet Trialists' Collaboration (1988) Secondary prevention of vascular disease by prolonged antiplatelet treatment. *Br. med. J.*, 296, 320–331

Antiplatelet Trialists' Collaboration (1994a) The aspirin papers. Aspirin benefits patients with vascular disease and those undergoing revascularisation. *Br. med. J.*, 308, 71–72

Antiplatelet Trialists' Collaboration (1994b) Collaborative overview of randomised trials of antiplatelet therapy I: Prevention of death, myocardial infarction, and stroke by prolonged antiplatelet therapy in various categories of patients. *Br. med. J.*, 308, 81–106

---

[1] For definitions of the italicized terms, see the Preamble, pp. 12–13.

Aonuma, S., Kohama, U. & Fujimoto, S. (1982) Studies on aspirin derivatives with very little side-effects. III. Absorption, distribution, excretion and metabolism of tritium-labeled aspirin-isopropylantipyrine (AIA) in rats. *J. Pharmacobiodyn.*, **5**, 252–258

Arvind, P., Papavassiliou, E.D., Tsioulias, G.J., Lovelace, C.I.P., Duceman, B. & Rigas, B. (1995) PGE2 down-regulates the expression of HLA-DR antigen in human colon adenocarcinoma cell lines. *Biochemistry*, **34**, 5604–5609

Arvind, P., Qiao, L., Papavassiliou, E.D., Goldin, E., Koutsos, M.I. & Rigas, B. (1996). Aspirin and aspirin-like drugs induce the expression of HLA-DR in HT29 colon adenocarcinoma cells. *Int. J. Oncol.*, **52**, 237–245

Aspirin Myocardial Infarction Study Research Group (1980) A randomized controlled trial of aspirin in persons recovered from myocardial infarction. *J. Am. med. Assoc.*, **243**, 661–669

Asymbekova G.U., Banartsev, P.D., Ochan, T.B., Rozenfeld, B.Ye., Sariyev, A.K., Folomeyeva I.Yu. & Pavlovich, S.V. (1995) Pharmacokinetics and pharmacodynamics of aspirin prophylactic doses in pregnant females at high risk placental insufficiency. *Exp. clin. Pharmacol.*, **58**, 35–39

Axelsen, R.A. (1976) Analgesic-induced renal papillary necrosis in the Gunn rat: The comparative nephrotoxicity of aspirin and phenacetin. *J. Pathol.*, **120**, 145–150

Axelsen, R.A. (1980) Nephrotoxicity of mild analgesics in the Gunn strain of rat. *Br. J. clin. Pharmacol.*, **10**, 309S–312S

Bansal, P. & Sonnenberg, A. (1996) Risk factors of colorectal cancer in inflammatory bowel disease. *Am. J. Gastroenterol.*, **91**, 44–48

Bartsch, H., Malaveille, C., Camus, A.-M., Martel-Planche, G., Brun, G., Hautefeuille, A., Sabadie, N., Barbin, A., Kuroki, T., Drevon, C., Piccoli, C. & Montesano, R. (1980) Validation and comparative studies on 180 chemicals with *S. typhimurium* strains and V79 Chinese hamster cells in the presence of various metabolizing systems. *Mutat. Res.*, **76**, 1–50

Bochner, F., Graham, G.G., Cham, E., Imhoff, D.M. & Haavisto, T.M. (1981) Salicylate metabolite kinetics after several salicylates. *Clin. Pharmacol. Ther.*, **30**, 266–275

Boettcher, F.L. & Salvi, R.J. (1991) Salicylate ototoxicity: Review and synthesis. *Am. J. Otolaryngol.*, **12**, 33–47

Bostrom, H., Berntsen, K. & Whitehouse, M.W. (1964) Biochemical properties of anti-inflammatory drugs. II. Some effects on sulphate-35S metabolism in vivo. *Biochem. Pharmacol.*, **13**, 413–420

Briggs, D.F., Coutts, R.T. & Walter, L.J. (1977) A note of the bioavailability of five Canadian brands of acetylsalicylic acid tablets. *Can. J. Pharmacol. Sci.*, **12**, 23

Britton, M., Helmers, C. & Samuelsson, K. (1987) High-dose acetylsalicylic acid after cerebral infarction — A Swedish co-operative study. *Stroke*, **18**, 325–334

Brouet, I. & Ohshima, H. (1995) Curcumin, an anti-tumour promoter and anti-inflammatory agent, inhibits induction of nitric oxide synthase in activated macrophages. *Biochem. biophys. Res. Commun.*, **206**, 533–540

Brouwers, J.R.B.J. & De Smet, P.A.G.M. (1994) Pharmacokinetic–pharmacodynamic drug interactions with nonsteroidal anti-inflammatory drugs. *Clin. Pharmacokinet.*, **27**, 462–485

Bruce, W.R. & Heddle, J.A. (1979) The mutagenic activity of 61 agents as determined by the micronucleus, Salmonella, and sperm abnormality assays. *Can. J. genet. Cytol.*, **21**, 319–334

Budavari, S., ed. (1989) *The Merck Index*, Rahway, NJ, Merck & Co., p. 870

Burrell, J.H., Yong, J.L. & Macdonald, G.J. (1991) Analgesic nephropathy in Fischer 344 rats: Comparative effects of chronic treatment with either aspirin or paracetamol. *Pathology*, **23**, 107–114

Cai, Y., Sohlenius, A.-K., Andersson, K., Sundberg, C. & DePierre, J.W. (1994) Effects of acetylsalicylic acid on parameters related to peroxisome proliferation in mouse liver. *Biochem. Pharmacol.*, **47**, 2213–2219

Cai, Y., Appelkvist, E.-L. & DePierre, J.W. (1995) Hepatic oxidative stress and related defences during treatment of mice with acetylsalicylic acid and other peroxisome proliferators. *J. Biochem. Toxicol.*, **10**, 87–94

CAPRIE Steering Committee (1996) A randomized, blinded trial of clopidogrel versus aspirin in patients at risk of ischemic events (CAPRIE). *Lancet*, **348**, 1329–1339

Carmichael, J. & Shankel, S.W. (1985) Effects of nonsteroidal anti-inflammatory drugs on prostaglandins and renal function. *Am. J. Med.*, **78**, 992–1000

Carson, S.S., Prazma, J., Pulver, S.H. & Anderson, T. (1989) Combined effects of aspirin and noise in causing permanent hearing loss. *Arch. Otolaryngol Head Neck Surg.*, **115**, 1070–1075

Chan, W.Y. (1983) Prostaglandins and nonsteroidal antiinflammatory drugs in dysmenorrhea. *Ann. Rev. Pharmacol. Toxicol.*, **23**, 131–149

Chow, W.H., McLaughlin, J.K., Linet, M.S., Niwa, S. & Mandel, J.S. (1994) Use of analgesics and risk of renal cell cancer. *Int. J. Cancer*, **59**, 467–470

CLASP (Collaborative Low-dose Aspirin Study in Pregnancy) Collaborative Group (1994) CLASP: A randomised trial of low-dose aspirin for the prevention and treatment of pre-eclampsia among 9364 pregnant women. *Lancet*, **343**, 619–629

CLASP Collaborative Group (1995) Low dose aspirin in pregnancy and early childhood development: Follow up of the collaborative low dose aspirin study in pregnancy. *Br. J. Obstet. Gynaecol.*, **102**, 861–868

Clissold, S.P. (1986) Aspirin and related derivatives of salicylic acid. *Drugs*, **32**, 8–26

Clive, D.M. & Stoff, J.S. (1984) Renal syndromes associated with non-steroidal anti-inflammatory drugs. *New Engl. J. Med.*, **310**, 563–572

Cohen, M. (1996) Platelet glycoprotein IIb/IIIa receptors in coronary artery disease. *Ann. intern. Med.*, **124**, 843–844

Coronary Drug Project Research Group (1976) Aspirin in coronary heart disease. *J. chron. Dis.*, **29**, 625–642

Costello, P.B., Caruana, J.A. & Green, F.A. (1984) The relative roles of hydrolases of the erythrocyte and other tissues in controlling aspirin survival *in vivo*. *Arthr. Rheumatol.*, **27**, 422-426

Craven, P.A. & DeRubertis, F.R. (1992) Effect of aspirin on 1,2-dimethylhdrazine-induced colonic carcinogenesis. *Carcinogenesis*, **13**, 541–546

Cummings, K.B. & Robertson, R.P. (1977) Prostaglandin: Increased production by renal cell carcinoma. *J. Urol.*, **118**, 720–723

D'Agati, V. (1996) Does aspirin cause acute or chronic renal failure in experimental animals and in humans? *Am. J. Kidney Dis.*, **28**, S24-S29

Davenport, H.W. (1967) Salicylate damage to the gastric mucosal barrier. *New Engl. J. Med.*, **276**, 1307–1312

Davis, A.E. & Patterson, F. (1994) Aspirin reduces the incidence of colonic carcinoma in the dimethylhydrazine rat animal model. *Aust. N.Z. J. Med.*, **24**, 301–303

Denda, A., Ura, H., Tsujiuchi, T., Tsutsumi, M., Eimoto, H., Takashima, Y., Kitazawa, S., Kinugasa, T. & Konishi, Y. (1989) Possible involvement of arachidonic acid metabolism in phenobarbital promotion of hepatocarcinogenesis. *Carcinogenesis*, **10**, 1929–1935

Denda, A., Tang, Q., Endoh, T., Tsujiuchi, T., Horiguchi, K., Noguchi, O., Mizumoto, Y., Nakae, D. & Konishi, Y. (1994) Prevention by acetylsalicylic acid of liver cirrhosis and carcinogenesis as well as generations of 8-hydroxydeoxyguanosine and thiobarbituric acid-reactive substances caused by a choline-deficient, L-amino acid-defined diet in rats. *Carcinogenesis*, **15**, 1279–1283.

Diamond, S. & Freitag, F.G. (1989) Do nonsteroidal anti-inflammatory agents have a role in the treatment of migraine headaches? *Drugs*, **37**, 755–760

Dubach, U.C., Rosner, B. & Sturmer, T. (1991) An epidemiologic study of abuse of analgesic drugs — Effects of phenacitin and salicylate on mortality and cardiovascular morbidity (1968 to 1987). *New Engl J. Med.*, **324**, 155–160

Dubovska, D., Piotrovskij, V.K., Gajdos, M., Krivosikova, Z., Spustova, V. & Trnovec, T. (1995) Pharmacokinetics of acetylsalicylic acid and its metabolites at low doses: A compartmental modeling. *Meth. Find. exp. Clin. Pharmacol.*, **17**, 67–77

Dunn, T.L., Gardiner, R.A., Seymour, G.J. & Lavin, M.F. (1987) Genotoxicity of analgesic compounds assessed by an in vitro micronucleus assay. *Mutat. Res.*, **189**, 299–306

Dutch TIA Trial Study Group (1991) A comparison of two doses of aspirin (30 mg vs. 283 mg a day) in patients after a transient ischemic attack or minor ischemic stroke. *New Engl. J. Med.*, **325**, 1261–1266

ECPPA (Estudo Colaborativo para Prevenção da Pré-eclampsia com Aspirina) Collaborative Group (1996) ECPPA: Randomised trial of low dose aspirin for the prevention of maternal and fetal complications in high risk pregnant women. *Br. J. Obstet. Gynaecol.*, **103**, 39–47

Eddy, L.B., Morgan, R.J. & Carney, H.C. (1976) Hearing loss due to combined effects of noise and sodium salicylate. *ISA Trans.*, **15**, 103–108

Editions du Vidal (1995) *Dictionnaire Vidal*, 72nd Ed., Paris, p. 125

Egan, K.M., Stampfer, M.J., Giovannucci, E., Rosner, B.A. & Colditz, G.A. (1996) Prospective study of regular aspirin use and the risk of breast cancer. *J. natl Cancer Inst.*, **88**, 988–993

Ehresmann, U., Alemany, J. & Loew, D. (1977) [Use of acetylsalicylic acid in the prevention of re-occlusion following revascularization interventions. Results of a double-blind long-term study.] *Med. Welt,* **28**, 1157–1162 (in German)

Elder, D.J.E., Hague, A., Hicks, D.J. & Paraskeva, C. (1996) Differential growth inhibition by the aspirin metabolite salicylate in human colorectal tumor cell lines: Enhanced apoptosis in carcinoma and *in vitro*-transformed adenoma relative to adenoma cell lines. *Cancer Res.*, **56**, 2273–2276

Eling, T.E., Thompson, D.C., Foureman, G.L., Curtis, J.F. & Hughes, M.F. (1990) Prostaglandin H synthase and xenobiotic oxidation. *Ann. Rev. Pharmacol. Toxicol.*, **30**, 1–45

Endoh, T., Tang, Q., Denda, A., Noguchi, O., Kobayashi, E., Tamura, K., Horiguchi, K., Ogasawara, H., Tsujiuchi, T., Nakae, D., Sugimura, M. & Konishi, Y. (1996) Inhibition by acetylsalicylic acid, a cyclo-oxygenase inhibitor, and p-bromophenacylbromide, a phospholipase A2 inhibitor, of both cirrhosis and enzyme-altered nodules caused by a choline-deficient, L-amino acid-defined diet in rats. *Carcinogenesis*, **17**, 467–475

Farivar, R.S. & Brecher, P. (1996) Salicylate is a transcriptional inhibitor of the inducible nitric oxide synthase in cultured cardiac fibroblasts. *J. biol. Chem.*, **271**, 31585–31592

Feng, Y., Papavassiliou, E.D., Arvind, P., Tsioulias, G.J. & Rigas, B. (1996) The effect of eicosanoids on the expression of MHC genes in cultured human colon cancer cells and mouse colonocytes in vivo. *Prostaglandins Leukotrienes Essential Fatty Acids*, **65**, 373–378

Fields, W.S., Lemak, N.A., Frankowski, R.F. & Hardy, R.J. (1978) Controlled trial of aspirin in cerebral ischemia. Part II: Surgical group. *Stroke*, **9**, 309–318

Findlay, J.W., DeAngelis, R.L., Kearney, M.F., Welch, R.N. & Findlay, J.M. (1981) Analgesic drugs in breast milk and plasma. *Clin. Pharmacol. Ther.*, **29**, 625–633

Fischer, A.R., Rosenberg, M.A., Lilly, C.M., Callery, J.C., Rubin, P., Cohn, J., White, M.V., Igarashi, Y., Kaliner, M.A., Drazen, J.M. *et al.* (1994) Direct evidence for a role of the mast cell in the nasal reponse to aspirin in aspirin-sensitive asthma. *J. Allergy clin. Immunol.*, **96**, 1046–1056

Flower, R.G., Moncada, S. & Vane, J.R. (1985) Analgesic-antipyretics and antiinflammatory agents: Drugs employed in the treatment of gout. In: Gilman, A.G., Goodman, L.S., Rall, T.W. & Murad, F., eds, *The Pharmacological Basis of Therapeutics*, 7th Ed., New York, Macmillan, pp. 680–686

Friedman, G.D. & Ury, H.K. (1980) Initial screening for carcinogenicity of commonly used drugs. *J. natl Cancer Inst.*, **65**, 723–733

Friedman, G.D. & Ury, H.K. (1983) Screening for possible drug carcinogenicity: Second report of findings. *J. natl Cancer Inst.*, **71**, 1165–1175

Fries, J.F., Williams, C.A., Bloch, D.A. & Michel, B.A. (1991) Nonsteroidal anti-inflammatory drug-associated gastropathy: Incidence and risk factor models. *Am. J. Med.*, **91**, 213–222

Fromm, D. (1976) Ion selective effects of salicylate on antral mucosa. *Gastroenterology*, **71**, 743–749

Fromm, D. & Kolis, M. (1982) Effects of sodium salicylate and acetylsalicylic acid on intramural pH and ulceration of rabbit antral mucosa. *Surgery*, **91**, 438–447

Funkhouser, G.M. & Sharp, G.B. (1995) Aspirin and the reduced risk of oesophageal carcinoma. *Cancer*, **76**, 1116–1119

Furst, D.E., Gupta, N. & Paulus, H.E. (1977) Salicylate metabolism in twins. Evidence suggesting a genetic influence and induction of salicylate formation. *J. clin. Invest.*, **60**, 32

Galante, R.N., Egoville, J.C., Visalli, A.J. & Patel, D.M. (1981) Simultaneous GLC analysis of aspirin and nonaspirin salicylates in pharmaceutical tablet formulations. *J. pharm. Sci.*, **70**, 167–169

Gann, P.H., Manson, J.E., Glynn, R.J., Buring, J.E. & Hennekens, C.H. (1993) Low-dose aspirin and incidence of colorectal tumors in a randomized trial. *J. natl Cancer Inst.*, **85**, 1220–1224

Garidou, A., Tzonou, A., Lipworth, L., Signarello, L.B., Kalapothaki, V. & Trichopoulos, D. (1996) Life-style factors and medical conditions in relation to oesophageal cancer by histologic type in a low-risk population. *Int. J. Cancer*, **68**, 295–299

Giovannucci, E., Rimm, E.G., Stampfer, M.J., Colditz, G.A., Ascherio, A. & Willett, W.C. (1994) Aspirin use and the risk for colorectal cancer and adenoma in male health professionals. *Ann. intern. Med.*, **121**, 241–246

Giovannucci, E., Egan, K.M., Hunter, D.J., Stampfer, M.J., Colditz, G.A., Willett, W.C. & Speizer, F.E. (1995) Aspirin and the risk of colorectal cancer in women. *New Engl. J. Med.*, **333**, 609–614

Giri, A.K. (1993) The genetic toxicology of paracetamol and aspirin: A review. *Mutat. Res.*, **296**, 199–210

Gladtke, E. & Schausiel, U. (1987) Reye syndrome. *Monatsschr. Kinderheilkd.*, **135**, 699–704

Glauert, H.P., Srinivasan, S., Tatum, V.L., Chen, L.-C., Saxon, D.M. & Travis Lay, L. (1992) Effects of the peroxisome proliferators ciprofibrate and perfluorodecanoic acid on hepatic cellular antioxidants and lipid peroxidation in rats. *Biochem. Pharmacol.*, **43**, 1353–1359

Goel, S.K., Lawani, N.D. & Reddy J.K. (1986) Peroxisome proliferation and lipid peroxidation in rat liver. *Cancer Res.*, **46**, 1324–1330

Gold, A. & Wilpizeski, C.R. (1966) Studies in auditory adaptation. The effects of sodium salicylate on evoked auditory potentials in cats. *Laryngoscope*, **76**, 674–685

Goldman, A.S. & Yakovac, W.C. (1963) The enhancement of salicylate teratogenicity by maternal immobilization in the rat. *J. Pharmacol. exp. Ther.*, **142**, 351–357

Goodman Gilman A., Rall, T.W., Nies, A.S. & Taylor, P., eds (1990) *The Pharmacological Basis of Therapeutics*, 8th Ed., Oxford, Pergamon Press, pp. 638–681

Graham, G.G., Champion, G.D., Day, R.O. & Paull, P.D. (1977) Patterns of plasma concentrations and urinary excretion of salicylate in rheumatoid arthritis. *Clin. Pharmacol. Ther.*, **22**, 410–420

Greenberg, E.R., Baron, J.A., Freeman, D.H., Jr, Mandel, J.S. & Haile, R. (1993) Reduced risk of large-bowel adenomas among aspirin users. *J. natl Cancer Inst.*, **85**, 912–916

Gridley, G., McLaughlin, J.K., Ekbom, A., Klareskog, L., Adami, H.-O., Hacker, D.G., Hoover, R. & Fraumeni, J.F., Jr (1993) Incidence of cancer among patients with rheumatoid arthritis. *J. natl Cancer Inst.*, **85**, 307–311

Grootveld, M. & Halliwell, B. (1988) Dihy-droxygenzoic acid is a product of human aspirin metabolism. *Biochem. Pharmacol.*, **37**, 271–280

Grufferman, S., Wang, H.H., Delong, E.R., Kimm, S.Y., Delzell, E.S. & Falletta, J.M. (1982) Environmental factors in the etiology of rhabdomyosarcoma in childhood. *J. natl Cancer Inst.*, **68**, 107–113

Gugler, R. & Allgayer, H. (1990) Effects of antacids on the clinical pharmacokinetics of drugs: An update. *Clin. Pharmacokinet.*, **18**, 210–219

Gupta, J.P. & Gupta, V. (1977) Serum aspirin esterase activity in women with habitual aspirin ingestion. *Clin. chim. Acta*, **81**, 261

Hall, S.M. (1990) Reye's syndrome and aspirin: A review. *Br. J. clin. Pract.*, **70** (Suppl.), 4–11

Hanif, R., Pittas, L., Feng, Y., Koutsos, M.I., Quao, L., Staiano-Coico, L., Shiff, S.I. & Rigas, B. (1996) Effects of nonsteroidal anti-inflammatory drugs on proliferation and induction of apoptosis in colon cancer cells by a prostaglandin-independent pathway. *Biochem. Pharmacol.*, **52**, 237–245

Harris, R.E., Namboodiri, K.K. & Farrar, W.D. (1995) Epidemiologic study of nonsteroidal anti-inflammatory drugs and breast cancer. *Oncol. Rep.*, **2**, 591–592

Harris, R.E., Namboodiri, K.K. & Farrar, W.D. (1996) Nonsteroidal antiinflammatory drugs and breast cancer. *Epidemiology*, **7**, 203–205

Hatori, A., Shigematsu, A. & Tsuya, A. (1984) The metabolism of aspirin in rats; localization, absorption, distribution and excretion. *Eur. J. Drug Metab. Pharmacokinet.*, **9**, 205–214

Hauth, J.C., Goldenberg, R.L., Parker, C.R., Philips, J.B., Copper, R.L., DuBard, M.B. & Cutter, G.R. (1993) Low-dose aspirin therapy to prevent preeclampsia. *Am. J. Obstet. Gynecol.*, **168**, 1083–1093

Hauth, J.C., Goldenberg, R.L., Parker, C.R., Jr, Cutter, G.R. & Cliver, S.P. (1995) Low-dose aspirin: Lack of association with an increase in abruptio placentae or perinatal mortality. *Obstet. Gynecol.*, **85**, 1055–1058

Hawkins, D., Pinckard, R.N. & Farr, R.S. (1968) Acetylation of human serum albumin by acetylsalicylic acid. *Science*, **160**, 780–781

Heinonen, O.P., Slone, D. & Shapiro, S. (1977) *Birth Defects and Drugs in Pregnancy*, Littleton, MA, Publishing Sciences Group

Hennekens, C.H., Buring, J.E., Sandercock, P., Gray, R., Collins, R., Wheatley, K., Doll, R. & Peto, R. (1990) Aspirin use and chronic diseases. *Br. med. J.*, **300**, 117–118

Hertz-Picciotto, I., Hopenhayn-Rich, C., Golub, M. & Hooper, K. (1990) The risks and benefits of taking aspirin during pregnancy. *Epidemiol. Rev.*, **12**, 108–148

Hess, H., Mietaschk, A. & Diechsel, G. (1985) Drug-induced inhibition of platelet function delays progression of peripheral occlusive arterial disease. A prospective double-blind arteriographically controlled trial. *Lancet*, **i**, 415–419

Hill, L., Murphy, M., McDowall, M. & Paul, A.H. (1988) Maternal drug histories and congenital malformations: Limb reduction defects and oral clefts. *J. Epidemiol. Community Health*, **42**, 1–7

Hirsh, J., Dalen, J.E., Fuster, V., Harker, L.B., Patrono, C. & Roth, G. (1995) Aspirin and other platelet-active drugs. The relationship among dose, effectiveness, and side effects. *Chest,* **108** (Suppl.), 247S–257S

Hurwitz, E.S. (1989) Reye's syndrome. *Epidemiol Rev.*, **11**, 249–253

Hutt, A.J., Caldwell, L. & Smith, R.L. (1986) The metabolism of aspirin in man: A population study. *Xenobiotica*, **16**, 239–249

Inoue, M., Morikawa, M., Tsuboi, M. & Sugiura, M. (1979a) Species difference and characterization of intestinal esterase of the hydrolysing activity of ester type drugs. *Jpn. J. Pharmacol.*, **29**, 9–16

Inoue, M., Morikawa, M., Tsuboi, M., Yamada, T. & Sigiura, M. (1979b) Hydrolysis of ester-type drugs by the purified esterase from human intestinal mucosa. *Jpn. J. Pharmacol.*, **29**, 17–25

Inoue, M., Morikawa, M., Tsuboi, M., Ito, Y. & Sugiura, M. (1980) Comparative study of human intestinal and hepatic esterases as related to the enzymatic properties and hydrolyzing activity for ester-type drugs. *Jpn. J. Pharmacol.*, **30**, 529–535

Ishidate, M., Jr (1988) *Data Book of Chromosomal Aberration Test In Vitro*, Rev. Ed., New York, Elsevier, p. 34

Isomäki, H.A., Hakulinen, T. & Joutsenlahti, U. (1978) Excess risk of lymphomas, leukemia, and myeloma in patients with rheumatoid arthritis. *J. chron. Dis.*, **31**, 691–696

Italian Study of Aspirin in Pregnancy (1993) Low-dose aspirin in prevention and treatment of intrauterine growth retardation and pregnancy-induced hypertension. *Lancet*, **341**, 396–400

Iwamoto, K., Takei, M. & Watanabe, J. (1982) Gastrointestinal and hepatic first-pass metabolism of aspirin in rats. *J. Pharm. Pharmacol.*, **34**, 176–180

Janakidevi, K. & Smith, M.J.H. (1970) Effects of salicylate on RNA polymerase activity and on the incorporation of orotic acid and thymidine into the nucleic acids of rat foetuses in vitro. *J. Pharm. Pharmacol.*, **22**, 249–252

Jasiewicz, M.L. & Richardson, J.C. (1987) Absence of mutagenic activity of benorylate, paracetamol and aspirin in the Salmonella/mammalian microsome test. *Mutat. Res.*, **190**, 95–100

Johnson, A.G., Nguyen, T.V. & Day, R.O. (1994) Do nonsteroidal anti-inflammatory drugs affect blood pressure? A meta-analysis. *Ann. intern. Med.*, **121**, 289–300

Joschko, M.A., Dreosti, I.E. & Tulsi, R.S. (1993) The teratogenic effects of salicylic acid on the developing nervous system in rats in vitro. *Teratology*, **48**, 105-114

Juul-Moller, S., Edvardsson, N., Jahnmatz, B., Rosen, A., Sorensen, S. & Omblus, R. (1992) Double-blind trial of aspirin in primary prevention of myocardial infarction in patients with stable chronic angina pectoris. *Lancet*, **340**, 1421–1425

Kauffman, G. (1989) Aspirin-induced gastric mucosal injury: Lessons learned from animal models. *Gastroenterology*, **96**, 606–614

Kawachi, T., Yahagi, T., Kada, T., Tazima, Y., Oshidate, M., Sasaki, M. & Sugiyama, T. (1980) Cooperative programme on short-term assays for carcinogenicity in Japan. In: Montesano, R., Bartsch, H. & Tomatis, L., eds, *Molecular and Cellular Aspects of Carcinogen Screening Tests* (IARC Scientific Publications No. 27), Lyon, IARC, pp. 323–330

Kim, D.-H., Yang, Y.-S. & Jakoby, W.B. (1990) Aspirin hydrolyzing esterases from rat liver cytosol. *Biochem. Pharmacol.*, **40**, 481–487

Kimmel, C.A., Wilson, J.G. & Schumacher, H.J. (1971) Studies on metabolism and identification of the causative agent in aspirin teratogenesis in rats. *Teratology*, **4**, 15–24

King, M.-T., Beikirch, H., Eckhardt, K., Gocke, E. & Wild, D. (1979) Mutagenicity studies with X-ray-contrast media, analgesics, antpyretics, anti-rheumatics and some other pharmaceutical drugs in bacterial, Drosophila and mammalian test systems. *Mutat. Res.*, **66**, 33–43

Klän, R., Knispel, H.H. & Meier, T. (1993) Acetylsalicyclic acid inhibition of *N*-butyl(4-hydroxybutyl)nitrosamine-induced bladder carcinogenesis in rats. *J. Cancer Res. clin Oncol.*, **119**, 482–485

Klebanoff, M.A. & Berendes, H.W. (1988) Aspirin exposure during the first 20 weeks of gestation and IQ at four years of age. *Teratology*, **37**, 249–255

Konturek, S.J., Piastucki, I., Brzozowski, T., Radecki, T., Dembinska-Kiec, A., Zucha, A. & Gryglewski, R. (1981) Role of prostaglandins in the formation of aspirin-induced gastric ulcers. *Gastroenterology*, **80**, 4–9

Koshakji, R.P. & Schulert, A.R. (1973) Biochemical mechanisms of salicylate teratology in the rat. *Biochem. Pharmacol.*, **22**, 407–416

Krauss, R.S. & Eling, T.E. (1985) Formation of unique arylamine-DNA adducts from 2-aminofluorene activated by prostaglandin H synthase. *Cancer Res.*, **45**, 1680–1686

Kuboyama, N. & Fujii, A. (1992) Mutagenicity of analgesics, their derivatives and anti-inflammatory drugs with S-9 mix of several animal species. *J. Nihon Univ. Sch. Dent.*, **34**, 183–195

Kune, G.A., Kune, S. & Watson, L.F. (1988) Colorectal cancer risk, chronic illnesses, operations, and medications: Case control results from the Melbourne Colorectal Cancer Study. *Cancer Res.*, **48**, 4399–4404

Kuo, Y. & Shanbour, L.L. (1976) Mechanism of action of aspirin on canine gastric mucosa. *Am. J. Physiol.*, **230**, 762–767

Kyle, M.E. & Kocsis, J.J. (1985) The effect of age on salicylate-induced nephrotoxicity in male rats. *Toxicol. appl. Pharmacol.*, **81**, 337–347

Laakso, M., Mutru, O., Isomäki, H. & Koota, K. (1986) Cancer mortality in patients with rheumatoid arthritis. *J. Rheumatol.*, **13**, 522–526

Laznicek, M. & Laznickova, A. (1994) Kidney and liver contributions to salicylate metabolism in rats. *Eur. J. Drug Metab. Pharmacokinet.*, **19**, 21–26

Legaz, M.E., Acitores, E. & Valverde, F. (1992) Determination of salicylic acid by HPLC in plasma and saliva from children with juvenile chronic arthritis. *Tokai J. exp. Med.*, **17**, 229–237

Lemak, N.A., Fields, W.S. & Gary, H.E., Jr (1986) Controlled trial of aspirin in cerebral ischemia: An addendum. *Neurology*, **36**, 705–710

Lev, R., Siegel, H.I. & Jerzy Glass, G.B. (1972) Effects of salicylates on the canine stomach: A morphological and histochemical study. *Gastroenterology*, **62**, 970–980

Levy, G. (1979) Pharmacokinetics of salicylate in man. *Drug Metab. Rev.*, **9**, 3–19

Levy, G. & Tsuchiya, T. (1972) Salicylate accumulation kinetics in man. *New Engl. J. Med.*, **287**, 430–432

Levy, G.N. & Weber, W.W. (1992) 2-Amino-fluorene–DNA adducts in mouse urinary bladder: Effect of age, sex, and acetylator status. *Carcinogenesis*, **13**, 159–164

Levy, G., Vogel, A. & Amsel, L. (1969) Capacity-limited salicylurate formation during prolonged administration of aspirin to healthy human subjects. *J. pharm. Sci.*, **58**, 503–504

Liberman, S.V. & Wood, J.H. (1964) Aspirin formulation and absorption rate II. Influence on serum levels of tablets, antacids and solutions. *J. pharm. Sci.*, **53**, 1492

Lindblad, B., Persson, N.H., Takolander, R. & Bergqvist, D. (1993) Does low-dose acetylsalicylic acid prevent stroke after carotid surgery? A double-blind, placebo-controlled randomized trial. *Stroke*, **24**, 1125–1128

Liu, Y., Levy, G.N. & Weber, W.W. (1995) Activation of 2-aminofluorene by prostaglandin endoperoxide H synthase-2. *Biochem. biophys. Res. Commun.*, **215**, 346–354

Logan, R.F.A., Little, J., Hawtin, P.G. & Hardcastle, J.D. (1993) Effects of aspirin and non-steroidal anti-inflammatory drugs on colorectal adenomas: Case–control study of subjects participating in the Nottingham faecal occult blood screening programme. *Br. med. J.*, **85**, 912–916

Lubawy, W.C. & Burriss Garrett, R.J. (1977) Effects of aspirin and acetaminophen on fetal and placental growth in rats. *J. pharm. Sci.*, **66**, 111–113

Manning, M.D. & Carroll, B.E. (1957) Some epidemiological aspects of leukemia in children. *J. natl Cancer Inst.*, **19**, 1087–1094

Manson, J.E., Stampfer, M.J., Colditz, G.A., Willett, W.C., Rosner, B., Speizer, F.E. & Hennekens, C.H. (1991) A prospective study of aspirin use and primary prevention of cardiovascular disease in women. *J. Am. med. Assoc.*, **266**, 521–527

Marnett, L.J. (1992) Aspirin and the potential role of prostagladins in colon cancer. *Cancer Res.*, **52**, 5575–5589

Martinez, M.E., McPherson, R.S., Levin, B. & Annegers, J.F. (1995) Aspirin and other non-steroidal anti-inflammatory drugs and risk of colorectal adenomatous polyps among endoscoped individuals. *Cancer Epidemiol. Biomarkers Prev.*, **4**, 703–707

McCredie, M., Pommer, W., McLaughlin, J.K., Stewart, J.H., Lindblad, P., Mandel, J.S., Melhemgaard, A., Schlehofer, B. & Niwa, S. (1995) International renal-cell cancer study. II. Analgesics. *Int. J. Cancer*, **60**, 345–349

McDonald, A.D. (1994) Therapeutic drugs in early pregnancy and congenital defects. *J. clin. Epidemiol.*, **47**, 105–110

McGarrity, C., Samani, N.J., Beck, F. & Gulamhusein, A. (1981) The effect of sodium salicylate on the rat embryo in culture: An in vitro model for the morphological assessment of teratogenicity. *J. Anat.*, **133**, 257–269

McGeer, P.L., Schulzer, M. & McGeer, E.G. (1996) Arthritis and anti-inflammatory agents as possible protective factors for Alzheimer's disease: A review of 17 epidemiologic studies. *Neurology*, **47**, 425–432

Meisner, L.F. & Inhorn, S.L. (1972) Chemically induced chromosome changes in human cells in vitro. *Acta cytol.*, **16**, 41–47

Menouer, M., Ghernati, H.M., Bouabdallah, F. & Guermouch, M.H. (1982) Optimal operating conditions for the separation of salicylic acid and acetylsalicylic acid by HPLC. Application to traces analysis of salicylic acid in aspirin. *Analysis*, **10**, 172–176

Mereto, E., Frencia, L. & Ghia, M. (1994) Effect of aspirin on incidence and growth of aberrant crypt foci induced in the rat colon by 1,2-dimethylhydrazine. *Cancer Lett.*, **76**, 5–9

Minchin, R.F., Ilett, K.F., Teitel, C.H., Reeves, P.T. & Kadlubar, F.F. (1992) Direct *O*-acetylation of *N*-hydroxyarylamines by acetylsalicylic acid to form carcinogen–DNA adducts. *Carcinogenesis*, **13**, 663–667

Miners, J.O. (1989) Drug interactions involving aspirin (acetylsalicylic acid) and salicylic acid (review). *Clin. Pharmacokinet.*, **17**, 327–344

Mitchell, J.A., Akarasereenont, P., Thiemermann, C., Flower, R.J. & Vane, J.R. (1994) Selectivity of nonsteroidal antiinflammatory drugs as inhibitors of constitutive and inducible cyclooxygenase. *Proc. natl Acad. Sci. USA*, **90**, 11693–11697

Mittman, N., Janis, R. & Schlondorff, D. (1985) Salicylate nephropathy in the Gunn rat: Potential role of prostaglandins. *Prostaglandins*, **30**, 511–525

Moncada, S. & Vane, J.R. (1979) Arachidonic acid metabolites and the interactions between platelets and blood-vessel walls. *New Engl J. Med*, **300**, 1142–1147

Morlans, M., Laporte, J.R., Vidal, X., Cabeza, D. & Stolley, P.D. (1990) End-stage renal disease and non-narcotic analgesics: A case-control study. *Br. J. clin. Pharmacol.*, **30**, 712–723

Muller, F., Hundt, H.K.L. & Muller, D.G. (1977) Pharmacokinetic and pharmacodynamic implications of long-term administration of non-steroidal anti-inflammatory agents. *Int. J. clin. Pharmacol.*, **15**, 397

Muller, L., Kasper, P. & Madle, S. (1991) Further investigations on the clastogenicity of paracetamol and acetylsalicylic acid in vitro. *Mutat. Res.*, **263**, 83–92

Müller, A.D., Sonnenberg, A. & Wasserman, I.H. (1994) Diseases preceding colon cancer. A case–control study among veterans. *Dig. Dis. Sci.*, **39**, 2480–2484

Murasaki, G., Zenser, T.V., Davis, B.B. & Cohen, S.M. (1984) Inhibition by aspirin of N-[4-(5-nitro-2-furyl)-2-thiazolyl]formamide-induced bladder carcinogenesis and enhancement of forestomach carcinogenesis. *Carcinogenesis*, **5**, 53–55

Murray, M.D. & Brater, D.C. (1993) Renal toxicity of the nonsteroidal anti-inflammatory drugs. *Ann. Rev. Pharmacol. Toxicol.*, **32**, 435–465

Muscat, J.E., Stellman, S.D. & Wynder, E.L. (1994) Nonsteroidal antiinflammatory drugs and colorectal cancer. *Cancer*, **74**, 1847–1854

Myers, E.N. & Bernstein, J.M. (1965) Salicylate ototoxicity. *Arch. Otolaryngol.*, **82**, 483–493

Needs, C.J. & Brooks, P.M. (1985) Clinical pharmacokinetics of the salicylates. *Clin. Pharmacokinet.*, **10**, 164–177

Nelson, M.M. & Forfar, J.O. (1971) Associations between drugs administered during pregnancy and congenital abnormalities of the fetus. *Br. med. J.*, **i**, 523–527

Ohe, K., Hayashi, K., Shirakawa, T., Yamada, K., Kawasaki, T. & Miyoshi, A. (1980) Aspirin- and taurocholate-induced metabolic damage in mammalian gastric mucosa in vitro. *Am. J. Physiol.*, **239**, G457–G462

Oldham, J.W., Preson, R.F. & Paulson, J.D. (1986) Mutagenicity testing of selected analgesics in Ames Salmonella strains. *J. appl. Toxicol.*, **6**, 237–243

Olson, G.A., Leffler, C.W. & Fletcher, A.M. (1985) Gastroduodenal ulceration in rabbits producing antibodies to prostaglandins. *Prostaglandins*, **29**, 475–480

Orlowski, J.P., Gillis, J., Kilham, H.A. (1987) A catch in the Reye. *Pediatrics*, **80**, 638–642

Orozco-Alcala, J.J. & Baum, J. (1979) Regular and enteric coated aspirin: A re-evaluation. *Arthrit. Rheumatol.*, **22**, 1034

Owen, R.A. & Heywood, R. (1986) Strain-related susceptibility to nephrotoxicity induced by aspirin and phenylbutazone in rats. *Toxicol. Pathol.*, **14**, 242–246

Padmanabhan, R., Wasfi, I.A. & Craigmyle, M.B. (1994) Effect of pre-treatment with aspirin on alcohol-induced neural tube defects in the TO mouse fetuses. *Drug Alcohol Depend.*, **36**, 175–186

Paganini-Hill, A. (1995) Aspirin and colorectal cancer: The Leisure World cohort revisited. *Prev. Med.*, **24**, 113–115

Paganini-Hill, A., Chao, A., Ross, R.K. & Henderson, B.E. (1989) Aspirin use and chronic diseases: A cohort study of the elderly. *Br. med. J.*, **299**, 1247–1250

Paganini-Hill, A., Hsu, G., Ross, R.K. & Henderson, B.E. (1991) Aspirin use and incidence of large-bowel cancer in a California retirement community (correspondence). *J. natl Cancer Inst.*, **83**, 1182–1183

Parazzini, F., Bortolus, R., Chatenoud, L., Restelli, S. & Benedetto, C. (on behalf of the Italian Study of Aspirin in Pregnancy) (1994) Follow-up of children in the Italian Study of Aspirin in Pregnancy. *Lancet*, **343**, 1235

Patel, D.K., Notarianni, L.J. & Bennett, P.N. (1990) Comparative metabolism of high doses of aspirin in man and rat. *Xenobiotica*, **20**, 847–854

Patierno, S.R., Lehman, N.L., Henderson, B.E. & Landolph, J.R. (1989) Study of the ability of phenacetin, acetaminophen, and aspirin to induce cytotoxicity, mutation, and morphological transformation in C3H/10T1/2 clone 8 mouse embryo cells. *Cancer Res.*, **49**, 1038–1044

Patrono, C. (1994) Aspirin as an antiplatelet drug. *New Engl. J. Med.*, **330**, 1287–1294

Paulus, H.E. Siegel, M., Mongan, E., Okun, N. & Calabro, J.J. (1971) Variations of serum concentrations and half life of salicylate in patients with rheumatoid arthritis. *Arthr. Rev.*, **14**, 527–532

Peleg, I.I., Maibach, H.T., Brown, S.H. & Wilcox, C.M. (1994) Aspirin and nonsteroidal anti-inflammatory drug use and the risk of subsequent colorectal cancer. *Arch. intern. Med.*, **154**, 394–399

Peleg, I.I., Lubin, M.F., Cotsonis, G.A., Clark, W.S. & Wilcox, C.M. (1996) Long-term use of non-steroidal antiinflammatory drugs and other chemopreventors and risk of subsequent colorectal neoplasia. *Dig. Dis. Sci.*, **41**, 1319–1326

Pereira, M.A., Barnes, L.H., Rassman, V.L., Kelloff, G.V. & Steele, V.E. (1994) Use of azoxymethane-induced foci of aberrant crypts in rat colon to identify potential cancer chemopreventive agents. *Carcinogenesis*, **15**, 1049–1054

Pernerger, T.V., Whelton, P.K. & Klag, M.J. (1994) Risk of kidney failure associated with the use of acetaminophen, aspirin and nonsteroidal antiinflammatory drugs. *New Engl. J. Med.*, **331**, 1675–1679

Peto, R., Gray, R., Collins, R., Wheatley, K., Hennekens, C., Jamrozik, K., Warlow, C., Hafner, B., Thompson, E., Norton, S., Gilliland, J. & Doll, R. (1988) Randomized trial of prophylactic daily aspirin in British male doctors. *Br. med. J.*, **296**, 313–316

Pinckard, R.N., Hawkins, D. & Farr, R.S. (1968) In vitro acetylation of plasma proteins enzymes and DNA by aspirin. *Nature*, **219**, 68–69

Pommer, W., Bronder, E., Greiser, E., Helmert, U., Jesdinsky, K., Klimpel, A., Borner, K. & Molzahn, M. (1989) Regular analgesic intake and the risk of end-stage renal failure. *Am. J. Nephrol*, **9**, 403–412

Preston-Martin, S., Yu, M.C., Benton, B. & Henderson, B.E. (1982) N-Nitroso compounds and childhood brain tumours: A case–control study. *Cancer Res.*, **42**, 5240–5245

Rabinowitz, J.L., Feldman, E.S., Weinberger, A. & Schumacher, H.R. (1982) Comparative tissue absorption of ^{14}C-aspirin and topical triethanolamine in human and canine knee joints. *J. clin. Pharmacol.*, **22**, 42–48

Rao, K.V.N., Detrisac, C.J., Steele, V.E., Hawk, E.T., Kelloff, G.J. & McCormick, D.L. (1996) Differential activity of aspirin, ketoprofen and sulindac as cancer chemopreventive agents in the mouse urinary bladder. *Carcinogenesis*, **17**, 1435–1438

Reddy, J.K. & Lalwani, N.D. (1983) Carcinogenesis by hepatic peroxisome proliferators: Evaluation of the risk of hypolipidemic drugs and industrial plasticizers to humans. *CRC crit. Rev. Toxicol.*, **12**, 1–58

Reddy, B.S., Rao, C.V., Rivenson, A. & Kelloff, G. (1993) Inhibitory effect of aspirin on azoxymethane-induced colon carcinogenesis in F344 rats. *Carcinogenesis*, **14**, 1493–1497

Redfern, J.S., Blair, A.J., Lee, E. & Feldman, M. (1987) Gastrointestinal ulcer formation in rabbits immunized with prostaglandin E2. *Gastroenterology*, **93**, 744–752

Reeves, M.J., Newcomb, P.A., Trentham-Dietz, A., Stoner, B.E. & Remington, P.L. (1996) Nonsteroidal anti-inflammatory drug use and protection against colorectal cancer in women. *Cancer Epidemiol. Biomarkers Prev.*, **5**, 955–960

Reynolds, J.E.F. & Prasad, A.B., eds (1982) *Martindale — The Extra Pharmacopoeia*, 28th Ed., London, The Pharmaceutical Press, pp. 234–246

Reynolds, J.E.F., ed. (1993) *Martindale, The Extra Pharmocopoeia*, 13th Ed., London, The Pharmaceutical Press, pp. 3–7

Richards, I.D.G. (1969) Congenital malformations and environmental influences in pregnancy. *Br. J. prev. soc. Med.*, **23**, 218–225

Rigas, B., Goldman, I.S. & Levine, L. (1993) Altered eicosanoid levels in human colon cancer. *J. Lab. clin. Med.*, **122**, 518–523

Rigas, B., Tsioulias. G.J., Allan, C., Walli, R. & Brasitus, T.A. (1994) The effect of bile acids and piroxicam on MHC antigen expression in rat colonocytes during colon cancer development. *Immunology*, **83**, 319–323

RISC Group (1990) Risk of myocardial infarction and death during treatment with low dose aspirin and intravenous heparin in men with unstable coronary artery disease. *Lancet*, **336**, 827–830

Roberts, J. & Caserio, M.C., eds (1965) *Basic Principles of Organic Chemistry*, New York, W.A. Benjamin, p. 953

Roberts, M.S., Rumble, R.H. & Brooks, P.M. (1978) Salivery salicylate secretion and flow rates. *Br. J. clin. Pharmacol.*, **6**, 429

Roberts, M., Rumble, R.H., Wanwimolruk, S., Thomas, D. & Brooks, P.M. (1983) Pharmacokinetics of aspirin and salicylate in elderly subjects and in patients with alcoholic liver disease. *Eur. J. clin. Pharmacol.*, **25**, 253–261

Rosenberg, L., Palmer, J.R., Zauber, A.G., Warshauer, M.E., Stolley, P.D. & Shapiro, S. (1991) A hypothesis: Nonsteroidal anti-inflammatory drugs reduce the incidence of large-bowel cancer. *J. natl Cancer Inst.*, **83**, 355–358

Ross, D.K., Paganini Hill, A., Landolph, J., Gerkins, V. & Henderson, B.E. (1989) Analgesics, cigarette smoking and other risk factors for cancer of the renal pelvis and ureter. *Cancer Res.*, **49**, 1045–1048

Ross Lee, L.M., Elms, M.J., Cham, B.E., Bochner, F., Bunce, I.H. & Eadie, M.J. (1982) Plasma levels of aspirin following effervescent and enteric coated tablets, and their effect on platelet function. *Eur. J. clin. Pharmacol.*, **23**, 545

Ross Lee, L.M., Eadie, M.J., Heazlewood, V., Bochner, F., Bunce, I.H. & Eadie, M.J. (1983) Aspirin pharmacokinetics in migraine. The effect of metoclopramide. *Eur. J. clin. Pharmacol.*, **24**, 777–785

Rothman, K.J,. Fyler, D.C. Goldblatt, A. & Kreidberg, M.B. (1979) Exogenous hormones and other drug exposures of children with congenital heart disease. *Am. J. Epidemiol.*, **109**, 433–439

Rowe, P.H., Sarlinger, M.J., Kasdon, E., Hollands, M.J. & Silen, W. (1987) Parenteral aspirin and sodium salicylate are equally injurious to the rat gastric mucosa. *Gastroenterology*, **93**, 863–871

Rowland, N., Harris, Riegelman, P.A., Sholkoff, S.D. & Eyring, E.J. (1967) Kinetics of acetylsalicylic acid disposition in man. *Nature*, **215**, 413–414

Rowland, N., Riegelman, S., Harris, P.A. & Sholkoff, S.D. (1972) Absorption kinetics of aspirin in man following oral administration of an aqueous solution. *J. pharm. Sci.*, **61**, 379–385

Rumble, R.H., Brooks, P.M. & Roberts, M.S. (1980) Metabolism of salicylate during chronic aspirin therapy. *Br. J. clin. Pharmacol.*, **15**, 397

Rumore, M.M., Aron, M. & Hiross, E.J. (1987) A review of mechanism of action of aspirin and its potential as an immunomodulating agent. *Med. Hypoth.*, **22**, 387–400

SALT Collaborative Group (1991) Swedish aspirin low-dose trial (SALT) of 75 mg aspirin as secondary prophylaxis after cerebrovascular ischaemic events. *Lancet*, **338**, 1345–1349

Sandler, D.P., Smith, J.C., Weinberg, C.R., Buckalew, V.M., Jr, Dennis, V.W., Blythe, W.B. & Burgess, W.P. (1989) Analgesic use and chronic renal disease. *New Engl. J. Med.*, **320**, 1238–1243

Saxén, I. (1975) Associations between oral clefts and drugs taken during pregnancy. *Int. J. Epidemiol.*, **4**, 37–44

Schoenfeld, A., Bar, Y., Merlob, P. & Ovadia, Y. (1992) NSAID's: Maternal and fetal considerations. *Am. J. Reprod. Immunol.*, **28**, 141–147

Schreinemachers, D.M. & Everson, R.B. (1994) Aspirin use and lung, colon and breast cancer incidence in a prospective study. *Epidemiology*, **5**, 138–146

Schwartzbaum, J.A. (1992) Influence of mother's prenatal drug consumption on risk of neuroblastoma in the child. *Am. J. Epidemiol.*, **135**, 1358–1367

Sechserova, N., Secher, T., Raskova, H., Ellis, J., Vanesec, J. & Polak, L. (1979) Ondogenic drug studies in calves. I. Age dependent salicylate levels and metabolism. *Arzneimittel.-forsch.*, **29**, 650–651

Selby, J.V., Friedman, G.D. & Fireman, B.H. (1989) Screening prescription drugs for possible carcinogenicity: Eleven to fifteen years of follow-up. *Cancer Res.*, **49**, 5736–5747

Shahar, E., Folsom, A.R., Romm, F.J., Bisgard, K.M., Metcalf, P.A., Crum, L., McGovern, P.G., Hutchinson, R.G. & Heiss, G. (1996) Patterns of aspirin use in middle-aged adults: The Atherosclerosis Risk in Communities (ARIC) study. *Am. Heart J.*, **131**, 915–922

Shapiro, S., Siskind, V., Monson, R.R., Heinonen, O.P., Kaufman, D.W. & Slone, D. (1976) Perinatal mortality and birthweight in relation to aspirin taken during pregnancy. *Lancet*, **i**, 1375–1376

Shiff, S.J., Koutsos, M.I., Qiao, L. & Rigas, B. (1996) Nonsteroidal antiinflammatory drugs inhibit the proliferation of colon adenocarcinoma cells: Effects on cell cycle and apoptosis. *Exp. Cell Res.*, **222**, 179–188

Sibai, B.M., Caritis, S.N., Thom, E., Klebanoff, M., McNellis, D., Rocco, L., Paul, R.H., Romero, R., Witter, F., Rosen, M., Depp, R. & the National Institute of Child Health and Human Development Network of Maternal–Fetal Medicine Units (1993) Prevention of preeclampsia with low-dose aspirin in healthy nulliparous pregnant women. *New Engl. J. Med.*, **329**, 1213–1218

Silagy, C. (1993) Aspirin and the elderly. *Drugs Ageing*, **3**, 301–307

Slattery, J., Warlow, C.P., Shorrock, C.J. & Langman, M.J. (1995) Risks of gastrointestinal bleeding during secondary prevention of vascular events with aspirin — Analysis of vascular events and gastrointestinal bleeding during the UK–MA trial. *Gut*, **37**, 509–511

Slone, D., Heinonen, O.P., Kaufman, D.W., Siskind, V., Monson, R.R. & Shapiro, S. (1976) Aspirin and congenital malformations. *Lancet*, **i**, 1373–1375

Spenney, G. (1978) Acetylsalicylic acid hydrolase of gastric mucosa. *Am. J. Physiol.*, **234**, E606–E610

Staton, G.W., Jr & Ingram, R.H. (1996) Asthma. In: Dale, D.C. & Federman, D.D., eds, *Scientific American Medicine*, New York, Scientific American, pp. 9–20

Steering Committee of the Physicians' Health Study Research Group (1989) Final report on the aspirin component of the ongoing Physicians' Health Study. *New Engl. J. Med.*, **321**, 129–135

Steineck, G., Wiholm, B.E. & Gerhardsson de Verdier, M. (1995) Acetaminophen, some other drugs, some diseases and the risk of transitional cell carcinoma. A population-based case–control study. *Acta oncol.*, **34**, 741–748

Stemmermann, G.N., Nomura, A.M.Y. & Grove, J.S. (1989) Aspirin and colonic epithelium (correspondence). *Gastroenterology*, **96**, 270–271

Stressguth, A.P., Treder, R.P., Barr, H.M., Shepard, T.H., Bleyer, W.A., Sampson, P.D. & Martin, D.C. (1987) Aspirin and acetaminophen use by pregnant women and subsequent IQ and attention decrments. *Teratology*, **35**, 211–219

Sturmer, T., Glynn, R.J., Lee, I.M., Manson, J.E., Hennekens, C.H. & Buring, J.E. (1996) Aspirin use and colorectal cancer incidence in the Physicians' Health Study (PHS) (Abstract). *Am. J. Epidemiol.*, *Suppl.* **143**, S62

Suh, O., Mettlin, C. & Petrelli, N.J. (1993) Aspirin use, cancer, and polyps of the large bowel. *Cancer*, **72**, 1171–1177

Sullivan Bolyai, J.Z. & Corey, L. (1981) Epidemiology of Reye syndrome. *Epidemiol Rev.*, **3**, 1–26

Szczeklik, A. (1994) Aspirin-induced asthma: An update and novel findings. *Adv. Prostaglandin Thromboxane Leukotriene Res.*, **22**, 185–198

Takahashi, M., Furukawa, F., Toyoda, K., Sato, H., Hasegawa, R., Imaida, K. & Hayashi, Y. (1990) Effects of various prostaglandin synthesis inhibitors on pancreatic carcinogenesis in hamsters after initiation with N-nitroso(2-oxo-propyl)amine. *Carcinogenesis*, **11**, 393–395

Tang, Q., Denda, A., Tsujiuchi, T., Tsutsumi, M., Toshihiro A., Murata, Y., Maruyama, H. & Konishi, Y. (1993) Inhibitory effects of inhibitors of arachidonic acid metabolism on the evolution of rat liver preneoplastic foci into nodules and hepatocellular carcinomas with or without phenobarbital exposure. *Jpn. J. Cancer Res.*, **84**, 120–127

Thun, M.J., Namboodiri, M.M. & Heath, C.W., Jr (1991) Aspirin use and reduced risk of fatal colon cancer. *New Engl. J. Med.*, **325**, 1593–1596

Thun, M.J., Calle, E.E., Namboodiri, M.M., Flanders, W.D., Coates, R.J., Byers, T., Boffetta, P., Garfinkel, L. & Heath, C.W., Jr (1992) Risk factors for fatal colon cancer in a large prospective study. *J. natl Cancer Inst.*, **84**, 1491–1500

Thun, M.J., Namboodiri, M.M., Calle, E.E., Flanders, D.W. & Heath, C.W., Jr (1993) Aspirin use and risk of fatal cancer. *Cancer Res.*, **53**, 1322–1327

Trasler, D.G. (1965) Aspirin-induced cleft lip and other malformations in mice. *Lancet*, **i**, 606–607

Uzan, S., Beaufils, M., Breart, G., Bazin, B., Capitant, C. & Paris, J. (1991) Prevention of fetal growth retardation with low-dose aspirin: Findings of the EPREDA trial. *Lancet*, **337**, 1427–1431

Vaca, C.E., Wilheim, J. & Hams-Ringdahl, X. (1988) Interaction of lipid peroxidation products with DNA. A review. *Mutat. Res.*, **195**, 137–149

Vane, J.R. (1971) Inhibition of prostaglandin synthesis as a mechanism of action for aspirin like drugs. *Nature New Biol.*, **231**, 232–235

Vane, J.R., Flaner, R.J. & Botting, R.M. (1990) History of aspirin and its mechanism of action. *Stroke*, **21**, 12–23

Vasilenko, N.M., Manzhelai, E.S. & Gnezdilova, A.I. (1979) Gonadotoxic action of acetylsalicylic acid. *Pharmacol. Toxicol.*, **42**, 421–423

Verbeeck, R.K. (1990) Pharmacokinetic drug interactions with nonsteroidal anti-inflammatory drugs. *Clin. Pharmacokinet.*, **19**, 44–66

Viinikka, L., Hartikainen-Sorri, A.L., Lumme, R., Hiilesmaa, V. & Ylikorkala, O. (1993) Low dose aspirin in hypertensive pregnant women: Effect on pregnancy outcome and prostacyclin–thromboxane balance in mother and new-born. *Br. J. Obstet. Gynaecol.*, **100**, 809–815

Vinson, J.A. & Kozak, D.M. (1978) Analysis of aspirin tablets using quantitative NMR. *Am. J. pharm. Educ.*, **42**, 290–291

Wargovich, M.J., Chen, C.D., Harris, C., Yang, E. & Velasco, M. (1995) Inhibition of aberrant crypt growth by non-steroidal anti-inflammatory agents and differentiation agents in the rat colon. *Int. J. Cancer*, **60**, 515–519

Warkany, J. & Takacs, E. (1959) Experimental production of congenital malformation in rats by salicylate poisoning. *Am. J. Pathol.*, **35**, 315–331

Watanabe, M. (1982) The cytogenic effects of aspirin and acetaminophen on in vitro human lymphocytes. *Jpn. J. Hyg.*, **37**, 673–685

Weatherall, J.A.C. & Greenberg, G. (1979) Maternal drug usage and congenital malformations: A case–control study. *Contr. Epidemiol. Biostatist.*, **1**, 71–77

Werler, M.M., Mitchell, A.A. & Shapiro, S. (1989) The relation of aspirin use during the first trimester of pregnancy to congenital cardiac defects. *New Engl. J. Med.*, **321**, 1639–1642

White, K.N. & Hope, D.B. (1984) Partial purification and characterization of a microsomal carboxylesterase specific for salicylate esters from guinea-pig liver. *Biochim. biophys. Acta*, **785**, 138–147

Wilson, J.T., Brown, R.D., Bocchini, J.A. & Kearns, G.I. (1982) Efficacy, disposition and pharmacodynamics of aspirin, acetaminophen and choline salicylates in young febrile children. *Ther. Drug Monit.*, **4**, 147–180

Windorfer, A., Kuenzer, W. & Urbanck, R. (1974) The influence of age on the activity of acetylsalicylic acid esterase and protein binding. *Eur. J. clin. Pharmacol.*, **7**, 227

Winship, K.A., Cahal, D.A., Weber, J.C.P. & Griffin, J.P. (1984) Maternal drug histories and central nervous system anomalies. *Arch. Dis. Child.*, **59**, 1052–1560

Yue, T.L. & Varma, D.R. (1982) Pharmacokinetics, metabolism and disposition of salicylate in protein-deficient rats. *Drug Metab. Disposition*, **10**, 147–152

Zapadnyuk, V.I., Korkushko, O.V., Bezverkhaya, I.S. & Bely, A.A. (1987) Age-related peculiarities of acetylsalicylic acid pharmacokinetics. *Pharmacol. Toxicol.*, **50**, 79–82

Zierler, S. & Rothman, K.J. (1985) Congenital heart disease in relation to maternal use of bendectin and other drugs in early pregnancy. *New Engl. J. Med.*, **313**, 347–352

Sulindac

1. Chemical and Physical Characteristics

1.1 Name

Chemical Abstracts Services Registry Number
38194-50-2

Chemical Abstracts Primary Name
Sulindac

IUPAC Systematic Name
1*H*-Indene-3-acetic acid, 5-fluoro-2-methyl-1-{[4-(methyl-sulfinyl)phenyl]methylene}

Synonyms
(Z)-5-Fluoro-2-methyl-1-{[4-(methyl-sulfinyl)-phenyl]methylene}-1*H*-indene-3-acetic acid; *cis*-5-fluoro-2-methyl-1-[*p*-(methylsulfinyl)-benzylidene]indene-3-acetic acid; MK-231

1.2 Structural and molecular formula and relative molecular mass

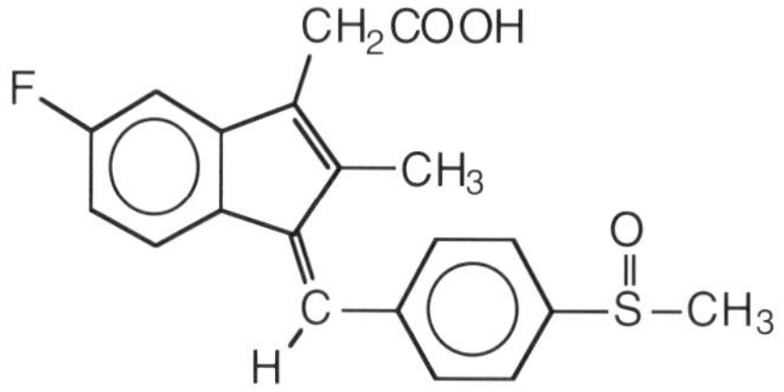

$C_{20}H_{17}FO_3S$ Relative molecular mass: 356.42

1.3 Physical and chemical properties

The data presented are for the pure substance and are taken from Budavari (1989) and Reynolds (1993), unless otherwise specified.

Description
Yellow, odourless crystals

Melting-point
182–185 °C

Solubility
A weak acid with a pK_a of 4.7 at 25 °C. Sparingly soluble in methanol and ethanol; slightly soluble in ethyl acetate; soluble in chloroform; practically insoluble in water at pH below 4.5. Solubility increases with rising pH to about 3.0 mg/ml at pH 7.

Spectroscopy data
Ultraviolet, infrared, nuclear magnetic resonance and mass spectra have been reported.

Stability
Stable in aquous solutions of acids and bases. In a solid state, stable for at least three days in air at 100 °C.

Stereoisomers
Sulindac is the Z isomer of 1*H*-indeno-3-acetic acid, 5-fluoro-2-methyl-1-{[4-(methyl-sulfinyl)-phenyl]methylene}.

1.4 Technical products

Trade names
Aflodac, Algocetil, Apo-Sulin, Arthrobid, Arthrocine, Artribid, Citireuma, Clinoril, Clisundac, Imbaral, Lyndak, Novosundac, Reumofil, Reumyl, Sudac, Sulartrene, Sulen, Sulic, Sulindal, Sulinol, Sulreuma.

2. Occurrence, Production, Use, Analysis and Human Exposure

2.1 Occurrence

Sulindac is not known to occur as a natural product.

2.2 Production

Sulindac is a synthetic product; it is manufactured in several countries. Accepted standard procedures for the synthesis of sulindac are described by Shen and Winter (1977). Technical details regarding its current commercial production were not available to the Working Group.

2.3   Use

Sulindac was introduced in the 1970s (Shen & Winter, 1977). It has analgesic, anti-inflammatory and antipyretic properties and is used in musculoskeletal and joint disorders, such as ankylosing spondylitis, osteoarthritis and rheumatoid arthritis, and also in the short-term management of conditions such as bursitis and tendinitis and acute gouty arthritis. The usual dose by mouth is 100–200 mg twice daily, taken with food (Reynolds, 1993).

Sulindac is a pro-drug, a pharmacologically inactive precursor that is converted *in vivo* to an active drug by metabolism or other physiological processes. Its sulfide metabolite inhibits cyclo-oxygenases. Some of its clinical properties may be attributable to the sulfone metabolite (Singh *et al.*, 1994).

2.4   Analysis

Sulindac has been measured in human plasma by high-performance liquid chromatography (Shimek *et al.*, 1981; Swanson & Boppana, 1981; Stubbs *et al.*, 1987), by combined isotope dilution radioimmunoassay (Hare *et al.*, 1977) and by differential pulse polarographic analysis (Zamboni *et al.*, 1983). Fluorescence detection combined with reversed-phase high-performance liquid chromatography has also been used to determine sulindac and its sulfone and sulfide metabolites in human serum (Siluveru & Stewart, 1995).

2.5   Human exposure

Estimates of the prevalence of sulindac use vary, but it is limited. Jones and Tait (1995) reported that sulindac accounted for less than 7% of NSAID prescriptions in 1014 cases identified in general practice in the United Kingdom.

Sulindac accounts for a minor proportion of NSAID use in the USA, as seen in the Tennessee Medicaid Programme (Griffin *et al.*, 1991).

3.   Metabolism, Kinetics and Genetic Variation

3.1   Human studies
3.1.1   Metabolism
Sulindac is an anti-inflammatory pro-drug which, after absorption, undergoes two major biotransformations in humans: reversible reduction to the sulfide metabolite, the most potent inhibitor of prostaglandin production, and irreversible oxidation to the sulfone metabolite, which is inactive as an antiinflammatory agent. Figure 1 shows the proposed metabolic scheme for sulindac. Approximately 88% of sulindac is absorbed in humans after oral administration of a 200-mg dose (Duggan *et al.*, 1977). In normal subjects and patients with surgical ileostomies, as much as 50% of the total sulfide was formed by gut bacteria (Strong *et al.*, 1985), probably from sulindac excreted in bile. It appears to undergo extensive reabsorption and enterohepatic recycling. Incubation of sulindac and its derivatives with over 200 strains of bacteria isolated from human faeces *in vitro* showed extensive reduction by both aerobes and anaerobes (Strong *et al.*, 1987).

3.1.2   Pharmacokinetics
After a single 200-mg oral dose of sulindac, the peak plasma concentration was 4.7 µg/ml after 1.6 h in one study (Strong *et al.*, 1985) and 5.4 µg/ml after 1 h in another (Duggan *et al.*, 1977). Sulindac binds tightly to human serum albumin (Russeva *et al.*, 1994) and has a mean half-life of 97 h (Strong *et al.*, 1985). The peak plasma concentration of the sulfide metabolite was about 2.7 mg/ml and was reached after 3.1 h. The half-life was 14 h in normal subjects and 2.6 h in patients with an ileostomy (Strong *et al.*, 1985). Sustained plasma levels of the sulfide metabolite are consistent with a prolonged anti-inflammatory action. The peak plasma concentration of the sulfone metabolite was about 1.5 mg/ml and was reached after 2.9 h. The half-life was 20 h in normal subjects and 5.4 h in patients with an ileostomy (Strong *et al.*, 1985).

The primary route of excretion in humans is via the urine, as both sulindac and its sulfone metabolite (free and as glucuronide conjugates). About 50% of an administered dose is excreted in the urine, the conjugated sulfone metabolite accounting for the major portion. No significant level of free or conjugated sulfide was detected in urine About 25% is found in the faeces, primarily as the sulfone and sulfide metabolites (Duggan *et al.,* 1977). The concentrations of these metabolites in the gut lumen and mucosa were not known to the Working Group.

Because sulindac is excreted in the urine primarily as biologically inactive forms, it may affect renal function to a lesser extent than other NSAIDs (Miller *et al.,* 1984); however, adverse renal effects have been reported (see section 7.1.1.(c)). Patients with end-stage renal failure had substantially lower total and free plasma concentrations of the active sulfide metabolite of sulindac (Ravis *et al.,* 1993). The apparent half-lives of sulindac and sulindac sulfide were similar in the two groups, but the half-life of the sulfone metabolite was longer in patients with renal failure.

Since many patients who take NSAIDs have rheumatoid arthritis and are also given methotrexate for their joint inflammation, a study was conducted to evaluate the potential interactions between methotrexate and sulindac. Sulindac had little effect on the disposition of methotrexate but a minor effect on the 7-OH-methotrexate metabolite (Furst *et al.,* 1990).

Sulindac and its active sulfide metabolite undergo placental transfer; however, the reduction of sulindac to the metabolite is decreased in the human fetus, and the process seems to be independent of gestational age (Kramer *et al.,* 1995).

3.2 Experimental models

The half-life of sulindac in plasma was 10 h in Sprague-Dawley rats, 3 h in beagle dogs and 0.5 h in rhesus monkeys (Hucker *et al.,* 1973). Rats had by far the highest plasma concentration (44.0 µg/ml) 1 h after an oral dose of 10 mg/kg bw; the concentrations were 0.8 µg/ml in dogs at 1 h, not detectable in rhesus monkeys 1 h after a dose of 3 mg/kg bw and 1.3 µg/ml in humans 1 h after a 50-mg oral dose. Rats and dogs eliminated the drug almost exclusively in faeces, whereas urinary excretion is favoured in monkeys and humans. The tissue distribution in rats indicated that the drug was

Figure 1. Sulindac and its sulfide and sulfone metabolites

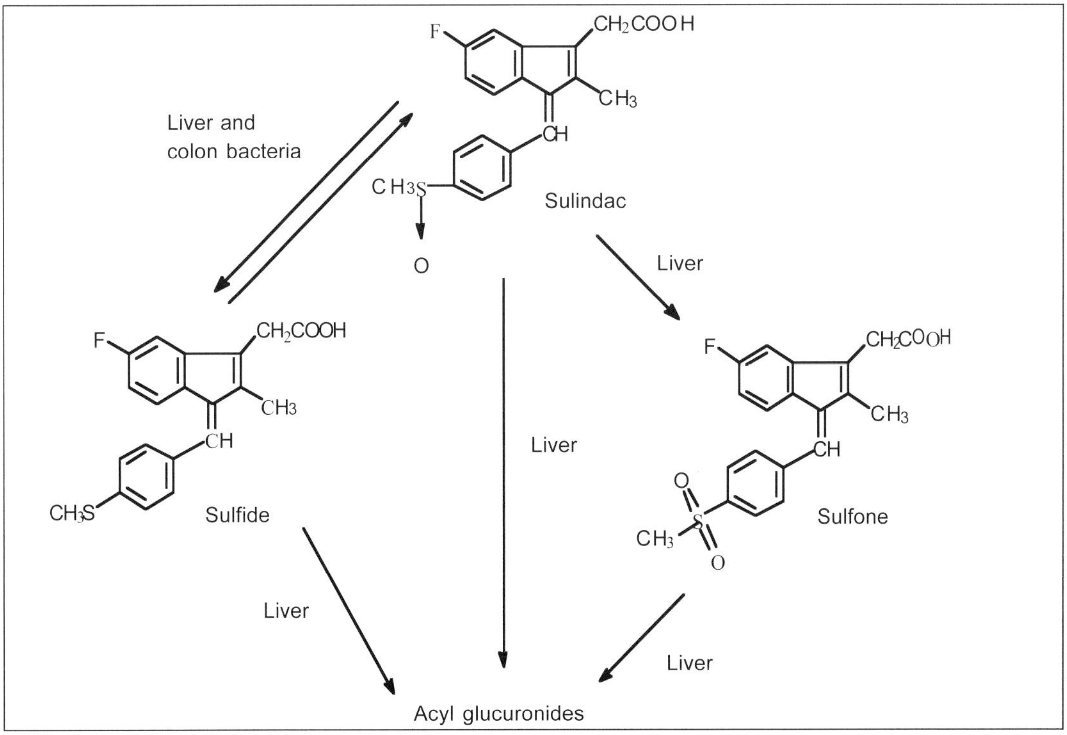

present at levels in the following order: plasma > liver > stomach > kidney > small intestine. The values increased after 4 h in stomach (37 µg/g), small intestine (17 µg/g) and large intestine (7.2 µg/g) but declined in all other tissues. In rats, 86% of the dose was recovered in bile 24 h after an intravenous dose of 10 mg/kg, whereas 53% was recovered after an equivalent oral dose. Bile collected from a dog given 10 mg/kg intravenously contained 93% of the dose. Administration of a large oral dose (100 mg/kg bw) to rats did not appreciably alter the excretion pattern. In rats, placental transfer is quite low. The concentrations of sulindac and the sulfide and sulfone metabolites found in rat milk were 10–20% of plasma levels.

Sulindac can be reduced to the sulfide by rat liver or kidney homogenates and by rat faecal contents (Lee & Renwick, 1995a,b).

3.3 Genetic variation
No data were available to the Working Group.

4. Cancer-preventive Effects

4.1 Human studies
4.1.1 Studies of adenomatous polyps in patients with familial adenomatous polyposis
The relationship between familial adenomatous polyposis (FAP) and colorectal cancer is discussed in the General Remarks.

(a) Non-randomized intervention studies
Thirteen non-randomized case series comprising a total of 128 patients with FAP have been studied to examine the efficacy of sulindac in preventing or inhibiting adenomatous polyps (Waddell & Loughry, 1983; Gonzaga et al., 1985; Waddell et al., 1989; Charneau et al., 1990; Friend, 1990; Rigau et al., 1991; Tonelli & Valanzano, 1993; Winde et al., 1993; Mäkelä & Laitinen, 1994; Spagnesi et al., 1994; Cerdán et al., 1995; Kadmon et al., 1995; Winde et al., 1995). Sulindac at doses of 100–400 mg daily, maintained for up to four years, results in a reduction in the number and size of colorectal polyps in comparison with those before treatment, regression of some adenomatous polpys on endoscopy and regression of some extra-colonic desmoid tumours. (Desmoid tumours are histologically benign, extracolonic, connective tissue tumours that affect FAP patients.) When treatment with sulindac was stopped, the polyps reappeared; when treatment was resumed, the polyps regressed again (Charneau et al., 1990; Labayle et al., 1991; Rigau et al., 1991; Mäkelä & Laitinen, 1994). In studies to establish optimal doses, in which sulindac was administered in rectal suppositories, sustained treatment with doses as low as 50 mg/day maintained polyp suppression in many patients. The maintenance of treatment with sulindac appeared to be more important for polyp inhibition than did the amount taken daily (Winde et al., 1993, 1995, 1997). Carcinoma of the rectum was, however, reported in three patients with FAP during sulindac therapy in whom regression of polyps had been observed (Niv & Fraser, 1994; Thorson et al., 1994; Lynch et al., 1995).

(b) Randomized trials
Three small randomized clinical trials have confirmed that sulindac reduces the number and size of colorectal polyps in patients with FAP (Table 1).

Labayle et al. (1991) conducted a randomized, placebo-controlled, double-blind cross-over study of 10 patients with FAP and rectal polyps, previously treated by colectomy and ileorectal anastamosis. One patient was excluded from treatment because of noncompliance. Nine patients received either sulindac, 300 mg/day (100 mg three times per day), or placebo during two four-month periods separated by one month. During sulindac treatment, the rectal polyps regressed completely in six patients and almost completely in three. During placebo treatment, the polyps increased in size in five patients, remained unchanged in two and decreased in two. The difference between the groups given sulindac and placebo was statistically significant ($p < 0.01$).

Giardiello et al. (1993) conducted a randomized, double-blind, placebo-controlled trial of 22 patients with FAP, including 18 who had not undergone colectomy. The patients received either sulindac at 300 mg/day (150 mg twice a day) or placebo for nine months and were evaluated by flexible sigmoidoscopy for the number and size of polyps every three months for one year. When sulindac treatment was stopped at nine months, the mean number of polyps had decreased to 44% of the original number (p = 0.014) and the diameter of the polyps to 35% of the original value (p < 0.001). No patient had complete resolution of polyps. Three months after treatment with sulindac was stopped, both the number and the size of the polyps in the sulindac-treated patients had increased, but the values remained significantly lower than the original ones.

Nugent et al. (1993) described a randomized, placebo-controlled trial of 24 patients with FAP, all of whom had duodenal polyps, and 14 with rectal polyps. Patients were randomized to sulindac at 400 mg/day (200 mg twice daily) or placebo for six months. Treatment was associated with a reduction in epithelial-cell proliferation, as measured by 5-bromo-2-deoxyuridine in the duodenum (median labelling index, 15.8 or 14.4%; p = 0.003) and some regression of duodenal polyps (p = 0.12). In the rectum, a larger reduction in cell proliferation (median labelling index, 8.5 vs. 7.4; p = 0.018) and a greater reduction in rectal polyps were seen. Debinski et al. (1995) later clarified that this trial showed a significant reduction in small (< 2 mm) duodenal polyps in the group given sulindac (9/11) versus the placebo group (4/12) but no reduction in

polyps ≥ 3 mm. [The Working Group noted that duodenal polyps in FAP patients may not be relevant to the situation of sporadic polyps and colon cancer, that cell proliferation in the duodenum may be less relevant to cancer than is proliferation in the colon or rectum and that the number of patients was not clearly stated for all end-points.]

(c)   Studies of biomarkers
Spagnesi et al. (1994) studied 20 FAP patients (six with ileorectal anastomoses and 14 with an intact colon) and examined three end-points: cell proliferation (by thymidine labelling), labelled cell distribution along the crypts and number of polyps. While administration of sulindac (100 mg twice a day for two months) induced a significant reduction in the number of polyps, there were no changes in the proliferation indices.

Winde et al. (1997) measured genetic biomarkers of epithelial proliferation in a non-randomized, dose-finding, intervention study of 38 patients with FAP. All of the patients had had a colectomy and ileoanastomosis. Twenty-eight were given sulindac by intrarectal suppository at an initial dose of 150 mg twice daily, which was reduced to a mean dose of 64 mg/day for up to four years. Ten control patients with FAP received no sulindac. The treated patients had a marked reduction in the number of rectal polyps (386 polyps in

Table 1. Published randomized clinical trials of sulindac and adenomatous polyps

Authors	Patients	Dosage	Design	Results
Labayle et al. (1991)	10 patients with FAP, colectomy and rectal polyps, France	300 mg/day or placebo, 4-month regimens, alternating	Randomized double-blind, cross-over	Polyps regressed completely in 6 patients, partly in 3 during sulindac treatment
Giardiello et al. (1993)	22 patients with FAP (18 without colectomy), USA	300 mg/day or placebo x 9 months	Randomized double-blind	Sulindac decreased number of polys by 56% (p = 0.014) and size by 65% (p < 0.001), in comparison with baseline
Nugent et al. (1993); Debinski et al. (1995)	24 patients with FAP and duodenal polyps, USA	400 mg/day or placebo x 6 months	Randomized double-blind	Duodenal polys < 2 mm regressed in 9 of 11 patients on sulindac vs 4 of 12 on placebo. No change in larger (≥ 3 mm) polyps

FAP, familial adenomatous polyposis

28 people originally; no polyps in 24 people treated for 11 months or longer). Mutant *ras* oncogene expression became undetectable after sulindac treatment for ≥ 6 months. The proliferative index was significantly (20%) lower in patients treated with sulindac for one year than at baseline. A significant decrease in the frequency of wild and mutant *p53* was seen only when antibodies with broad specificity were used but not with those more specific to mutant *p53*. Immunohistochemical overexpression of the apoptosis-blocking protein BCL-2 was correlated inversely to mutant p53 staining in adenomatous tissue.

4.1.2 Randomized clinical trial of sporadic adenomatous polyps

Ladenheim *et al.* (1995) randomized 44 adults to either sulindac (150 mg twice a day for four months) or placebo to assess the effect on regression of sporadic polyps that were originally < 1 cm. The patients were selected from 162 asymptomatic people aged ≥ 50, who were screened by flexible sigmoidoscopy at three hospitals. People with adenomatous polyps > 1 cm or contraindications to taking NSAIDs were excluded. Treatment of four of the 22 patients given sulindac was stopped because of side-effects (anaemia in two patients, heartburn in one) or complications (urogenital sepsis in one patient), thought to be unrelated to treatment. No significant difference in the number or the mean size of polyps was seen among the sulindac-treated patients. Five polyps in patients given sulindac had disappeared in comparison with three in the group given placebo; nine adenomas remained in the group given sulindac and 12 in controls. [The Working Group noted the low statistical power of the study.]

4.1.3 Case studies of treatment for desmoid tumours

Regression of desmoid tumours during treatment with sulindac has been reported in some studies (Belliveau & Graham, 1984; Waddell & Kirsch, 1991; Kadmon *et al.*, 1995; Izes *et al.*, 1996) but not in all (Klein *et al.*, 1987).

4.2 Experimental models

4.2.1 Experimental animals

(a) Colon
Short-term studies. Groups of 14 male Fischer 344 rats, seven weeks of age, were fed AIN-76A diets containing sulindac at concentrations of 0, 200 or 400 µg/g diet [0, 200 or 400 ppm]. After seven days of feeding sulindac, all rats were given weekly subcutaneous injections of 15 mg/kg bw azoxymethane for two weeks. Formation of aberrant colonic foci was determined eight weeks after the second weekly treatment. The numbers of foci per colon were 181 in controls, 118 in rats at 200 ppm (7.7% inhibition) and 81 in those at 400 ppm (37% inhibition; $p < 0.05$) (Pereira *et al.*, 1994). In a similar study, dietary administration of sulindac at 320 ppm in the diet suppressed the number of foci per colon by 59% ($p < 0.05$) (Reddy *et al.*, 1996).

Long-term studies. These studies are summarized in Table 2.

Two groups of 48 female Balb/c mice, six to eight weeks of age, were injected subcutaneously with 25 mg/kg bw 1,2-dimethylhydrazine dissolved in 0.4% ethylenediamine tetraacetic acid in normal saline, pH 6.5, once weekly with or without sulindac for up to 25 weeks. Sulindac [purity unspecified] was administered in drinking-water at a concentration [unspecified] such that each animal received about 5 mg/kg bw per day. In a second experiment, 48 female Balb/c mice were treated with 1,2-dimethylhydrazine for 17 weeks and then randomized to control (22 rats) or sulindac (23 rats). The control group received water. Those given sulindac received a solution in drinking-water for up to 11 weeks, as described above. Body weights were not given.

In the first study, which was designed to investigate the efficacy of sulindac administered simultaneously with 1,2-dimethylhydrazine, 38 animals in each group survived until the end of the study. Of the tumours observed macroscopically, 96% were adenomas and the rest were adenocarcinomas. Microadenomas developed in 92% of control animals and 47% of those given sulindac

($p < 0.0001$), and colon tumours developed in 89% (34/38) of control animals and 42% (16/38) treated with sulindac (odds ratio, 12; 95% CI, 3.5–40). The overall colon tumour burden, the number of tumours per mouse and the number of tumours per tumour-bearing mouse were significantly reduced in the group given sulindac as compared with the control group ($p < 0.022$–0.0001). In the second study, in which sulindac was administered after the carcinogen, it did not inhibit colon carcinogenesis (numbers of animals with tumours, 17/18 and 18/18) (Moorghen et al., 1988).

A group of 18 male Sprague-Dawley rats, weighing 400–500 g (age unspecified), was given 1,2-dimethylhydrazine dihydrochloride subcutaneously at a dose of 20 mg/kg bw once weekly (equivalent to 10 mg/kg bw 1,2-dimethylhydrazine) for 20 weeks. The site and diameter of each colon tumour were determined by laporotomy and colonoscopy. The rats were then randomized into two groups, receiving either 10 mg/kg bw sulindac (eight rats) or the vehicle, 0.5% methylcellulose (10 rats), twice daily by intragastric administration for four weeks. The animals given sulindac developed no additional tumours, whereas the controls had 13 additional colon tumours. Furthermore, the mean size of the 14 tumours in animals treated with sulindac was significantly smaller (9.3 mm) than that of the 39 tumours in the controls (57 mm; $p = 0.026$). In this model system, predominantly carcinomas were induced (Skinner et al., 1991).

Groups of 30 male Fischer 344 rats (age unspecified) were given subcutaneous injections of 15 mg/kg bw azoxymethane once weekly for two weeks. Two weeks after the second injection, 30 animals were fed AIN-76A diet containing 0.04% [400 ppm] sulindac for 31 weeks. These animals showed a 27% reduction in the number of colon tumours per rat in comparison with controls (Alberts et al., 1995). [The Working Group noted that the actual numbers of colon tumours were not given and statistical significance was not reported.]

In a preliminary study, the MTD of sulindac in male Fischer 344 rats was shown to be about 400 ppm. In a preclinical efficacy study, groups of 36 male Fischer 344 rats, five weeks of age,

were fed AIN-76A diet containing 0, 160 or 320 ppm sulindac (purity, > 98%). At seven weeks of age, all animals were given two weekly subcutaneous injections of 15 mg/kg bw azoxymethane per week. Animals intended for studying the post-initiation effects of sulindac were given the compound in the diet at 320 ppm, starting 14 weeks after the second azoxymethane injection. Treatment was continued in all groups until termination of the study 52 weeks after azoxymethane treatment. All of the colonic tumours were evaluated histopathologically. No differences in body weight were seen among the groups. Inhibition of the incidence (percentage of animals with tumours) and multiplicity (tumours per animal) of invasive and non-invasive adenocarcinomas of the colon in rats during the initiation and post-initiation phases was seen to be dose-dependent ($p < 0.001$–0.0001). Furthermore, administration of sulindac post-initiation significantly suppressed the incidence ($p < 0.0001$) and multiplicity ($p < 0.0001$) of colon adenocarcinomas (see Table 2). Oral administration of sulindac also reduced the colon tumour volume by more than 52% ($p < 0.01$) (Rao et al., 1995).

Genetically altered mice. Sulindac has been tested in the Min/+ mouse model, which is described in the General Remarks. These studies are summarized in Table 2.

Groups of 10 female C57Bl/6J-Min/+ mice, five to six weeks of age, were fed AIN-76A diet and given sulindac at 160 mg/ml [160 ppm] in the drinking-water (estimated to provide 0.5 mg/animal per day). Control animals were given the diet alone. No differences in body weights or food intake were seen among the study groups. All animals were killed at 110 days of age. Multiple intestinal tumours were seen in all control animals, whereas only one mouse treated with sulindac had an adenoma of the colon. The control Min/+ mice had 12 intestinal tumours per mouse, and those given sulindac had 0.1 tumour/mouse ($p < 0.001$). Ninety percent of the tumours were located in the ileum and jejunum (Boolbol et al., 1996).

In another study, groups of 32–36 male and female Min/+ mice, 28 days of age, were given

Table 2. Chemopreventive activity of sulindac against tumourigenesis in the colon and small intestine of experimental animals

Site	Strain, species, sex and basal diet	Carcinogen, doses, route of administration	Sulindac dose, route and duration of administration	Tumour incidence (% animals with tumours)		Tumour multiplicity (tumours/animals)		Reference
				Control	Sulindac	Control	Sulindac	
Colon	Mice, Balb/c, female, standard chow	DMH, s.c., 25 mg/kg bw once weekly for 25 weeks	5 mg/kg bw, daily in drinking-water during and after carcinogen treatment	89	42 $p < 0.05$	NR	NR	Moorghen et al. (1988)
Colon	Mice, Balb/c, female, standard chow	DMH, s.c., 25 mg/kg bw, once weekly for 17 weeks	5 mg/kg bw, daily in drinking-water during and after carcinogen treatment	94	100 $p > 0.05$	NR	NR	Moorghen et al. (1988)
Colon	Rats, Sprague-Dawley, male, standard chow	DMH, s.c., 10 mg/kg bw, once weekly for 20 weeks	10 mg/kg bw, daily by gavage for 4 weeks after carcinogen treatment	100	100 $p > 0.05$	39	14 $p < 0.012$	Skinner et al. (1991)
Colon	Rats, F344, male, AIN-76A diet	AOM, 15 mg/kg bw, once weekly for 2 weeks	0.4 mg/g diet, daily two weeks after carcinogen treatment	Reduced to 39% of control		Reduced to 27% of control		Alberts et al. (1995)
Colon	Rats, F344, male, AIN-76A diet	AOM, 15 mg/kg bw, once weekly for 2 weeks	0.16 mg/g diet, daily one week before, during and after carcinogen treatment	81	42 $p < 0.01$	1.5	0.68 $p < 0.001$	Rao et al. (1995)
Colon	Rats, F344, male, AIN-76A diet	AOM, 15 mg/kg bw, once weekly for 2 weeks	0.16 mg/g diet, daily one week before, during and after carcinogen treatment	81	55 $p < 0.001$	1.5	0.44 $p < 0.001$	Rao et al. (1995)
Colon	Rats, F344, male, AIN-76A diet	AOM, 15 mg/kg bw, once weekly for 2 weeks	0.32 mg/g diet, beginning 14 weeks after carcinogen treatment	81	68 $p < 0.0001$	1.5	0.29 $p < 0.0001$	Rao et al.(1995)

Table 2 (contd)

Site	Strain, species, sex, and basal diet	Carcinogen, doses, route of administration	Sulindac dose, route and duration of administration	Tumour incidence (% animals with tumours)		Tumour multiplicity (tumours/animals)		Reference
				Control	Sulindac	Control	Sulindac	
Small intestine	Mice, C57Bl/6J-Min, female, AIN-76A diet	No treatment	0.5 mg/mouse per day in drinking-water daily	100	10	12	0.1 $p < 0.001$	Boolbol et al. (1996)
Small intestine	Mice, C57Bl/6J-Min, male, AIN-76A diet	No treatment	21 mg/l in drinking-water daily	100	100	49	52 $p < 0.05$	Beazer-Barclay et al. (1996)
Small intestine	Mice, C57Bl/6J-Min, male, AIN-76A diet	No treatment	84 mg/l in drinking-water daily	100	100	49	30 $p < 0.001$	Beazer-Barclay et al. (1996)
Small intestine	Mice, C57Bl/6J-Min, male, AIN-76A diet	No treatment	0.17 mg/g diet daily	100	100	33	12 $p < 0.0001$	Beazer-Barclay et al. (1996)
Small intestine	Mice, C57Bl/6J-Min, male, AIN-76A diet	No treatment	0.33 mg/g diet daily	100	100	33	9.8 $p < 0.00001$	Beazer-Barclay et al. (1996)

NR

DMH, 1,2-dimethylhydrazine; s.c., subcutaneous; bw, body weight; NR, not reported; AOM, azoxymethane sulindac in the drinking-water at 21 or 84 mg/litre [5 and 20 mg/kg bw per day] or in AIN-76A diet at 167 or 334 µg/g [40 and 80 mg/kg bw per day] for about 50 days. Administration of sulindac had no effect on body-weight gains, but the numbers of intestinal tumours were significantly suppressed by treatment with sulindac in drinking-water at 84 mg/litre or in the diet at either dose (Beazer-Barclay *et al.*, 1996).

(b)   Mammary gland
These studies are summarized in Table 3.

Groups of 30 female Sprague-Dawley rats, 50 days old, were given a single intraperitoneal injection of N-methyl-N-nitrosourea at 50 mg/kg bw and fed AIN-76A diet containing 0 or 0.06% [600 ppm] sulindac [purity unspecified] beginning seven days after the carcinogen treatment. Sulindac had no effect on body-weight gain. After 24 weeks of treatment with sulindac, all mammary tumours were examined histopathologically. The tumour incidence was not significantly different in the controls (93%; 28/30) and those treated with sulindac (87%; 26/30) groups; however, the tumour multiplicity and burden were significantly inhibited in animals fed sulindac as compared with those fed the control diet ($p < 0.05$). The mean numbers of mammary tumours (± SE) were 4.2 ± 0.5 in the control group and 2.7 ± 0.4 in the sulindac-treated group; the tumour burdens in grams ± SE were 15.8 ± 2.5 in the control group and 5.7 ± 1.8 in the sulindac-treated group. Mammary tumour latency was longer in the rats given sulindac than in controls ($p < 0.02$) (Thompson *et al.*, 1995).

Female Sprague-Dawley rats, 50 days of age, were injected with either 12.5 or 37.5 mg/kg bw N-methyl-N-nitrosourea to induce mammary tumours. Seven days later, the metabolite of sulindac, sulindac sulfone, was incorporated into AIN-76A diet at a concentration of 0.03 or 0.06% (w/w) [300 or 600 ppm]. Thirty rats were assigned to each dietary group treated with the high dose of carcinogen and 44 rats to each group treated with the low dose. Sulindac sulfone significantly reduced the incidence and the number of tumours per rat, irrespective of the dose of carcinogen injected. Its preventive activity was comparable to that of sulindac. Tumour latency was prolonged significantly by sulindac sulfone, particularly at the low dose of carcinogen, when it was prolonged by more than eight weeks (Thompson *et al.*, 1997).

(c)   Oesophagus
This study is summarized in Table 3. Groups of 15 male Fischer 344 rats [age unspecified] received three subcutaneous injections of 1 mg/kg bw N-nitrosomethylbenzylamine per week for five weeks. Two weeks before the start of this treatment, 15 rats received sulindac (purity, > 99%) in the diet at a concentration of 125 mg/g [125 ppm]; another group received sulindac one week after completion of carcinogen treatment, up to 25 weeks. There were no differences in mean body weights among the groups. The oesophageal tumours observed in this study were primarily exophytic, pedunculated lesions which proved to be squamous-cell papillomas. Neither the tumour incidence (100, 93 and 93%) nor the tumour multiplicity (2.9, 2.3 and 2.3 tumours/rat) was significantly inhibited when sulindac was administered before and during or after carcinogen treatment, respectively (Siglin et al., 1995). [The Working Group noted that the tumour yield induced by N-nitrosomethylbenzylamine was high and that the dose of sulindac may have been insufficient to inhibit these oesophageal tumours.]

(d)   Urinary bladder
This study is summarized in Table 3. Groups of 75 male B6D2F1 mice, five to six weeks of age, received sulindac in the diet a doses of 200 or 400 mg/g [200 and 400 ppm] one week before the first of eight weekly oral doses of 7.5 mg N-nitroso(4-hydroxybutyl)amine in ethanol:water. The study was terminated 24 weeks after administration of the carcinogen. The survival of animals at termination ranged from 93 to 100% in both groups, and administration of sulindac had a minimal effect on terminal body weights. Sulindac induced a dose-related decrease in the incidence of nitrosamine-induced urinary bladder cancer: control, 20/74 (27%); 200 ppm sulindac, 6/73 (8.2%); and 400 ppm sulindac, 2/75 (2.7%). There was no significant difference

Table 3. Chemopreventive activity of sulindac against carcinogenesis in other organs of experimental animals

Site	Strain, species, sex and basal diet	Carcinogen, doses, route of administration	Sulindac, dose, route and duration of administration	Tumour incidence (% animals with tumours)		Tumour multiplicity (tumours/animal)		Reference
				Control	Sulindac	Control	Sulindac	
Mammary gland	Rats, Sprague-Dawley, female, AIN076A diet	MNU, i.p., 50 mg/kg bw, single dose	600 ppm in diet for 24 weeks	93	87	4.2	2.7 $p < 0.05$	Thompson et al. (1995)
Mammary gland	Rats, Sprague-Dawley, female, AIN 76A diet	MNU, i.p., 12.5 mg/kg bw, single dose	Sulindac sulfone, 300 ppm diet 1 week after carcinogen treatment	100	39 $p < 0.05$	16	9 $p < 0.05$	Thompson et al. (1997)
Mammary gland			600 ppm in diet 1 week after carcinogen treatment	100	55 $p < 0.05$	16	8 $p < 0.05$	Thompson et al. (1997)
Mammary gland	Rats, Sprague-Dawley, female, AIN 76A diet	MNU, i.p., 37.5 mg/kg bw, single dose	300 ppm diet, 1 week after carcinogen treatment	100	100	126	103	Thompson et al. (1997)
			600 ppm in diet, 1 week after carcinogen treatment	100	100	126	68 $p < 0.005$	
Oesophagus	Rats, F344, male, AIN-76A diet	NMBzA, s.c., 1.0 mg/kg bw, 3 doses/week for 5 weeks	125 ppm diet before, during and after carcinogen for 25 weeks	100	93	2.9	2.3	Siglin et al. (1995)
Urinary bladder	Mice, B6D2F1, AIN-76A diet	OH-BBN, oral, 7.5 mg/week for 8 weeks	200 ppm diet for 24 weeks	27	8.2 $p < 0.01$	NR	NR	Rao et al. (1996)
			400 ppm diet for 24 weeks	27	2.7 $p < 0.01$	NR	NR	
Lung	Mice, A/J AIN-76A diet	NNK, 9.1 mg/mouse, in drinking-water for 7 weeks	130 ppm diet for 2 weeks before carcinogen and until termination at 16 weeks	100	92	15.7	7.4 $p < 0.01$	Castonguay et al. (1991); Pepin et al. (1992)
Lung	Mice, A/J, AIN-76A diet	NNK, 9.1 mg/animal in drinking-water for 7 weeks	123 ppm diet −2 → 23 weeks	100	100	8.44	4.12 $p < 0.001$	Jalbert & Castonguay (1992)
			−2 → 7 weeks	100	100	8.44	6.04 $p < 0.05$	
			+7 → 23 weeks	100	100	8.44	7.41 $p > 0.05$	

MNU, N-methyl-N-nitrosourea; i.p., intraperitoneal; bw, body weight; NMBzA, N-nitrosomethylbenzylamine; s.c., subcutaneously; OH-BBN, N-nitrosobutyl(4-hydroxybutyl)amine; NR, not reported; NNK, 4-N-nitrosomethylamino)-1-(3-pyridyl)-1-butanone in the histopathology of the lesions, including the degree of malignancy (Rao *et al.*, 1996).

(e)   Lung
These studies are summarized in Table 3.

Groups of 23–28 female A/J mice, six to seven weeks of age, were fed sulindac (purity, 99%) at 0 or 130 mg/g diet [130 ppm]. Two weeks later, 4-(N-nitrosomethylamino)-1-(3-pyridyl)-1-butanone (NNK) (purity, 98.5%), which is present in tobacco smoke, was administered in the drinking-water for seven weeks (total dose, 9.0–9.2 mg/mouse). All animals were necropsied 16 weeks after the end of carcinogen treatment. Dietary administration of sulindac had no effect on body-weight gain or food consumption. The incidence of lung adenomas in the carcinogen-treated group was 90%, and the multiplicity was 15.7 tumours per mouse. Administration of sulindac reduced the tumour multiplicity to 7.4 tumours per mouse (53% inhibition; $p < 0.001$), without affecting tumour incidence (Castonguay *et al.*, 1991; Pepin *et al.*, 1992).

In a further study, NNK was administered by the same protocol as described above, but three groups of mice were given sulindac (123 ppm) on weeks –2 to +23, –2 to +7 or +7 to +23. Treatment with NNK alone induced 8.4 lung adenomas per mouse; the treatments with sulindac reduced the multiplicity (± SE) of lung adenomas to 4.12 ± 0.44 ($p < 0.001$), 6.04 ± 0.43 ($p < 0.05$) and 7.41 ± 0.82 ($p > 0.05$), respectively. The authors concluded that the efficacy of sulindac given during and after initiation was additive (Jalbert & Castonguay, 1992).

4.2.2 In-vitro models
No data were available to the Working Group.

4.3   Mechanisms of chemoprevention
Sulindac was the first NSAID reported to be useful for the treatment of FAP (Waddell & Loughry, 1983). Administration of sulindac to affected individuals induced polyp regression, which was reversed on cessation of treatment. These findings have been confirmed in several subsequent studies (Belliveau & Graham, 1984;

Waddell *et al.*, 1989; Labayle *et al.*, 1991; Rigau *et al.*, 1991; Giardiello *et al.*, 1993). The efficacy of sulindac may be related to its unique pharmacokinetic properties, which lead to high concentrations of its active metabolite, sulindac sulfide, in the colonic lumen (Hucker *et al.*, 1973; Duggan *et al.*, 1977; Shen & Winter, 1977).

4.3.1   Effects on cell proliferation and apoptosis
Numerous studies of the human colon cancer line HT-29 have shown that sulindac sulfide and sulfone can inhibit cell growth and stimulate apoptosis (Piazza *et al.*, 1995; Shiff *et al.*, 1995; Hanif *et al.*, 1996; Shiff *et al.*, 1996). In these studies, the cultured HT-29 cells were exposed to various concentrations of the sulindac metabolites, and several indices of growth regulation and/or apoptosis were evaluated. Both compounds inhibited cell growth and stimulated apoptosis, but in many of the studies only at concentrations in the range 0.5–1.2 mmol/litre. Therefore, the biological significance of these findings is uncertain.

Sulindac sulfone, when administered at pharmacological doses rather than the doses that result from the metabolism of sulindac, has no effect on cyclooxygenase (COX)[1] activity but inhibits cell proliferation and stimulates apoptosis (Thompson *et al.*, 1995), indicating that these effects are not related to COX activity (Shiff *et al.*, 1995; Hanif *et al.*, 1996; Schnitzler *et al.*, 1996). Another non-prostaglandin-related effect of sulindac sulfide and sulfone is to reduce the levels of cell-cycle regulatory proteins such as cdc2 (Shiff *et al.*, 1996), which may be related to the ability of these metabolites to inhibit cell proliferation.

A study of another colon cancer cell line, LIM 1215, with very sensitive polymerase chain reaction assay techniques, demonstrated that both sulindac sulfide and sulfone at doses of about 10 mmol/litre can induce the expression of *APC* mRNA (Schnitzler *et al.*, 1996). Since the *APC* gene has been shown to play a key role in colorectal carcinogenesis in both humans and

---

[1] Used as a synonym for prostaglandin endoperoxide synthase (PGH synthase)

animal models, this could have some significance; however, the investigators did not determine whether the increase in *APC* mRNA resulted in an increase in the amount of the functional APC protein. A question raised by this study is that, if the *APC* gene has already been inactivated by a mutation leading to premature chain termination, which occurs in 50% of spontaneous human colorectal adenocarcinomas, what benefit would there be in increasing the mRNA levels of this detective tumour suppressor gene?

Some NSAIDs cause apoptosis when applied to *v-src*-transformed chicken embryo fibroblasts (Lu *et al.*, 1995); however, sulindac had no effect on morphological inhibition of transformation. This study was the first to indicate that cells which overexpress *COX-2* may be somewhat resistant to programmed cell death, and that this can be reversed by addition of an NSAID.

Few nontransformed intestinal epithelial cell lines are available for in-vitro studies. Several groups have evaluated the mechanisms of growth control of a rat intestinal epithelial-1 (RIE-1) cell line in culture (DuBois *et al.*, 1995). Sulindac sulfide can inhibit mitogenesis of these cells (DuBois *et al.*, 1994a). Additionally, the cells express the inducible COX-2 enzyme after treatment with cytokines and growth factors (DuBois *et al.*, 1994b), and the increased expression of *COX-2* in these cells makes them resistant to apoptosis (Tsujii & DuBois, 1995). Treatment of the cells with relatively low doses of sulindac sulfide (5–10 mmol/litre), however, reversed these phenotypic changes, indicating that a potential mechanism for the chemopreventive effect of sulindac may be its ability to inhibit COX-2.

4.3.2   Effects on oncogene expression

See the General Remarks for a discussion of the role of the *ras* oncogene in colon cancer.

Groups of six male Fischer 344 rats were fed a diet containing 320 ppm sulindac and were given azoxymethane dissolved in normal saline subcutaneously at a dose of 15 mg/kg bw per week for two weeks. Vehicle control groups received an equal volume of normal saline. The animals were sacrificed 52 weeks after treatment and their colonic mucosa and tumours were analysed for mutations in codons 12 and 13 of *K-ras* and for expression of *ras p21*. Azoxymethane-induced G to A transitions were observed at the second nucleotide of codon 12 of *K-ras*, in which the amino acid aspartic acid replaced wild-type glycine. Sulindac not only suppressed the selective amplification of initiated cells with azoxymethane-induced mutated *K-ras* codon 12, but significantly inhibited the azoxymethane-induced expression of total and mutant *ras p21* (Singh & Reddy, 1995). The important finding of this study is that sulindac, which has been reported to induce polyp regression in patients with FAP and to inhibit carcinogen-induced colon carcinogenesis in experimental animals, significantly suppressed *ras* activation at both the DNA and protein level.

5.   Other Beneficial Effects

No data were available to the Working Group.

6.   Carcinogenicity

6.1   Humans

The Working Group was not aware of any epidemiological studies of the carcinogenicity of sulindac or its metabolites

6.2   Experimental animals

No study of adequate duration to evaluate carcinogenicity was available to the Working Group.

7. Other Toxic Effects

7.1   Adverse effects
7.1.1   Humans

See also the General Remarks and the chapter on sulindac. Relatively few studies refer specifically to the toxicity of sulindac. In many studies of the possible toxicity of NSAIDs, distinction was made only between aspirin and NSAIDs of other types. In common with other non-aspirin NSAIDs, sulindac is used at anti-inflammatory doses and inhibits COX-1 and COX-2; therefore, data on the toxicity of non-aspirin NSAIDs are relevant to the assessment of the toxicity of sulindac.

(a) Gastrointestinal tract toxicity

NSAIDs can damage the oesophagus and can exacerbate gastro-oesophageal reflux disease (Heller *et al.*, 1982; Kikendale, 1991). Gastrointestinal bleeding and ulceration are potentially serious side-effects of all NSAIDs, as discussed in the chapter on aspirin. In the meta-analysis of Henry *et al.* (1996), described in the General Remarks, the risks for serious complications in the upper gastrointestinal tract after use of sulindac were similar to those of most other NSAIDs. In a ranking analysis, sulindac ranked 7 (1 being the most and 12 the least toxic) of 12 NSAIDs analysed. The pooled estimated RRs for NSAID users in comparison with ibuprofen users were between 1.6 and 2.7. Given the baseline risk for ulcer disease, which ranges from 0.5 per 1000 per year in young adults (Garcia Rodriguez *et al.*, 1992) to 4 per 1000 in older adults (Smalley *et al.*, 1995), the rates of serious ulcer complications among sulindac users can be estimated to be about 2 per 1000 in young adults and 15 per 1000 in people over the age of 65.

NSAIDs other than aspirin have also been associated with other deleterious effects on the small intestine, including inflammation resulting in blood and protein loss (Bjarnasson *et al.*, 1987), stricture (Matsuhashi *et al.*, 1992), perforation and diarrhoea (Kwo & Tremaine, 1995). Large-bowel perforation and haemorrhage are also associated with use of non-aspirin NSAIDs (Langman *et al.*, 1985).

(b) Hepatotoxicity

Acute hepatotoxicity due to NSAIDs other than aspirin is an uncommon complication (Friis & Andreasen, 1992; Tarazi *et al.*, 1993; Rodriguez *et al.*, 1994). The incidence of acute liver injury was 3.7 per 100 000 NSAID users, or 1.1 per 100 000 NSAID prescriptions, among 625 307 persons who were prescribed any of 12 NSAIDs by a defined group of general practitioners in England between 1987 and 1991 (Rodriguez *et al.*, 1994).

(c) Nephrotoxicity

Acute renal toxicity due to NSAIDs can result from allergic interstitial nephritis, concurrent exposure to phenacetin, urate obstruction or haemodynamic alterations in patients with underlying kidney disease (Murray & Brater, 1993; Murray *et al.*, 1995).

In a study of patients with chronic glomerular disease who were treated with therapeutic doses of sulindac, no effect was found on renal blood flow, glomerular filtration rate or urinary excretion of prostaglandins (Eriksson *et al.*, 1991); however, in a study of healthy volunteers and patients with liver disease (Laffi *et al.*, 1986), sulindac was found to blunt the renal responses to intravenous furosemide (Patrono, 1986).

Many experimental studies have shown that a large proportion of patients with conditions such as congestive heart failure, dehydration and cirrhosis, which result in a dependence on prostaglandins to maintain renal perfusion, suffer a decline in renal function when exposed to specific NSAIDs (Murray & Brater, 1990; Whelton *et al.*, 1990). There is some debate over whether all NSAIDs have a similar deleterious effect and, specifically, whether sulindac is less likely to cause a deterioration in renal function (Whelton & Hamilton, 1991). It is clear, however, that all such drugs, including sulindac, can both decrease renal prostaglandin production and cause a deterioration in renal function under conditions of decreased effective circulating volume (Brater *et al.*, 1985, 1986; Kleinknecht *et al.*, 1986; Stillman & Schlesinger, 1990).

The decline in renal function is usually reversible with discontinuation of the drugs. The frequency of the effect varies with the population studied, but may reach 13% in frail, elderly patients in nursing homes (Gurwitz *et al.*, 1990) and is much less frequent in healthier populations. In the general population, hospitalizations for acute renal failure are rare. Use of non-aspirin NSAIDs increases the risk by about fourfold, from a rate among non-users of about 2 per 100 000 yearly. The increase in risk is dose-dependent and highest during the first month of use (Perez-Gutthann *et al.*, 1996).

The data on NSAIDs and chronic renal failure are sparse. Typical analgesic nephropathy is widely accepted to be caused by phenacetin (Dubach *et al.*, 1991), but there is also evidence that acetaminophen (Sandler *et al.*, 1989; Pernerger *et al.*, 1994) and NSAIDs (Adams *et al.*, 1986; Pernerger *et al.*, 1994) produce a similar type of kidney damage and/or other types of chronic renal failure.

(d)   Blood pressure

Non-aspirin NSAIDs as a group interfere with the efficacy of antihypertensive drugs (Wong *et al.*, 1986; Radack & Deck, 1987; Chrischilles & Wallace, 1993; Johnson *et al.*, 1994), raise blood pressure in hypertensive subjects (Radack & Deck, 1987; Pope *et al.*, 1993) and may result in the initiation of antihypersensitive treatment in older persons (Gurwitz *et al.*, 1994).

In a meta-analysis of 50 randomized, place-bo-controlled trials, use of NSAIDs for periods of weeks raised supine mean blood pressure by 5 mm Hg (range 1.2–8.7) (Johnson *et al.*, 1994). All NSAIDs appeared to have this effect, but the most marked increases in blood pressure were observed with piroxicam, indomethacin and ibuprofen; however, the numbers were too small to demonstrate statistically significant differences.

(e)   Reproductive and developmental effects

The reported adverse effects of NSAID treatment during pregnancy and labour include: (i) prolongation of pregnancy and labour, (ii) increased maternal blood loss associated with delivery and (iii) anaemia. Use of sulindac during the third trimester of pregnancy is contraindicated because of potential premature closure of the ductus arteriosus, pulmonary hypertension and haemostatic abnormalities causing bleeding. Reductions in fetal urine output and in the volume of amniotic fluid are other possible adverse effects of NSAID therapy (Ostensen, 1994). At least one case report has indicated that ingestion of sulindac during pregnancy can lead to toxic epidermal necrolysis in newborns (Roupe *et al.*, 1986).

7.1.2 Experimental animals

The values for the short-term TD_{50} (a comparative measure of toxicity) for intestinal ulceration and perforation in rats are 27 and 71 mg/kg bw (0.08 and 0.2 mmol/kg bw), respectively (Shen & Winter, 1977). Rats given split daily doses of 0.28 mmol/kg bw per day sulindac intragastrically for four days (17.5 times the maximum human daily dose) developed medium and severe gastrointestinal ulceration with some evidence of perforation (Venuti *et al.*, 1989). In 90-day studies, rats given a dose of 40 mg/kg bw per day had ulcerative enteritis (reviewed by Shen & Winter, 1977). Dogs showed hepatic changes at 20 mg/kg bw per day, without concomitant gastrointestinal ulceration. Microscopic examination revealed portal fibrosis, bile-duct proliferation and inflammatory cell infiltration. Monkeys also showed no gastointestinal ulceration, but they had hepatic effects similar to those seen in dogs.

Sulindac increases intestinal permeability in rats about five times less than indomethacin (Davies *et al.*, 1994), indicating that it may cause less small intestinal ulceration than indomethacin. Although the clinical literature suggests that the sulfone metabolite does not cause gastric ulcer formation, it exacerbated ulcer formation due to stress in rodents (Glavin & Sitar, 1986).

Long-term administration of sulindac at a dose of 40 mg/kg bw per day resulted in one death related to ulcer in 30 animals. No occult blood was detected in faeces at any dose, but at autopsy, on termination of the experiment, ulcerative enteritis was detected in about one-third of the rats at the highest dose. Only minor effects on liver and kidney function have been reported in rats, mice, dogs and monkeys, and only at a maximum dose of 40 mg/kg bw per day (Shen & Winter, 1977).

7.2   Genetic and related effects

No data were available to the Working Group.

8.   Summary of data

8.1   Chemistry, occurrence and human exposure

Sulindac, a non-steroidal anti-inflammatory drug introduced in the 1970s, has analgesic, anti-inflammatory and anti-pyretic properties. It has limited use. The usual dose for muscu-loskeletal and joint disorders is 100–200 mg twice daily.

8.2 Metabolism and kinetics

Therapeutic doses of sulindac are almost totally absorbed by humans after oral administration. The peak plasma concentrations of sulindac and its sulfide metabolite are achieved within a few hours. Sulindac undergoes extensive enterohepatic recyling. The primary route of excretion in humans is via the urine as both sulindac and its sulfone metabolite.

8.3 Cancer-preventive effects

8.3.1 Humans

Randomized trials have shown conclusively that daily doses of 300–400 mg sulindac reduce the number and size of adenomatous colorectal polyps in patients with familial adenomatous polyposis. One observational study suggested that suppression of adenomas can be maintained with a daily intrarectal dose of 60 mg. Tumour inhibition may be incomplete: Three patients in whom polyps were suppressed by treatment with sulindac developed carcinoma of the rectum despite continuing therapy.

One small randomized trial of sulindac with low statistical power showed no regression of small (< 1 cm) adenomatous polyps in patients without familial adenomatous polyposis. Thus, the efficacy of sulindac against sporadic polyps remains to be established.

No adequate data were available to address the effect of sulindac on the risk for colorectal cancer.

8.3.2 Experimental animals

In seven studies in mouse and rat models, sulindac administered with or subsequent to carcinogens inhibited the development of preneoplastic and neoplastic lesions in the colon. In mice predisposed to intestinal malignancy by a germ-line mutation in the *Apc* gene, sulindac reduced the incidence of spontaneous intestinal tumours.

In single studies on the effects of sulindac on urinary bladder and lung carcinogenesis in mouse models, sulindac administered during and after the carcinogen inhibited tumour development. In two studies on mammary carcinogenesis in rats, sulindac and its metabolite sulindac sulfone, given one week after carcinogen treatment, inhibited tumour development.

8.3.3 Mechanism of action

The precise mechanism for the chemopreventive action of sulindac is currently unknown. In human transformed intestinal epithelial cells in culture, doses of sulindac sulfide and sulindac sulfone higher than those that could be achieved pharmacologically inhibited cell growth and stimulated programmed cell death. In cells that overexpress the *Cox-2* gene, sulindac can reverse the tumorigenic phenotype by inhibiting *Cox-2*. Sulindac suppresses *ras* activation in colon mucosal cells of azoxymethane-treated rats.

8.4 Other beneficial effects

No data were available to the Working Group.

8.5 Carcinogenicity

No data were available to the Working Group.

8.6 Toxic effects

8.6.1 Humans

In common with other NSAIDs, sulindac increases the risk for gastrointestinal toxicity, including complications of ulcer, in a dose-dependent manner and increases the risks for toxic effects on the liver and kidney.

8.6.2 Experimental animals

Sulindac is well tolerated at high doses in rats, mice, dogs and rhesus monkeys. Minor effects occur in liver and kidney. Ulcerative enteritis is seen at very high doses in rats. The toxicity of the major human metabolites in these experimental models has not been reported.

9. Recommendations for research

Research to define the relative importance of the two metabolites, sulindac sulfide and sulindac sulfone, in the prevention of tumorigenesis in given human organs is of high priority. Better understanding of the chemopreventive action of sulindac in humans would require long-term studies of patients with familial adenomatous polyposis or large epidemiological studies in the general population.

10. Evaluation[1]

10.1 Cancer-preventive activity
10.1.1 Humans
There is *limited evidence* that sulindac has cancer-preventive activity in patients with familial adenomatous polyposis. This evaluation is based on clear demonstration of the inhibition and regression of adenomatous polyps.

There is *inadequate evidence* that sulindac has cancer-preventive activity in people without familial adenomatous polyposis.

10.1.2 Experimental animals
There is *sufficient evidence* that sulindac has cancer-preventive activity in experimental animals. This evaluation is based on models of cancers of the colon, urinary bladder, lung and mammary gland.

10.2 Overall evaluation
Randomized controlled trials in humans provide *limited evidence* that sulindac prevents colorectal cancer by suppressing adenomatous polyps in patients with familial adenomatous polyposis. There is no evidence for the prevention of cancers at other sites. Experimental animal models provide *sufficient evidence* that sulindac prevents cancers of the colon, mammary gland, lung and urinary bladder. These findings indicate the need for further evaluation of the cancer-preventive activity of sulindac against colorectal cancer in persons at high risk for the disease but are not applicable to the general population. The adverse effects of sulindac in humans comprise dose-dependent upper gastrointestinal bleeding and ulceration and hepatic and renal toxicity. If sulindac were to be used as a chemopreventive agent in large populations, the evidence of benefit would have to be clear and the benefits themselves significant.

11. References

Adams, D.H., Howie, A.J., Michael, J., McConkey, B., Bacon, P.A. & Adu, D. (1986) Non-steroidal anti-inflammatory drugs and renal failure. *Lancet*, **i**, 57–60

Alberts, D.S., Hixson, L., Ahnen, D., Bogert, C., Einspahr, J., Paranka, N., Brendel, K., Gross, P.H., Pamukcu, R. & Burt, R.W. (1995) Do NSAIDs exert their colon cancer chemoprevention activities through the inhibition of mucosal prostaglandin synthethase? *J. cell. Biochem.*, **22**, 18–23

Beazer-Barclay, Y., Levy, D.B., Moser, A.R., Dove, W.F., Hamilton, S.R., Vogelstein, B. & Kinzler, K.W. (1996) Short communication: Sulindac suppresses tumorigenesis in the min mouse. *Carcinogenesis*, **17**, 1757–1760

Belliveau, P. & Graham, A.M. (1984) Mesenteric desmoid tumor in Gardner's syndrome treated by sulindac. *Dis. Colon Rectum*, **27**, 53–54

Bjarnasson, I., Zanelli, G., Prouse, P., Smethurst, P., Smith, T., Levi, S., Gumpel, M.J. & Levi, A.J. (1987) Blood and protein loss via small-intestinal inflammation induced by non-steroidal anti-inflammatory drugs. *Lancet*, **ii**, 711–714

Boolbol, S.K., Dannenberg, A.J., Chadburn, A., Martucci, C., Guo, X.-J., Ramonetti, J.T., Abreu-Goris, M., Newmark, H.L., Lipkin, M.L., DeCosse, J.J. & Bertagnolli, M.M. (1996) Cyclooxygenase-2 overexpression and tumor formation are blocked by sulindac in a murine model of familial adenomatous polyposis. *Cancer Res.*, **56**, 2556–2560

Brater, D.C., Anderson, S., Baird, B. & Campbell, W.B. (1985) Effects of ibuprofen, naproxen and sulindac on prostaglandins in men. *Kidney Int.*, **27**, 66–73

Brater, D.C., Anderson, S.A., Brown Cartwright, D. & Toto, R.D. (1986) Effects of nonsteroidal antiinflammatory drugs on renal function in patients with renal insufficiency and in cirrhotics. *Am. J. Kidney Dis.*, **8**, 351–355

Budavari, S., ed. (1989) *The Merck Index*, Rahway, NJ, Merck & Co., p. 8964

Castonguay, A., Pepin, P. & Stoner, G.D. (1991) Lung tumorigenicity of NNK given orally to A/J mice: Its application to chemopreventive efficacy studies. *Exp. Lung Res.*, **17**, 485–499

---

[1] For definitions of the italicized terms, see the Preamble, pp. 12–13

Cerdán, F.J., Torres-Melero, J., Martínez, S., Gutiérrez del Olmo, A. & Balibrea, J.L. (1995) [Treatment with sulindac of adenomatous polyps in familial polyposis.] *Rev. esp. Enferm. Dig.*, **87**, 574–576 (in Spanish)

Charneau, J., D'Aubigny, N., Burtin, P., Person, B. & Boyer, J. (1990) [Rectal micropolyps after total colectomy for familial polyposis: Efficacity of sulindac.] *Gastroenterol. clin. biol.*, **14**, 153–157 (in French)

Chrischilles, E.A. & Wallace, R.B. (1993) Non-steroidal anti-inflammatory drugs and blood pressure in an elderly population. *J. Gerontol.*, **48**, 91–6

Davies, N.M., Wright, M.R. & Jamali, F. (1994) Antiinflammatory drug-induced small intestinal permeability: The rat is a suitable model. *Pharm. Res.*, **11**, 1652–1656

Debinski, H.S., Trojan, J., Nugent, K.P., Spigelman, A.D. & Phillips, R.K.S. (1995) Effect of sulindac on small polyps in familial adenomatous polyposis. *Lancet*, **345**, 855–856

Dubach, U.C., Rosner, B. & Sturmer, T. (1991) An epidemiological study of abuse of analgesic drugs: Effects of phenacetin and salicylate on mortality and cardiovascular morbidity. *New Engl J. Med.*, **324**, 155–160

Dubois, R.N., Awad, J., Morrow, J., Roberts, L.J. & Bishop, P.R. (1994a) Regulation of eicosanoid production and mitogenesis in rat intestinal epithelial cells by transforming growth factor α and phorbol ester. *J. clin. Invest.*, **93**, 493–498

DuBois, R.N., Bishop, P., Awad, J.A., Makita, K. & Lanhan, A. (1994b) Cloning and characterization of a growth factor-inducible cyclooxygenase gene from rat intestinal epithelial cells. *Am. J. Physiol.*, **266**, G8922–G827

Duggan, D.E., Hare, L.E., Ditzler, C.A., Lei, B.W. & Kwan, K.C. (1977) The disposition of sulindac. *Clin. Pharmacol. Ther.*, **21**, 326–335

Eriksson, L.O., Sturfelt, G., Thysell, H. & Wollheim, F.A. (1991) Effects of sulindac and naproxen on prostaglandin excretion in patients with impaired renal function and rheumatoid arthritis. *Am. J. Med.*, **89**, 313–321

Friend, W.G.. (1990) Sulindac suppression of colorectal polyps in Gardner's syndrome. *Am. Family Phys.*, **41**, 891–894

Friis, H. & Andreasen, P.B. (1992) Drug-induced hepatic injury: An analysis of 1100 cases reported to the Danish Committee on Adverse Drug Reactions between 1978 an 1987. *J. intern. Med.*, **232**, 133–138

Furst, D.E., Herman, R.A., Koehnke, R., Ericksen, N., Hash, L., Riggs, C.E., Porras, A. & Veng-Pedersen, P. (1990) Effect of aspirin and sulindac on methotrexate clearance. *J. pharm. Sci.*, **79**, 782–786

Garcia Rodriguez, L.A., Walker, A.M. & Perez Gutthann, S. (1992) Nonsteroidal antiinflammatory drugs and gastrointestinal hospitalizations in Saskatchewan: A cohort study. *Epidemiology*, **3**, 337–342

Giardiello, F.M., Hamilton, S.R., Krush, A.J., Piantadosi, S., Hylind, L.M., Celano, P., Booker, S.V., Robinson, C.R. & Offerhaus, G.J.A. (1993) Treatment of colonic and rectal adenomas with sulindac in familial adenomatous polyposis. *New Engl. J. Med.*, **328**, 1313–1316

Glavin, G.B. & Sitar, D.S. (1986) The effects of sulindac and its metabolites on acute stress-induced gastric ulcers in rats. *Toxicol. appl. Pharmacol.*, **83**, 386–389

Gonzaga, R.A.F., Lima, F.R., Carneiro, S., Maciel, J. & Aramante, M., Jr (1985) Sulindac treatment for familial polyposis coli (Letter to the Editor). *Lancet*, **i**, 751

Griffin, M.R., Piper, J.M., Dougherty, J.R., Snowden, W. & Ray, W.A. (1991) Non-steroidal anti-inflammatory drug use and increased risk for peptic ulcer disease in elderly persons. *Ann. intern. Med.*, **114**, 257–263

Gurwitz, J.H., Avorn, J., Ross Degnan, D. & Lipsitz, L.A. (1990) Nonsteroidal anti-inflammatory drug associated azotemia in the very old. *J. Am. med. Assoc.*, **264**, 471–475

Gurwitz, J.H., Avorn, J., Bohn, R.L., Glynn, R.J., Monane, M. & Mogun, H. (1994) Initiation of antihypertensive treatment during nonsteroidal anti-inflammatory drug therapy. *J. Am. med. Assoc.*, **272**, 781–786

Hanif, R., Pittas, A., Feng, Y., Koutsos, M.I., Quao, L., Staiano-Coico, L., Shiff, S.I. & Rigas, B. (1996) Effects of nonsteroidal anti-inflammatory drugs on proliferation and on induction of apoptosis in colon cancer cells by a prostaglandin-independent pathway. *Biochem. Pharmacol.*, **52**, 237–245

Hare, L.E., Ditzler, C.A., Hichens, M., Rosegay, A. & Duggan D.E. (1977) Analysis of sulindac and metabolites by combined isotope dilution—radioimmunoassay. *J. pharm. Sci.*, **66**, 414–417

Heller, S.R., Fellow, I.W & Ogilvie, A.L. (1982) Non-steroidal anti-inflammatory drugs and benign oesophageal stricture. *Br. med. J.*, **285**, 167–168

Henry, D., Lim, L.L., Garcia Rodriguez, L.A., Perez Gutthann, S., Carson, J.L., Griffin, M., Savage, R., Logan, R., Moride, Y., Hawkey, C., Hill, S.L. & Fries, J.T. (1996) Variability in risk of gastrointestinal complications with individual non-steroidal anti-inflammatory drugs. Results of a collaborative meta-analysis. *Br. med. J.*, **312**, 1563–1566

Hucker, H.B., Stauffer, S.C., White, S.D., Rhodes, R.E., Arison, B.H., Umbenhauer, E.R., Bower, R.J. & McMahon, F.G. (1973) Physiologic disposition and metabolic fate of a new anti-inflammatory agent, cis-5-fluoro-2-methyl-1-[p-(methylsulfinyl)-benzylidenyl]indeno-3-acetic acid in the rat, dog, rhesus monkey, and man. *Drug Metab. Disposition*, **1**, 721–736

Izes, J.K., Zinman, L.N. & Larsen, C.R. (1996) Regression of large pelvic desmoid tumor by tamoxifen and sulindac. *Urology*, **47**, 756–759

Jalbert, G. & Castonguay, A. (1992) Effects of NSAIDs on NNK-induced pulmonary and gastric tumorigenesis in A/J mice. *Cancer Lett.*, **66**, 21–28

Johnson, A.G., Nguyen, T.V. & Day, R.O. (1994) Do nonsteroidal anti-inflammatory drugs affect blood pressure? A meta-analysis. *Ann. intern. Med.*, **121**, 289–300

Jones, R.H. & Tait, C.L. (1995) Gastrointestinal side-effects of NSAIDs in the community. *Br J. clin. Pract.*, **49**, 67–70

Kadmon, M., Möslein, G., Buhr, H.J. & Herfarth, C. (1995) [Desmoids in patients with familial polyposis (FAP).] *Klin. ther. Beobachtung. Heidelberger Polyposis-Reg. Chirurg.*, **66**, 997–1005 (in German)

Kikendale, J.W. (1991) Pill-induced oesophageal injury. *Gastroenterol. Clin. North Am.*, **20**, 835–846

Klein, W.A., Miller, H.H., Anderson, M. & DeCosse, J.J. (1987) The use of indomethacin, sulindac, and tamoxifen for the treatment of desmoid tumors associated with familial polyposis. *Cancer*, **60**, 2863–2868

Kleinknecht. D., Landais, P. & Goldfarb, B. (1986) Analgesic and non-steroidal anti-inflammatory drug associated acute renal failure: A prospective collaborative study. *Clin. Nephrol.*, **25**, 275–281

Kramer, W.B., Saade, G., Ou, C.N., Rognerud, C., Dorman, K., Mayes, M. & Moise, K.J. (1995) Placental transfer of sulindac and its active sulfide metabolite in humans. *Am. J. Obstet. Gynecol.*, **172**, 886–890

Kwo, P.Y. & Tremaine, W.J. (1995) Nonsteroidal anti-inflammatory drug-induced enteropathy: Case discussion and review of the literature. *Mayo Clin. Proc.*, **70**, 55–61

Labayle, D., Fischer, D., Vielh, P., Drouhin, F., Pariente, A., Bories, C., Duhamel, O., Trousset, M. & Attali, P. (1991) Sulindac causes regression of rectal polyps in familial adenomatous polyposis. *Gastroenterology*, **101**, 635–639

Ladenheim, J., Garcia, G., Titzer, D., Herzenberg, H., Lavori, P., Edson, R. & Omary, M.B. (1995) Effect of sulindac on sporadic colonic polyps. *Gastroenterology*, **108**, 1083–1087

Laffi, G., Daskalopoulos, G., Kronborg, I., Hsueh, W., Gentilini, P. & Zipser, R.D. (1986) Effects of sulindac and ibuprofen in patients with cirrhosis and ascites. An explanation for the renal-sparing effect of sulindac. *Gastroenterology*, **90**, 182–187

Langman, M.J., Morgan, L. & Worrall, A. (1985) Use of anti-inflammatory drugs by patients admitted with small or large bowel perforations and haemorrhage. *Br med. J.*, **290**, 347–349

Lee, S.C. & Renwick, A.G. (1995a) Sulphoxide reduction by rat intestinal flora and by *Escherichia coli in vitro*. *Biochem. Pharmacol.*, **49**, 1567–1576

Lee, S.C. & Renwick, A.G. (1995b) Sulphoxide reduction by rat and rabbit tissues in vitro. *Biochem. Pharmacol.*, **49**, 1557–1565

Lu, X., Xie, W., Reed, D., Bradshaw, W.S. & Simmons, D.L. (1995) Nonsteroidal anti-inflammatory drugs cause apoptosis and induce cyclooxygenase in chicken embryo fibroblasts. *Proc. natl Acad. Sci. USA*, **92**, 7961–7965

Lynch, H.T., Thorson, A.G. & Smyrk, T. (1995) Rectal cancer after prolonged sulindac chemoprevention. A case report. *Cancer*, **75**, 936–938

Mäkelä, J.T. & Laitinen, S. (1994) Sulindac therapy for familial adenomatous polyposis after colectomy and ileorectal anastomosis. *Ann. chir. gynaecol.*, **83**, 265–267

Matsuhashi, N., Yamada, A., Hiraishi, M., Konishi, T., Minota, S., Saito, T., Sugano, K., Yazaki, Y., Mori, M. & Shiga, J. (1992) Multiple strictures of the small intestine after long-term nonsteroidal anti-inflammatory drug therapy. *Am. J. Gastroenterol.*, **87**, 1183–1186

McManus, P., Primrose, JG., Henry, D.A., Birkett, D.J., Lindner, J. & Day, R.O. (1996) Pattern of non-steroidal anti-inflammatory drug use in Australia 1990–1994. A report from the Drug Utilization Sub-committee of Pharmaceutical Benefits Advisory Committee. *Med. J. Aust.*, **164**, 589–592

Miller, M.J., Bednar, M.M. & McGiff, J.C. (1984) Renal metabolism of sulindac: Functional implications. *J. Pharmacol. exp. Ther.*, **231**, 449–456

Moorghen, M., Ince, P., Finney, K.J., Sunter, J.P., Appleton, D.R. & Watson, A.J. (1988) A protective effect of sulindac against chemically-induced primary colonic tumours in mice. *J. Pathol.*, **156**, 341–347

Murray, M.D. & Brater, D.C. (1990) Adverse effects of nonsteroidal anti-inflammatory drugs on renal function. *Ann. intern. Med.*, **112**, 559–560

Murray, M.D. & Brater, D.C. (1993) Renal toxicity of the nonsteroidal anti-inflammatory drugs. *Ann. Rev. Pharmacol. Toxicol.*, **33**, 435–465

Murray, M.D., Black, P.K., Kuzmik, D.D., Haag, K.M., Manatunga, A.K., Mullin, M.A., Hall, S.D. & Brater, D.C. (1995) Acute and chronic effects of nonsteroidal antiinflammatory drugs on glomerular filtration rate in elderly patients. *Am. J. med. Sci.*, **310**, 188–197

Niv, Y. & Fraser, G.M. (1994) Adenocarcinoma in the rectal segment in familial polyposis coli is not prevented by sulindac therapy. *Gastroenterology*, **107**, 854–857

Nugent, K.P., Farmer, K.C.R., Spigelman, A.D., Williams, C.B. & Phillips, R.K.S. (1993) Randomized controlled trial of the effect of sulindac on duodenal and rectal polyposis and cell proliferation in patients with familial adenomatous polyposis. *Br. J. Surg.*, **80**, 1618–1619

Ostensen, M. (1994) Optimisation of anti-rheumatic drug treatment in pregnancy. *Clin. Pharmacokinet.*, **27**, 486–503

Patrono, C. (1986) Inhibition of renal prostaglandin synthesis in man: Methodological and clinical implications. *Scand. J. Rheumatol.*, **Suppl. 62**, 14–25

Pepin, P., Bouchard, L., Nicole, P. & Castonguay, A. (1992) Effects of sulindac and oltipraz on the tumorigenicity of 4-(methylnitrosamino)-1-(3-pyridyl)-1-butanone in A/J mouse lung. *Carcinogenesis*, **13**, 341–348

Pereira, M.A., Barnes, L.H., Rassman, V.L., Kelloff, G.V. & Steele, V.E. (1994) Use of azoxymethane-induced foci of aberrant crypts in rat colon to identify potential cancer chemopreventive agents. *Carcinogenesis*, **15**, 1049–1054

Perez-Gutthann, S., Garcia Rodriguez, L.A., Raiford, D.S., Duque-Oliart, A. & Ris-Romeu, J. (1996) Nonsteroidal anti-inflammatory drugs and the risk of hospitalization for acute renal failure. *Arch. intern. Med.*, **156**, 2433–2439

Pernerger, T.V., Whelton, P.K. & Klag, M.J. (1994) Risk of kidney failure associated with the use of acetaminophen, aspirin and nonsteroidal antiinflammatory drugs. *New Engl. J. Med.*, **331**, 1675–1679

Piazza, G.A., Rahm, A.L., Krutzsch, M., Sperl, G., Paranka, N.S., Gross, P.H., Brendel, K., Burt, R.W., Alberts, D.S., Pamukcu, R. & Ahnen, D.J. (1995) Antineoplastic drugs sulindac sulfide and sulfone inhibit cell growth by inducing apoptosis. *Cancer Res.*, **55**, 3110–3116

Pope, J.E., Anderson, J.J. & Felson, D.T. (1993) A meta-analysis of the effects of nonsteroidal anti-inflammatory drugs on blood pressure. *Arch. intern. Med.*, **153**, 477–484

Radack, K. & Deck, C. (1987) Do nonsteroidal anti-inflammatory drugs interfere with blood pressure control in hypotensive patients? *J. gen. intern. Med.*, **2**, 108–112

Rao, C.V., Rivenson, A., Simi, B., Zang, E., Kelloff, G., Steele, V. & Reddy, B.S. (1995) Chemo-prevention of colon carcinogenesis by sulindac, a non-steroidal anti-inflammatory agent. *Cancer Res.*, **55**, 1464–1472

Rao, K.V.N., Detrisac, C.J., Steele, V.E., Hawk, E.T., Kelloff, G.J. & McCormick, D.L. (1996) Differential activity of aspirin, ketoprofen and sulindac as cancer chemopreventive agents in the mouse urinary bladder. *Carcinogenesis*, **17**, 1435–1438

Ravis, W.R., Diskin, C.J., Campagna, K.D., Clark, C.R. & McMillian, C.L. (1993) Pharmacokinetics and dialyzability of sulindac and metabolites in patients with end-stage renal failure. *J. clin. Pharmacol.*, **33**, 527–534

Reddy, B.S., Rao, C.V., & Seibert, K. (1996) Evaluation of cyclooxygenase-2 inhibitor for potential chemopreventive properties in colon carcinogenesis. *Cancer Res.*, **56**, 4566-4569.

Reynolds, J.E.F., ed. (1993) *Martindale, The Extra Pharmocopoeia*, 13th Ed., London, The Pharmaceutical Press, pp. 34–35

Rigau, J., Pigué, J.M., Rubio, E., Planas, R., Tarrech, J.M. & Bordas, J.M. (1991) Effects of long-term sulindac therapy on colonic polyposis. *Ann. intern. Med.*, **115**, 952–954

Rodriguez, L.A.G., Williams, R., Derby, L.E., Dean, A.D. & Jick, H. (1994) Acute liver injury associated with nonsteroidal anti-inflammatory drugs and the role of risk factors. *Arch. intern. Med.*, **154**, 311–316

Roupe, G., Ahlmen, M., Fagerberg, B. & Suurkula, M. (1986) Toxic epidermal necrolysis with extensive mucosal erosions of the gastrointestinal and respiratory tracts. *Int. Arch. Allergy appl. Immunol.*, **80**, 145–151

Russeva, V., Stavreva, N., Rakovska, R. & Michailova, D. (1994) Binding of sulindac to human serum albumin studied by circular dichroism. *Arzneimittel.-forsch./Drug Res.*, **44**, 159–162

Sandler, D.P., Smith, J.C., Weinberg, C.R., Buckalew, V.M., Dennis, V.W., Blythe, W.B. & Burgess, W.P. (1989) Analgesic use and chronic renal disease. *New Engl. J. Med.*, **320**, 1238–1243

Schnitzler, M., Dwight, T. & Robinson, B.G. (1996) Sulindac increases the expression of APC mRNA in malignant colonic epithelial cells: An in vitro study. *Gut*, **38**, 707–713

Shen, T.Y. & Winter, C.A. (1977) Chemical and biological studies on indomethacin, sulindac and their analogs. *Adv. Drug Res.*, **12**, 89–295

Shiff, S.J., Tsai, L.-L., Qiao, L. & Rigas, B. (1995) Sulindac sulfide inhibits proliferation, causes cell cycle quiescence, and induces apoptosis in HT29 human colon adenocarcinoma cells. *J. clin. Invest.*, **96**, 491–503

Shiff, S.J., Koutsos, M.I., Qiao, L. & Rigas, B. (1996) Nonsteroidal antiinflammatory drugs inhibit the proliferation of colon adenocarcinoma cells: Effects on cell cycle and apoptosis. *Exp. Cell. Res.*, **222**, 179–188

Shimek, J.L., Rao, N.G.S. & Khalil, S.K.W. (1981) High-performance liquid-chromatographic analysis of tolmetin, indomethacin and sulindac in plasma. *J. liq. Chromatogr.*, **4**, 1987–2013

Siglin, J.C., Barch, D.H. & Stoner, G.D. (1995) Effects of dietary phenethyl isothiocyanate, ellagic acid, sulindac and calcium on the induction and progression of *N*-nitrosomethylbenzylamine-induced esophageal carcinogenesis in rats. *Carcinogenesis*, **16**, 1101–1106

Siluveru, M. & Stewart, J.T. (1995) Determination of sulindac and its metabolites in human serum by reversed-phase high-performance liquid chromatography using on-line post-column ultraviolet irradiation and fluorescence detection. *J. Chromatogr.*, **673**, 91–96

Singh, J. & Reddy, B.S. (1995) Molecular markers in chemoprevention of colon cancer. Inhibition of expression of ras-p21 and p53 by sulindac during azoxymethane induced colon carcinogenesis. *Ann. N.Y. Acad. Sci.*, **768**, 205–209

Singh, J., Rao, C.V., Kulkarni, N., Simi, B. & Reddy, B.S. (1994) Molecular markers as intermediate end-points in chemoprevention of colon cancer: Modulation of *ras* activation by sulindac and phenyl hexylisothiocyanate during colon carcinogenesis. *Int. J. Oncol.*, **5**, 1009–1018

Skinner, S.A., Penney, A.G. & O'Brien, P.E. (1991) Sulindac inhibits the rate of growth and appearance of colon tumors in the rat. *Arch. Surg.*, **126**, 1094–1096

Smalley, W.E., Ray, W.A., Daugherty, J.R. & Griffin, M.R. (1995) Nonsteroidal anti-inflammatory drugs and the incidence of hospitalizations for peptic ulcer disease in elderly persons. *Am J. Epidemiol.*, **141**, 539–545

Spagnesi, M.T., Tonelli, F., Dolara, P., Caderni, G., Valanzano, R., Anastasi, A. & Bianchini, F. (1994) Rectal proliferation and polyp occurrence in patients with familial adenomatous polyposis after sulindac treatment. *Gastroenterology*, **106**, 362–366

Stillman, M.T. & Schlesinger, P.A. (1990) Non-steroidal anti-inflammatory drug nephrotoxicity. Should we be concerned? *Arch. intern. Med.*, **150**, 268–270

Strong, H.A., Warner, N.J., Renwick, A.G. & George, C.F. (1985) Sulindac metabolism: The importance of an intact colon. *Clin. Pharmacol. Ther.*, **38**, 387–393

Strong, H.A., Renwick, A.G., George, C.F., Liu, Y.F. & Hill, M.J. (1987) The reduction of sulphinpyrazone and sulindac by intestinal bacteria. *Xenobiotica*, **17**, 685–696

Stubbs, R.J., Ng, L.L., Entwistle, L.A. & Bayne W.F. (1987) Analysis of sulindac and metabolites in plasma and urine by high-performance liquid chromatography. *J. Chromatogr.*, **413**, 171–180

Swanson, B.N. & Boppana, V.K. (1981) Measurement of sulindac and its metabolites in human plasma and urine by high-performance liquid chromatography. *J. Chromatogr.*, **225**, 123–130

Tarazi, E.M., Harter, J.G., Zimmerman, H.J., Oshak, K.G. & Eaton, R.A. (1993) Sulindac-associated hepatic injury: Analysis of 91 cases reported to the Food and Drug Administration. *Gastroenterology*, **104**, 569–574

Thompson, H.J., Briggs, S., Paranak, N.S., Piazza, G.A., Brendel, K., Gross, P.H., Sperl, G.J., Pamukcu, R. & Ahnen, D.J. (1995) Brief communications: Inhibition of mammary carcinogenesis in rats by sulfone metabolite of sulindac. *J. natl Cancer Inst.*, **87**, 1259–1260

Thompson, H.J., Jiang, C., Lu, J., Mehta, R.G., Piazza, G.A., Paranka, N.S., Pamukcu, R. & Ahnen, D.J. (1997) Sulfone metabolite of sulindac inhibits mammary carcinogenesis. *Cancer Res.*, **57**, 267–271

Thorson, A.G., Lynch, H.T. & Smyrk, T.C. (1994) Rectal cancer in FAP patients after sulindac. *Lancet*, **343**, 180

Tonelli, F. & Valanzano, R. (1993) Sulindac in familial adenomatous polyposis (Letter to the Editor). *Lancet*, **342**, 1120

Tsujii, M. & DuBois, R.N. (1995) Alterations in cellular adhesion and apoptosis in epithelial cells overexpressing prostaglandin endoperoxide synthase-2. *Cell*, **83**, 493–501

Venuti, M.C., Young, J.M., Maloney, P.J., Johnson, D. & McGreevy, K. (1989) Synthesis and biological evaluation of omega-(N,N,N-tri-alkylammonium) alkyl esters and thioesters of carboxylic acid nonsteroidal antiinflammatory agents. *Pharm. Res.*, **6**, 867–873

Waddell, W.R. & Kirsch, W.M. (1991) Testolactone, sulindac, warfarin, and vitamin K_1 for unresectable desmoid tumors. *Am. J. Surg.*, **161**, 416–421

Waddell, W.R. & Loughry, R.W. (1983) Sulindac for polyposis of the colon. *J. surg. Oncol.*, **24**, 83–87

Waddell, W.R., Ganser, G.F., Cerise, E.J. & Loughry, R.W. (1989) Sulindac for polyposis of the colon. *Am. J. Surg.*, **157**, 175–179

Whelton, A. & Hamilton, C.W. (1991) Nonsteroidal anti-inflammatory drugs: Effects on kidney function. *J. clin. Pharmacol.*, **31**, 588–598

Whelton, A., Stout, R.L., Spilman, P.S. & Klassen, D.K. (1990) Renal effects of ibuprofen, piroxicam and sulindac in patients with asymptomatic renal failure. A prospective, randomized, crossover comparison. *Ann. intern. Med.*, **112**, 568–576

Winde, G., Gumbinger, H.G., Osswald, H., Kemper, F. & Bünte, H. (1993) The NSAID sulindac reverses rectal adenomas in colectomized patients with familial adenomatous polyposis: Clinical results of a dose-finding study on rectal sulindac administration. *Int. J. colorectal Dis.*, **8**, 13–17

Winde, G., Schmid, K.W., Schlegel, W., Fischer, R., Osswald, H. & Bünte, H. (1995) Complete reversion and prevention of rectal adenomas in colectomized patients with familial adenomatous polyposis by rectal low-dose sulindac maintenance treatment. Advantages of a low-dose nonsteroidal anti-inflammatory drug regimen in reversing adenomas exceeding 33 months. *Dis. Colon Rectum*, **38**, 813–830

Winde, G., Schmid, K.W., Brandt, B., Müller, C. & Osswald, H. (1997) Clinical and genomic influence of sulindac on rectal mucosa in familial adenomatous polyposis (FAP). *Dis. Colon Rectum* (in press)

Wong, D.G., Spence, J.D., Lamki, L., Freeman, D. & McDonald, J.W. (1986) Effect of non-steroidal anti-inflammatory drugs on control of hypotension by beta-blockers and diuretics. *Lancet*, **i**, 997–1001

Zamboni, R., Corti, P. & Nucci, L. (1983) Polarographic analysis of sulindac in pharmaceutical products and differential pulse polarographic analysis of sulindac and its metabolites in plasma. *Boll. Chim. Farm.*, **122**, 505–511

Piroxicam

1. Chemical and Physical Characteristics

1.1 Name

Chemical Abstracts Services Registry Number
36322-90-4

Chemical Abstracts Primary Name
Piroxicam

IUPAC Systematic Name
4-Hydroxy-2-methyl-N-2-pyridinyl-2H-1,2-benzo-thiazino-3-3-carboxamide-1,1-dioxide

Synonyms
3,4-Dihydro-2-methyl-4-oxo-N-2-pyridyl-2H-1,2–benzothiazine-3-carboxamide 1,1-dioxide

1.2 Structural and molecular formulae and relative molecular mass

$C_{15}H_{13}N_3O_4S$ Relative molecular mass: 331.35

1.3 Physical and chemical properties

From Budavari *et al.* (1996), unless otherwise specified

Description
Crystals

Melting-point
198–200 °C

Solubility
Piroxicam may be crystallized from methanol; has a pK_a of 6.3 in solution (2:1 dioxane:water)

Spectroscopy data
The ultraviolet, infrared, [1]H- and ^{13}C-nuclear magnetic resonance and mass spectra of the compound have been determined (Mihalic *et al.*, 1982).

Stability
Stable at 40 °C in the dark for up to 24 months (Mihalic *et al.*, 1982). The three main degradation products are 2-aminopyridine, 2-methyl-2H-1,2-benzothiazine-4-(3H)one 1,1-dioxide and N-methyl-N'-(2-pyridinyl)ethanediamide (Tománkova & Sabartová, 1989).

1.4 Technical products

2-Aminopyridine may be present as an impurity in the final product (Tománková & Sabartová, 1989).

2. Occurrence, Production, Use, Analysis and Human Exposure

2.1 Occurrence

Piroxicam is not known to occur in nature.

2.2 Production

The synthesis of piroxicam has been described (Lombardino & Wiseman, 1972; Lombardino *et al.*, 1973), but technical details of its current commercial production were not available to the Working Group.

2.3 Use

Piroxicam was introduced in 1980 as an analgesic, anti-inflammatory and antipyretic agent. It is generally taken in single or divided doses of 10–40 mg. In Sweden, a single daily dose of 20 mg accounted for 90% of piroxicam prescriptions (Wessling *et al.*, 1990). Piroxicam is used primarily for the treatment of rheumatoid arthritis and osteoarthritis. Other conditions for which it is used include juvenile rheumatoid arthritis, anklylosing spondylitis and acute gout. It has been administered for musculoskeletal disorders, minor sports injuries and post-partum pain (Brogden *et al.*, 1981).

2.4 Analysis

Methods for the determination of piroxicam in pharmaceutical preparations and in biological fluids are refined continually, and the appropriate references should be consulted for the most recent developments. Most procedures are based on high-performance liquid chromatography (HPLC), but methods involving thin-layer chromatography and spectrophotometry have also been described. Piroxicam has been determined by HPLC in serum (Twomey *et al.*, 1980) and plasma (Edno *et al.*, 1995). A method for the determination of piroxicam and its major metabolites in human plasma, urine or bile by HPLC has been described (Milligan, 1992).

2.5 Human exposure

Piroxicam is one of the commoner NSAIDs in use (Guess *et al.*, 1988; Langman *et al.*, 1994). Usage has tended to decline as a consequence of the toxicity of piroxicam to the gastrointestinal tract (McManus *et al.*, 1996).

3. Metabolism, Kinetics and Genetic Variation

3.1 Humans

3.1.1 Metabolism

Piroxicam is extensively metabolized by the liver. The metabolic pathway in humans is shown in Figure 1. The primary route of biotransformation, however, involves hydroxylation to form the primary metabolite, 5'-hydroxypiroxicam (Hobbs, 1986; Verbeeck *et al.*, 1986a). The metabolites have little or no anti-inflammatory activity (Calin, 1988). A single cytochrome P450 monooxygenase enzyme, the CYP2C subfamily, is thought to catalyse hepatic oxidation and may be responsible for the considerable interindividual that has been observed. Polymorphism of the CYP2C gene family has been noted in humans (Zhao *et al.*, 1992; Leemann *et al.*, 1993).

3.1.2 Pharmacokinetics

The piroxicam molecule has four functional groups that significantly affect its pharmacokinetics: the enol group, the sulfate group, the N-methyl group and the hetrocyclic side-chain (Calin, 1988). The enol group has a low pK$_a$ and is completely ionized, therefore prolonging the activity of the drug. The sulfate group is lipopholic, which enhances absorption in the gut. The N-methyl group increases absorption and slows hydroxylation, thereby prolonging the effect of the drug. Finally, the heterocyclic side-chain increases the effectiveness of the agent by strongly inhibiting prostaglandin synthesis. Overall, the pharmacokinetics of piroxicam are linear (Calin, 1988).

(a) Absorption

Piroxicam is well absorbed after oral administration (Hobbs, 1986). It is more completely absorbed after oral or rectal administration than after intravenous injection; rectal absorption was slower than oral absorption, however, with a peak at 5.6 h (Verbeeck *et al.*, 1986a). Food has been shown to slow the rate of oral absorption, increasing the mean time from 2.8 to 4.3 h. It does not, however, apparently affect the extent to which the drug is absorbed (Ishizaki *et al.*, 1979; Verbeeck *et al.*, 1986a).

After absorption, piroxicam, like other anti-inflammatory drugs is extensively bound to human serum albumin (Hobbs, 1986) and may displace other protein-bound agents. About 99% of all circulating piroxicam is protein bound (Richardson *et al.*, 1987; Calin, 1988). While the maximum plasma concentrations are generally reached within 2 h, this time can vary between 1 and 6 h (Hobbs, 1986; Calin, 1988). The plasma concentrations are generally within 20% of peak levels about 1 h after ingestion of a single oral dose. Multiple peaks are observed in the concentration–time profile of piroxicam in plasma 2–12 h after dosing, which may indicate enterohepatic recirculation (Verbeeck *et al.*, 1986a), as discussed below. As the mean plasma half-life is about 50 h, the drug can be administered once per day; however, there is considerable interindividual variability (> 36%) in the half-life (Hobbs, 1986).

After repeated daily oral doses of 20 mg, the plasma concentrations increase gradually and

Figure 1. Metabolism of piroxicam in humans

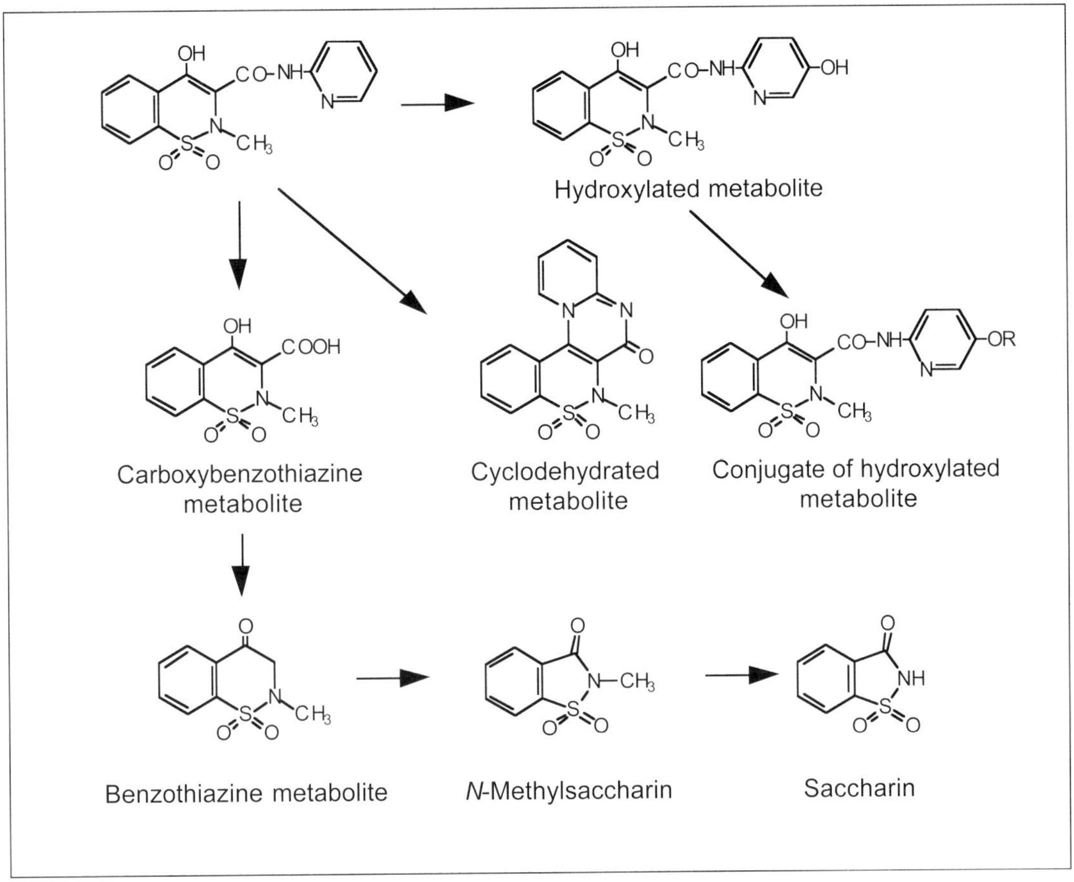

Hydroxylated metabolite

Carboxybenzothiazine metabolite

Cyclodehydrated metabolite

Conjugate of hydroxylated metabolite

Benzothiazine metabolite

N-Methylsaccharin

Saccharin

From Hobbs (1986)

reach a steady-state concentration of approximately 7 µg/ml (peak range, 4.5–7.2 µg/ml; trough range, 3.9–5.6 µg/ml) within 7–12 days (Hobbs, 1986; Calin, 1988). The volume of distribution is approximately 8 litres (Hobbs, 1986).

After administration of 20 mg/day to six healthy young volunteers for 15 days, the trough steady-state level of piroxicam was 5.5 mg/ml, and the half-life was 55 h. An average of 1% remained unbound. An average of 25% of the dose was recovered in urine as 5'-hydroxypiroxicam and 17% in the form of the glucuronide conjugate. The average steady-state level of piroxicam in plasma was 7.0 µg/ml (Richardson et al., 1987).

(b)   Distribution

Since about 99% of a dose of piroxicam is bound to protein, its distribution is limited primarily to the extracellular spaces. Nevertheless, it readily penetrates the synovial fluid and is found in concentrations that are approximately 40% (Verbeeck et al., 1986a; Calin, 1988) or 50% (Trnavska et al., 1984) of those in plasma. The extent of binding of piroxicam to protein in synovial fluid was approximately the same as that in plasma.

The apparent volume of distribution is reportedly small, 0.14 litre/kg, a value typical for most NSAIDs (Verbeeck et al., 1986a). The volume of distribution is 0.10–0.20 litre/kg (Olkkola et al., 1994).

In a study of four lactating women undergoing long-term treatment with piroxicam for arthritis, the concentrations in breast milk were 1–3% of those in plasma (Ostensen *et al.*, 1988). No accumulation of piroxicam in milk relative to that in plasma was seen after 52 days of treatment. The investigators concluded that the daily dose ingested by breast-fed infants is only 3.5% (maximum 6.3%) of the weight-related maternal dose of piroxicam.

(c)   Elimination

No more than 5% of a dose of piroxicam is excreted intact in the urine (Hobbs, 1986). At steady-state, 75% of a dose is excreted in approximately equal proportions in urine and faeces as 5'-hydroxypiroxicam and its glucuronide conjugate (Verbeeck *et al.*, 1986a).

Since renal clearance is so low, the kinetics of piroxicam are usually not altered in patients with renal impairment (Table 1). Piroxicam could, however, accumulate in patients with pronounced renal impairment and/or in patients receiving longer courses of therapy (Whelton *et al.*, 1990). Rudy *et al.* (1994) found that the time to reach the maximum concentration was shorter and unbound clearance was approximately 11% higher in elderly individuals with renal impairment than in younger individuals.

The total body clearance of piroxicam is extremely low (2–3 ml/min) (Verbeeck *et al.*, 1986a). As a consequence, the plasma half-life is long, ranging from 30 to 60 h in healthy subjects (Calin, 1988). Total plasma clearance has been determined to be 0.002–0.003 litre/kg bw per hour (Olkkola *et al.*, 1994).

A summary of the pharmacokinetic parameters of piroxicam is provided in Table 2.

(d)   Enterohepatic recirculation

Enterohepatic recirculation of NSAIDs has been proposed as a major factor in the development of intestinal lesions, such as ulceration of the duodenum and jejunum. To assess the extent of enteroheptic recirculation, the pharmacokinetics of piroxicam were compared in six healthy volunteers, with and without concomitant treatment with cholestyramine, in a randomized cross-over study. The participants were given either 20 mg piroxicam once daily, alone or with a dose of 24 g/day of cholestyramine, each for four days. Cholestyramine increased the elimination of piroxicam by about twofold (half-time, 50 vs 28 h). Simultaneous administration of piroxicam and cholestyramine increased the clearance of piroxicam by 58%. The investigators concluded that piroxicam is eliminated to a large extent in the bile (Benveniste *et al.*, 1990). The effect of 12–16 g/day cholestyramine or 15–70 g/day activated charcoal on the binding of piroxicam in the intestine, thus preventing its enterohepatic circulation, has been studied further (Laufen & Leitold, 1986; Ferry *et al.*, 1990). Significant reductions in the half-life of piroxicam were seen during treatment. Charcoal had a slightly smaller effect (control half-life of 53 h reduced

Table 1. Effect of renal impairment on the kinetics of piroxicam

No. of subjects	Age range (years)	Impairment	Conclusion	Reference
18 (26 controls)	30–80	Mild: elevated *N*-acetyl-β–glucosaminidase, urea or creatine level	No change in half-life, clearance or steady-state level	Darragh *et al.* (1985)
19	27–94	Mild to moderate: creatinine clearance, 22–88 ml/min	No correlation between creatinine clearance and kinetics	Woolf *et al.* (1983)
6 (6 controls)	23–72	Mild to moderate: creatinine clearance, 13–48 ml/min	Normal half-life (17–59 h)	Dupont *et al.* (1982)

Modified from Hobbs (1986)

Table 2. Principal pharmacokinetic parameters of piroxicam after oral administration

Study participants	Dose (mg)	C_{max} (mg/ml)	C_{av}^{ss} (g/ml)	T_{max} (h)	V_d (l/kg)	Protein binding (%)	$T_{1/2}\beta$ (h)	Reference
Young adult volunteers	20 sd	1.5–3		2–3	0.1–0.2	99	30–70	Darragh et al. (1985)
Young adult volunteers	30 sd	3–5						Hobbs & Twomey (1979)
Young adult volunteers	60 sd	6–8						Ishizaki et al. (1979)
Young adult volunteers	20 od md		5–8		0.1–0.2		30–70	Mäkelä et al. (1991); Richardson et al. (1985)
Elderly volunteers	20 sd	1.5–3		1.5–3	0.1–0.2		40–70	Rogers et al. (1981)
Children	0.4 mg/kg bw per day; md	5–10	3–8		0.12–0.25		21–40	Tilstone et al. (1981); Woolf et al. (1983)

Modified from Olkkola et al. (1994)

C_{max}, maximum plasma concentration; C_{av}^{ss} average steady-state plasma concentration; T_{max}, time to achieve maximum plasma concentration; V_d, volume of distribution; $T_{1/2}\beta$, half-life; sd, single dose; od, daily dose; md, multiple doses

to 40 h) than cholestyramine (control half-life of 47 h reduced to 28 h).

(e) Effects of age and sex

The pharmacokinetics of piroxicam do not appear to be related to age or sex (Table 3). No significant difference was found in the mean elimination half-time for old and young subjects (Campbell et al., 1985); however, sig-nificant interindividual variation was seen, the measured steady-state levels being three times higher in subjects with slow clearance than in those with more rapid clearance. Furthermore, patients with slow drug clearance required three weeks to achieve steady-state. The slow clearance of these individuals may give cause for concern, since side-effects have been shown to be dose-related.

Plasma concentrations, elimination half-life, the concentration–time relationship and the volume of distribution were not influenced by age or sex (Woolf et al., 1983; Edwards et al., 1985; Hundal et al., 1993). Additionally, mild to moderate renal impairment had no observable effect (Darragh et al., 1985).

Some studies have shown differences between young and elderly individuals in the pharmacokinetics of piroxicam. In a study of 23 patients aged 27–79 years given a standard dose of 20 mg/day for six weeks, the clearance, half-life and steady-state concentrations of piroxicam were modestly correlated with the age of the patients. Thus, patients over 60 years eliminated piroxicam more slowly than younger patients, their clearance values were lower, and the steady-state concentrations were higher (Blocka et al., 1988). In a further series of patients, aged 57–71 years, a twofold increase in the concentration–time relationship and a 53% reduction in clearance were found (Caldwell, 1994).

Table 3. Effect of age on the kinetics of piroxicam

Study type	No. of subjects	Age range (years)	Influence of age	Reference
Single dose	25	20–75	Clearance significantly lower in elderly females only	Richardson *et al.* (1985)
	24	19–86	No significant effect	Campbell *et al.* (1985)
	44	20–80	No significant effect	Darragh *et al.* (1985)
Multiple doses	23	27–79	Significant effect	Verbeeck *et al.* (1986b)
	44	20–80	No significant effect	Darragh *et al.* (1985)
	19	27–94	No significant effect	Woolf *et al.* (1983)
Kinetic monitoring	254	21–83	No significant effect	Hobbs & Gordon (1984)
	635	24–90	Mean levels significantly higher in elderly females only; small effect	Rugstad *et al.* (1986)

Modified from Hobbs (1986)

In a study of 10 children with rheumatic disease, aged 7–16 years, the maximum concentration was 3.6–9.8, the volume of distribution was 0.12–0.25 litre/kg (mean, 0.16 litre/kg), and the total body clearance was 2.1–5.0 ml/kg bw per hour, with a mean of 3.4 ml/kg bw per hour. The clearance was higher and the half-life shorter than those reported in other studies (Mäkelä *et al.*, 1991).

Healthy elderly women eliminate piroxicam more slowly than healthy young women (Richardson *et al.*, 1985). Although plasma protein binding was not affected by age or sex, body clearance was 33% lower in elderly women than in young women, yielding higher steady-state plasma concentrations.

In patients with osteoarthritis, the plasma concentration increased significantly with increasing age, and women had higher concentrations than men (Rugstad *et al.*, 1986).

3.2 Experimental models

The kinetics and metabolism of piroxicam in laboratory animals have been reviewed extensively (Wiseman & Hobbs, 1982; Ando & Lombardino, 1983; Brogden *et al.*, 1981).

3.2.1 Metabolism

The biotransformation of piroxicam has been studied in rats, rabbits, dogs and rhesus monkeys. In Sprague–Dawley rats, rhesus monkeys and beagle dogs, hydroxylation of the pyridyl ring at the 5' site was the primary route of metabolism. The metabolic pathways were qualitatively the same in all three species, but an additional hydroxylation of the benzothiazine ring was seen in rats (Hobbs & Twomey, 1981). The primary metabolite of piroxicam metabolism is the same in humans as in these three animal species.

3.2.2 Pharmacokinetics

(a) Absorption

The kinetics of piroxicam (at 3 and 10 mg/kg bw) in plasma of rabbits was similar after oral and rectal administration (Schianterelli *et al.*, 1981). Half-lives of 2–9 h in rabbits, rats and rhesus monkeys and 45 h in beagle dogs have been measured (Wiseman *et al.*, 1976; Hobbs & Twomey, 1979).

After intravenous administration of 10 mg/kg bw to fasted, male Wistar rats, the volume of distribution was lower than the physiological volume (232 ml/kg bw at steady-state and 234 ml/kg bw at the terminal phase) (Fernandez-Troconis *et al.* 1991). Plasma clearance was 22 ml/h per kg bw and blood clearance was 35 ml/h per kg bw. The extraction ratio was 0.0006, the intrinsic clearance 1140 ml/h per kg bw and the half-life 7.5 h.

Studies conducted with tritiated piroxicam in the beagle dog indicate that piroxicam is well absorbed after oral administration (Hobbs & Twomey, 1981). In three young male and three young female beagle dogs, piroxicam showed a high level of bioavailability after oral administration (Galbraith & McKellar, 1991).

The elimination half-life in dogs is similar to that in humans (approximately 45 h), and the LD_{50} for piroxicam is 700 mg/kg bw. The half-life after intravenous injection of 0.3 mg/kg bw was 40 h; the volume of distribution was 0.29 litre/kg (± 0.018), and the clearance was 0.66 litre/h. After oral administration of 0.3 mg/kg bw, the maximum concentration was 1.35 µg/ml (± 0.12), and the time to achieve that concentration was 3.1 h (± 1.0) (Galbraith & McKellar, 1991). The plasma concentration showed successively lower peaks and troughs, strongly suggesting that the drug had undergone enterohepatic cycling, as has also been postulated in humans. If this is the case, piroxicam may accumulate when administered daily. Further studies are required to determine the extent to which the drug accumulates before steady-state levels are reached, to ensure that dogs tolerate repeated treatments. Different breeds of dogs may differ in measured pharmacokinetic parameters.

(b)   Distribution
In two model systems, piroxicam was preferentially distributed in inflamed tissue: in urate-inflamed knee joints of dogs and in the region of carrageenan-induced paw oedema in mice (Noguchi et al., 1984).

(c)   Elimination
CD Sprague-Dawley rats given an oral dose of 20 mg/kg bw excreted 86% of the dose in the urine within 48 h. Beagle dogs given an oral dose of 20 mg/kg bw of piroxicam excreted 72% of the dose over 168 h, equally divided between the urine and faeces. This finding is consistent with the measured long half-life in this species. Rhesus monkeys given an oral dose of 20 mg/kg bw of piroxicam excreted 86% of the dose during the initial 72 h, equally divided between the urine and faeces (Hobbs & Twomey, 1981).

(d)   Effects of age and sex
After intravenous doses of 0.50 and 5.0 mg/kg bw piroxicam to Sprague-Dawley rats, the half-life was 13 h in males and 41 h in females.

It was concluded that the dose had no effect on the disposition of piroxicam, but the sex of the animals had a marked effect on the pharmacokinetics. The mean total clearance of 0.0062 litre/h per kg bw in females was more than three times greater than the value in males. Males thus had a larger free fraction, and females had a higher association constant for binding to serum proteins. The free piroxicam clearance differed twofold (0.76 litre/h per kg bw in males and 0.42 litre/h per kg bw in females). The steady-state volume of distribution, however, appeared to be unaffected by the sex of the animals. It is believed that protein binding explains some of the sex-dependent disposition of piroxicam and that sex-dependent metabolism may be a primary consideration (Roskos & Boudinot, 1990).

In a study of the effect of age on the pharmacokinetics of piroxicam in rats, male Fischer 344 rats, aged 5 and 24 months, were given 1 mg/kg bw piroxicam per day intravenously for five days. Statistically significant, age-related differences in pharmacokinetics were seen. For example, the half-life of piroxicam was 5.9 ± 0.7 h in young rats and 31 ± 9.9 h in older rats — nearly five times longer. Total clearance was faster in the young rats, with a value of 0.048 ± 0.012 litre/h per kg bw, while the older rats had a clearance rate of only 0.021 ± 0.003 litre/h per kg bw. The steady-state volume of distribution was 0.42 ± 0.05 litre/kg bw in the young rats and 0.56 ± 0.10 in the older rats (Boudinot et al., 1993).

3.3   Genetic variation
No data were available to the Working Group.

4.   Cancer-preventive Effects

4.1   Human studies
The only available data on the effects of piroxicam on cancer risk are derived from case series. One case report (Gowen, 1996) described a 73-year-old man with a history of rectal carcinoma who subsequently was found to have two villous adenomas of the caecum. Since the patient refused surgery, piroxicam was given, at 10 mg

three times per week and the patient was urged to reduce his alcohol intake and adhere to a bland diet. Both adenomas regressed within three months. In another study, two patients with three adenomas were followed by regular endoscopy. One polyp appeared to have shrunk from 12 to 8 mm in diameter after six months, and two others of 4 and 10 mm remained unchanged in size (Hixson *et al.*, 1993). [The Working Group noted that these limited data provide little information about the chemopreventive potential of piroxicam.]

Piroxicam at 20 mg/day had no effect on rectal mucosal proliferation in seven patients with a history of colorectal adenoma, a finding with limited statistical power. Piroxicam did, however, induce a dose-related decrease in mucosal prostaglandin E_2 levels; a modest decrease was seen at 5 mg/kg bw, which was not significantly different from the baseline value. A dose of 10 mg daily reduced the prostaglandin E_2 levels by about 30%, and 20 mg/day reduced the levels by more than 50% (Earnest *et al.*, 1990).

4.2   Experimental models
4.2.1   Experimental animals

(a)   Colon
Short-term studies. Groups of five to eight Fischer 344 rats were given a diet containing 125 ppm piroxicam for 35 days. Azoxymethane was given at a dose of 30 mg/kg bw as a single subcutaneous injection seven days after the start of piroxicam treatment. All rats were killed 35 days after the end of the experimental period, and the numbers of aberrant crypt foci were counted under a microscope. The numbers of foci per colon were 25.8 ± 2.2 in controls and 15.7 ± 2.8 in those given piroxicam. Piroxicam also significantly reduced the numbers of aberrant crypts per focus ($1.84 + 0.10$) as compared with those in the control group (2.04 ± 0.04) ($p < 0.05$) (Pereira *et al.*, 1994).

Groups of 5–10 male Fischer 344 rats, weighing 100–125 g, were given azoxymethane at a dose of 15 mg/kg bw by subcutaneous injection once a week for two weeks. Two weeks after the second injection of azoxymethane, rats were given AIN-76A diet containing 0, 200

or 400 ppm piroxicam (40% and 80% of the maximum tolerated dose (MTD) determined in an eight-week study) for four weeks and were then killed. No significant growth retardation was observed. Piroxicam reduced not only the total numbers of foci per colon but also those containing more than three crypts per focus, in a dose-dependent manner ($p < 0.05$) (Wargovich *et al.*, 1995).

Long-term studies. Seven randomized groups of eight weanling C57Bl/6J-Min/+ mice were fed AIN-93 diets containing 0, 50, 100 or 200 ppm piroxicam. All animals were killed after six weeks, and the intestinal adenomas were counted. Tumour multiplicity was decreased in a dose-dependent manner, from 17.3 ± 2.7 in the controls to 2.1 ± 1.1 in mice fed 200 ppm piroxicam ($p < 0.001$); the tumour multiplicity was 5.2 ± 1.2 in animals at 50 ppm and 4.5 ± 1.0 in those at 100 ppm ($p < 0.001$) (Jacoby *et al.*, 1996).

Groups of 9–10 Lobund inbred Sprague-Dawley weanling rats received intrarectal administrations of N-methyl-N-nitrosourea at a dose of 0.5 ml of a 0.8% solution, three times every two days (total dose, 12 mg/rat). One week after the last administration of carcinogen, rats were given 0 (control) or 130 mg/kg of diet [130 ppm] piroxicam [purity and source unspecified] in L-485 all-grain diet for 19 weeks and then killed. The experiment was repeated using the same protocol. The animals were examined for intestinal tumours macroscopically and histologically. Piroxicam did not retard the growth of the rats significantly during the experimental period, but the number of rats that died during this time was not given. The incidences of tumours of the small intestine and colon were 9/9 (100%) in the control groups in both the first and second experiments and 5/10 (50%) and 3/9 (33%) in piroxicam-treated groups in the two experiments. [The method used for deriving p values was not described.] Most of the tumours were adenocarcinomas. The numbers of small intestinal tumours were 33 in controls and three in piroxicam-treated animals in the first experiment and one in controls and none in piroxicam-treated animals in the second experiment;

the numbers of colon tumours were 28 in controls and six in piroxicam-treated animals in the first experiment and 33 in controls and three in piroxicam-treated animals in the second experiment. Piroxicam significantly decreased the total numbers of intestinal tumours per rat in both the first ($p < 0.0001$) and second ($p < 0.001$) experiments (Pollard & Luckert, 1984).

Groups of 21–25 male Sprague-Dawley rats, weighing 100–125 g each, were given azoxymethane subcutaneously at a dose of 8 mg/kg bw once a week for eight weeks and 0, 65 or 130 mg/kg of diet [65 and 130 ppm] piroxicam in the diet during and after carcinogen treatment for 26 weeks; they were then killed. The basal diet used in this experiment was a semisynthetic, dextrose- and casein-based diet. Intestinal tumours were counted macroscopically, and 10 tumours from each group were examined histologically. No significant growth retardation was observed. The incidences and numbers of tumours per rat in the small and large intestines were not significantly different in control and piroxicam-treated groups; however, the total numbers of intestinal tumours per rat were 3.4 ± 2.3 in controls, 3.2 ± 1.9 in those given 65 ppm piroxicam and 2.3 ± 1.6 in those given 130 ppm piroxicam, showing a significant reduction as compared with the control group ($p < 0.05$) (Nigro et al., 1986).

Groups of 36 male Fischer 344 rats, seven weeks of age, were given a single subcutaneous injection of azoxymethane at a dose of 29.6 mg/kg bw. Piroxicam was mixed with basal NIH-07 diet at concentrations of 0 (control), 25, 50, 75 or 150 mg/kg of diet [25, 50, 75 or 150 ppm] and was fed to the rats one, 13 and 23 weeks after carcinogen treatment; the stability of piroxicam in the diet for seven days was > 92%. All of the rats were killed 40 weeks after azoxymethane treatment, and intestinal tumours were examined macroscopically and histologically. No significant growth retardation was observed. The incidences of colon tumours (percentage of animals with tumours) were inhibited in a dose-dependent manner in rats fed diets containing piroxicam ($p < 0.001$) one or 13 weeks after carcinogen treatment, with incidences in animals fed diets containing

0, 25, 50, 75 and 150 ppm piroxicam of 89, 61, 58, 50 and 39%, respectively, when starting at one week (Table 4) and 89, 69, 69, 44 and 33% respectively, when starting at 13 weeks. The numbers of tumours per animal were also significantly inhibited in these animals ($p < 0.01$–0.0001). When the diets containing piroxicam were fed 23 weeks after carcinogen treatment, the colon tumour incidences were significantly inhibited ($p < 0.05$) in groups fed 25 or 150 ppm piroxicam (Reddy et al., 1987).

Groups of 20–23 male Lobund Sprague-Dawley rats, six weeks of age, were given a single subcutaneous injection of methylazoxymethanol acetate at a dose of 30 mg/kg bw, followed by an L-485 diet containing 0 or 130 mg/kg of diet [130 ppm] piroxicam [purity unspecified] starting one or 20 weeks after carcinogen treatment. Control animals were killed after 20 and 40 weeks, and those given piroxicam were killed after 40 weeks of carcinogen treatment. Intestinal tumours were examined macroscopically and histologically. No significant growth retardation was observed. The combined incidences of tumours of the small and large intestine were 19/21 (90%) in control rats killed at 20 weeks, 19/20 (95%) in controls killed at 40 weeks, 9/21 (43%) in animals given piroxicam one week after carcinogen treatment and 17/23 (74%) in rats started at 20 weeks. The numbers of intestinal tumours were 2.8/rat in controls at 20 weeks, 2.7/rat in those killed at 40 weeks, 0.6/rat in animals given piroxicam starting at one week and 1.4/rat in those started at 20 weeks (Pollard & Luckert, 1989).

Groups of 30 male Fischer 344 rats, seven weeks of age, were given a single subcutaneous injection of azoxymethane at a dose of 29.6 mg/kg bw, followed one week later by piroxicam mixed with AIN-76A basal diet at concentrations of 0 (control), 25, 75 or 150 ppm. All rats were sacrificed 56 weeks after azoxymethane treatment, and intestinal tumours were examined macroscopically and histologically. None of the rats died during the experimental period, and no significant growth retardation was observed. The incidences and numbers of colon adenocarcinomas, but not colon adenomas or small intestinal tumours, were reduced in rats receiving piroxicam at

Table 4. Effects of piroxicam on azoxymethane (AOM)-induced colon tumourigenesis when given one week after carcinogen treatment for 39 weeks to groups of 36 male Fischer 344 rats

Treatment	Incidence (%)			No. of tumours/rat (mean ± SD)		
(dose, ppm)	Total	Adenoma	Adeno-carcinoma	Total	Adenoma	Adeno-carcinoma
AOM alone	89	69	56	2.4 ± 1.4	1.3 ± 1.0	1.1 ± 0.9
AOM + piroxicam (25)	61*	61*	28*	1.3 ± 1.4*	1.0 ± 1.3	0.3 ± 0.6*
AOM + piroxicam (5)	58*	44*	25*	0.9 ± 1.1*	0.6 ± 0.7*	0.3 ± 0.6*
AOM + piroxicam (75)	50*	31*	25*	0.8 ± 1.1*	0.4 ± 0.7*	0.4 ± 0.7*
AOM + piroxicam (150)	39*	25*	22*	0.5 ± 0.6*	0.3 ± 0.4*	0.2 ± 0.4*

From Reddy et al. (1987)
*Significantly different from group receiving AOM alone ($p < 0.05$–0.001)

25 or 75 ppm ($p < 0.05$). The incidences of adenocarcinomas were 17/30 (57%) in controls, 10/30 (33.3%) in those receiving 25 ppm piroxicam, 6/30 (20%) in rats receiving 75 ppm piroxicam and 7/30 (23%) in those given 150 ppm piroxicam. The numbers of tumours/rat (mean ± SD) were 0.73 ± 0.14, 0.37 ± 0.10, 0.20 ± 0.09 and 0.30 ± 0.11 in the four groups, respectively (Reddy et al., 1990).

Groups of 36 male Fischer 344 rats, five weeks of age, were given a modified AIN-76A diet containing piroxicam at concentrations of 0 (control), 200 or 400 ppm (40 and 80% of the MTD, determined in a six-week study) throughout the experimental period. Two weeks after the diets were begun, azoxymethane was given by subcutaneous injection at a dose of 15 mg/kg bw once a week for two weeks. All rats were killed 52 weeks after the azoxymethane treatment, and intestinal tumours were examined macroscopically and histologically. No significant growth retardation was observed. The incidences and numbers of both small intestinal and colon adenocarcinomas, but not those of adenomas, were dose-dependently reduced. The incidences of colon adenocarcinomas were 72% in controls, 31% in rats at 200 ppm piroxicam and 22% in those given 400 ppm piroxicam ($p < 0.001$). The numbers of tumours per rat were 1.14 ± 0.18, 0.31 ± 0.07 and 0.29 ± 0.09 in the three groups, respectively ($p < 0.001$) (Rao et al., 1991).

Groups of 36 male Fischer 344 rats, six weeks of age, were given diets containing 0, 200 or 400 ppm piroxicam (40 and 80% of the MTD, determined in a six-week study) throughout the experimental period. Azoxymethane was given by subcutaneous injection at a dose of 15 mg/kg bw once a week for two weeks, starting one week after the beginning of the diet. All rats were killed 50 weeks after the second azoxymethane injection, and colon tumours were examined macroscopically and histologically. No significant growth retardation was observed. The numbers of colon adenocarcinomas, but not of adenomas, were reduced in the groups given piroxicam ($p < 0.05$–0.01). The reduction in incidence was dose-related: by 45% at 200 ppm piroxicam ($p < 0.05$) and by 64% at 400 ppm ($p < 0.01$) (Table 5; Reddy et al., 1992).

Groups of 20–32 male Fischer 344 rats, weighing 90–130 g were given an AIN-76 diet containing 75 ppm piroxicam throughout the experimental period. Azoxymethane was given by subcutaneous injection at a dose of 15 mg/kg bw once a week for two weeks starting two weeks after the diet was begun. All of the rats were killed 28 weeks after the first carcinogen treatment, and colon tumours were examined macroscopically and histologically. No significant growth retardation was observed. The incidences of colon tumours were 10/20 (50%) in controls and 9/32 (28%) in those given piroxicam ($p < 0.05$). The

Table 5. Effects of piroxicam on azoxymethane (AOM)-induced colon tumourigenesis when given before, during and after carcinogen treatment for 52 weeks to groups of 36 male Fischer 344 rats

Treatment	Incidence (%)			No. of tumours (mean ± SD)		
(dose ppm)	Total	Adenoma	Adeno-carcinoma	Total	Adenoma	Adeno-carcinoma
AOM alone	61	5.6	58	1.03 ± 1.14	0.05 ± 0.22	0.98 ± 1.1
AOM + piroxicam (200)	33*	8.3	33*	0.47 ± 0.68*	0.08 ± 0.2	0.39 ± 0.59*
AOM + piroxicam (400)	22*	2.8	19*	0.38 ± 0.72*	0.09 ± 0.36	0.29 ± 0.50*

From Reddy et al. (1992)
* Significantly different from group receiving AOM alone ($p < 0.05$–0.001)

numbers of tumours per tumour-bearing rat were not significantly reduced (Earnest et al., 1994).

(b)   Liver
Groups of 19 male inbred ACI/N rats, six weeks of age, were given a diet containing 0 or 130 ppm piroxicam for 18 weeks, followed by basal diet for a further 19 weeks. 2-Acetylamino-fluorene was added to the diet at a dose of 200 ppm starting one week after the diet containing piroxicam had been started, for 16 weeks. Rats were killed serially 17 (three rats), 21 (three rats), 25 (three rats) and 37 weeks (10 rats) after the beginning of the experiment, and the livers were examined macroscopically. No significant growth regardation was observed. The numbers of iron-excluding altered liver cell foci were significantly decreased by piroxicam at all times. By 37 weeks, the numbers of altered liver-cell foci (mean ± SD) were 42.6 ± 6.7 in controls and 24.2 ± 5.2 in rats given piroxicam. The incidences of hepatocellular adenomas and carcinomas were 10/10 (100%) in controls and 1/10 (10%) in rats given pirox-icam, and the numbers of tumours per rat were 4.0 ± 2.4 in controls and 0.10 ± 0.30 with pirox-icam. Piroxicam significantly decreased the numbers of foci ($p < 0.05$) and the incidences ($p < 0.0001$) and numbers ($p < 0.001$) of hepatic tumours (Tanaka et al., 1993).

(c)   Urinary bladder
Groups of 50–72 male B6D2F$_1$ mice, seven to eight weeks of age, were given a diet containing 0, 15 or 30 ppm piroxicam (40 and 80% of

the MTD, determined in 6–8-week studies) throughout the experimental period. The experiments with the low and high doses of piroxicam were performed separately. One week after the start of the diet containing piroxicam, mice were given doses of 7.5 mg N-nitrosobutyl(4-hydroxybutyl)amine in 20% ethanol once a week for eight weeks and were killed six months after the first treatment. Urinary bladder carcinomas were examined histologically. No significant growth retarda-tion was observed, and the survival rate was more than 80%. The incidences of transitional-cell carcinomas were 25/63 (40%) in controls and 5/69 (7%) at the low dose of piroxicam, and 28/65 (43%) in controls and 7/56 (13%) at the high dose. Both doses of piroxicam inhib-ited urinary bladder carcinogenesis ($p < 0.0001$ and $p < 0.001$, respectively) (Moon et al., 1993).

(d)   Mammary gland
Groups of 18–22 female Sprague-Dawley rats, 40 days old, were given a single intragastric intubation of 5 mg 7,12-dimethylbenz[a]-anthracene [solvent unspecified]. One week later, high- or low-fat diets containing 0 or 100 ppm piroxicam were given for 19 weeks. All rats were killed 20 weeks after carcinogen treatment, and the mammary carcinomas were examined macroscopically and histo-logically. Significant growth retardation was seen with the high-fat diet containing piroxicam. Piroxicam did not significantly affect the incidences or numbers of mammary adenocarcinomas (Kitagawa & Noguchi, 1994).

(e)   Lung

Two groups of 25 female A/Jg mice, six to seven weeks old, were given a total dose of 9.1 mg per animal of 4-(N-nitrosomethylamino)-1-(3-pyridyl)-1-butanone (NNK) in drinking-water between weeks 0 and 7. One group received AIN-76 diet without piroxicam and the other received piroxicam at 25 mg/kg diet. All mice were killed 16 weeks after the end of NNK treatment, and lung adenomas larger than 1 mm were counted under a dissecting microscope. The numbers of lung tumours were 8.44 ± 1.01 in controls and 5.88 ± 0.82 in those given piroxicam ($p < 0.05$) (Jalbert & Castonguay, 1992).

4.2.2 In-vitro models

(a)   Canine tumour cells

Four canine tumour cell lines, established from spontaneously arising canine tumours, were used to evaluate the effects of piroxicam and other NSAIDs against transitional-cell carcinoma, squamous-cell carcinoma, melanoma and soft-tissue sarcoma (Knapp *et al.*, 1995). Piroxicam was tested at concentrations of 0, 3, 30, 100, 250, 500, 750 and 1000 µmol/litre. The 50% inhibitory concentration, measured in short-term assays for growth rate, was 530 µmol/litre, a concentration more than 10 times the serum concentration that could be achieved safely *in vivo*. When piroxicam was combined with zileuton, a lipoxygenase inhibitor, the 50% inhibitory concentration was not significantly different from that of zileuton alone; combinations with the chemotherapeutic agents cisplatin (1.5 µmol/litre) and carboplatin (6.1 µmol/litre) had similar effects as when administered without piroxicam. Piroxicam is therefore not cytotoxic at concentrations that can be achieved safely *in vivo*, and the authors concluded that the antitumour activity of piroxicam is unlikely to be attributable to direct cytotoxicity against the tumour.

(b)   HT-29 colon adenocarcinoma cells

Shiff and colleagues (1996) evaluated the effects of piroxicam and other NSAIDs on cell proliferation, cell cycle phase distribution and the development of apoptosis in HT-29 colon adenocarcinoma cells *in vitro*. To evaluate the effect of piroxicam on cell proliferation, a monolayer of HT-29 cells was grown for 72 h in culture medium supplemented with 0, 100, 300, 600 or 900 µmol/litre piroxicam. The cells treated with piroxicam showed a significant, apparently concentration-dependent reduction in the rate of proliferation: at 100 µmol/litre, piroxicam had no significant effect but at 300 and 600 mmol/litre proliferation was reduced by 4.3–4.5-fold at 72 h; at 900 µmol/litre, cell proliferation was reduced by 18-fold.

A nonlinear, concentration-dependent effect was seen on the distribution of cells in different stages of the cell cycle. After 48 h of treatment with piroxicam, the number of cells in G_0/G_1 phase was increased and the proportion of those in the S phase was consequently decreased, indicating that piroxicam either inhibits the progression of cells through the G_1 phase or from G_1 into the S phase. Piroxicam, unlike other NSAIDs tested, did not reduce the proportion of cells in the G_2/M phase of the cell cycle.

Although the anti-proliferative effect of piroxicam can be partially accounted for by the observed effects on the cell cyle, the investigators also evaluated the effect of piroxicam on the rate of cell death, by studying the DNA content of HT-29 cells treated with piroxicam. Chromatin condensation was observed after treatment with 900 µmol/litre piroxicam for 72 h, and a rough correlation was seen between apoptosis reduction and the ability of piroxicam to suppress cell proliferation.

Piroxicam also induced distinctive morphological changes in the HT-29 colon adenocarcinoma cell line. After growth at a plate density of 0.5×10^6 for 72 h, untreated cells grew in aggregates, with individual cells assuming polygonal or rectangular shapes. After treatment with piroxicam at a concentration of 1500 µmol/litre, however, the cells grew in small groups, with individual cells assuming irregular shapes. These morphological changes were seen at 24 h and reached a maximum at 72 h.

The effects observed on cell proliferation, cell growth cycle distribution, rate of apoptosis and cell morphology are in agreement with results obtained in studies of the effects of sulindac sulfide on colon cancer cells (Shiff *et al.*, 1995) and of other NSAIDs on the proliferation of non-intestinal cultured cells (Neupert & Muller, 1975; Hial *et al.*, 1977; Bayer *et al.*, 1979).

(c)   Human breast cancer line
The effect of piroxicam, with or without linoleic acid, on a human breast cancer cell line, MDA-MS-231, was evaluated by Noguchi *et al.* (1995). Linoleic acid was included because, theoretically, it can be converted to arachidonic acid, which can in turn be converted into prostaglandins. The addition of linoleic acid alone to the cell culture at a concentration of 625 ng/ml promoted prostaglandin synthesis and thymidine incorporation. In the absence of linoleic acid, piroxicam suppressed cell growth and thymidine incorporation. Although piroxicam reduced the secretion of prostaglandin in the absence of linoleic acid, concentrations in excess of 100 µmol/litre were required to suppress prostaglandin secretion in the presence of linoleic acid. These results suggest that cyclooxygenase (COX[1]) inhibition, and therefore piroxicam administration, could play an active role in the suppression of cell growth.

(d)   Antimutagenicity in short-term tests
In addition to being important mediators of the inflammatory response, reactive oxygen species have been shown to induce mutations, malignant transformation and sister chromatid exchange in cultured mammalian cells (Weitzman & Stossel, 1981; Weitzman *et al.*, 1985). In addition, there is evidence that the intermediate formation of reactive oxygen species plays a role in the mechanism of action of several tumour promoters (Kenzler & Trush, 1984). For example, receptor binding by 12-*O*-tetradecanoylphorbol 13-acetate (TPA) results in activation of phospholipase A_2 and stimulation of the arachidonic acid cascade (Emerit & Cerutti, 1982), which progresses in part through COX to form oxygen-centred free radicals and malondialdehyde as well as

prostaglandins. TPA-induced chromosomal breakage can be prevented by inhibitors of arachidonic acid metabolism (Emerit *et al.*, 1983). Weitberg (1988) showed that piroxicam, which inhibits arachidonic acid metabolism by COX, prevents generation of sister chromatid exchange in Chinese hamster ovary cells when incubated with TPA-stimulated human blood leukocytes as the source of COX and the resulting reactive oxygen species and lipid peroxidation. The results support the concept that intermediates of lipid peroxidation play a role in DNA damage induced by free radicals and that NSAIDs like piroxicam and indomethacin may exert a protective or anticancer effect by decreasing the amount of free radical and toxic lipid peroxidation products resulting from COX metabolism of arachidonic acid.

4.3   Mechanisms of chemoprevention
(see also General Remarks)

4.3.1 Preneoplastic lesions
Inhibition of colon cancer by piroxicam is directly related to the ingested dose and occurs regardless of whether the drug is given one week or 23 or more weeks after the carcinogen in a 40-week tumour development protocol (Reddy *et al.*, 1987). In this model, the earliest phenotypic changes in colonic mucosa that correlate with ultimate cancer formation are aberrant crypt foci (McLellan *et al.*, 1991). These microscopic clusters of abnormal crypts have been shown to contain mutations similar to those occurring in human adenomatous polys and tumours and to grow over time after carcinogen administration (McLellan *et al.*, 1991; Pretlow *et al.*, 1993). Piroxicam administered in the diet of azoxymethane-treated rats both decreased the formation of aberrant crypt foci and caused them to regress (Pereira *et al.* 1996). Thus, piroxicam appears to suppress cancer development at both early and later stages after carcinogen exposure.

4.3.2 Inhibition of carcinogen activation
Piroxicam and other NSAIDs decrease activation of procarcinogens in colonic mucosa and reduce production of reactive oxygen species

---

[1] COX is used as a synonym for prostaglandin endoperoxide synthase (PGH synthase)

and malondialdehyde. Peroxyl free radicals and malondialdehyde are produced as by-products of the COX reaction and may directly contribute to tumour initiation and promotion (Mukai & Goldstein, 1976; Marnett, 1990). The peroxidase activity of COX can also result in oxidation and activation of environmental carcinogens, including dietary mutagens, which potentially play a role in causing colon cancer (Petry et al., 1989; Smith et al., 1991). Thus, piroxicam and other NSAIDs may decrease the risk for colon cancer by suppressing non-prostaglandin effects of COX.

4.3.3 Effects on cell proliferation and apoptosis

An important question raised by the results of the study of Shiff et al. (1996; see p. 138) is whether the antiproliferative and apoptotic effects of piroxicam on tumour cells are due to inhibition of prostaglandin synthesis via an effect on COX. Some evidence which suggests that the effect is independent of prostaglandin synthesis is provided by results of a study by Hanif et al. (1996). Two human colon cancer cell lines were studied: HT-29 which produces prostaglandins and HCT-15 which does not. Culture medium from the HCT-15 cells was thus devoid of prostaglandins, while that from HT-29 contained prostaglandins E_2, $F_{2\alpha}$ and I_2. When the culture medium was supplemented with serum, the HCT-15 cell medium had prostaglandins only at the levels found in the scrum, but the HT 29 cells had an additional amount owing to synthesis by these cells. Stimulation of prostaglandin synthesis by A23187, arachidonic acid and mellitin could not increase prostaglandin production by the HCT-15 cells but resulted in three- to fivefold increases in prostaglandin production by the HT-29 cells. COX-1 and COX-2 mRNA could not be demonstrated by reverse transcriptase–polymerase chain reaction in HCT-15 cells, while the messages for both were clearly present in HT-29 cells. Proliferation of HCT-15 cells was only modestly affected by addition of prostaglandin E_2 or $F_{2\alpha}$ (25% increase) but was severely reduced by incubation with piroxicam or sulindac and also severely reduced by addition of exogenous prostaglandin, sulindac or piroxicam. Thus, both piroxicam and sulindac exerted their antiproliferative and pro-apoptotic effects independently of prostaglandin synthesis (Hanif et al., 1996). It should be noted that the concentrations of NSAIDs used in these studies were significantly higher than those that could be achieved in vivo.

A variety of other factors potentially related to the development of colon cancer have also been shown to be affected by piroxicam. The cause for most is unclear. For example, colon tumour-suppressing doses of piroxicam in azoxymethane-treated rats exert a significant inhibitory effect on the expression of certain cancer-promoting oncogenes, such as ras p21 (Singh et al., 1994). Components of cellular signal transduction pathways may also be altered by NSAID treatment (Kantor & Hampton, 1978): pirixocam affects the cellular distribution of protein kinase C isoforms in colon tumour epithelial cells harvested from azoxymethane-treated rats (Roy et al., 1995). A similar change in protein kinase C isoform distribution was observed after oral treatment with ursodeoxycholic acid, a colon cancer-preventive agent in rats that is structurally unrelated to piroxicam (Wali et al., 1995). This observation suggests an effect of piroxicam on protein kinase C-related signalling pathways that may modify cell growth and differentiation. Further evaluation of this effect would be of interest.

4.3.4 Immune surveillance

Suppression of colon cancer in rats by piroxicam is accompanied by a reduction in prostaglandin concentrations in the colon mucosa (Kulkarni et al., 1992). Piroxicam and other NSAIDs may modify cancer development and progression by reducing the concentrations of prostaglandin E_2 in tissue, resulting from the up-regulation of COX-2. For example, immune cell surveillance and killing of malignant cells can be suppressed by high tissue levels of prostaglandin E_2, whereas immune cell responses are generally enhanced by drugs that decrease prostaglandin E_2 synthesis (Goodwin, 1984).

NSAIDs, and piroxicam in particular, have also been found to modify neutrophil activation and affect other inflammatory and immunological events (Calin, 1988). Abramson *et al.* (1991) postulated that the anti-inflammatory effects of piroxicam and other NSAIDs may be due to inhibition of neutrophil activation, possibly due to their effects on a guanosine-5′-triphosphate-binding protein within the plasma membrane of the neutrophil. In fact, Rosenstein *et al.* (1994) demonstrated that piroxicam modulates the production of various cytokines, causing elevated levels of interleukin-2, decreased levels of interleukins 1 and 6, tumour necrosis factor α and interferon-γ, but no effect on interleukin-4.

5.   Other beneficial effects

No data were available to the Working Group.

6.   Carcinogenicity

6.1   Humans
No data were available to the Working Group.

6.2   Experimental animals
No study of adequate duration to evaluate carcinogenicity was available to the Working Group.

7.   Other Toxic Effects

7.1   Adverse effects
7.1.1   Humans

(a)   Gastrointestinal tract toxicity
In a meta-analysis, the risks for serious upper gastrointestinal complications after use of piroxicam were statistically indistinguishable from those of most other NSAIDs. Within individual studies, however, piroxicam was consistently associated with higher risks for such complications, and in a ranking analysis it ranked 4 (1 being most and 12 least toxic) of 12 NSAIDs analysed. The pooled relative risk estimates for piroxicam users were 2.7–5.2 in comparison with ibuprofen users (Henry *et al.*, 1996). Given the baseline risk of ulcer disease, which ranges from 0.5 per 1000 per year in young adults (Garcia Rodriguez *et al.*, 1992) to 4 per 1000 in older

adults (Smalley *et al.*, 1996), the rates of serious ulcer complications among piroxicam users can be estimated to be about 2 per 1000 in younger adults and 15 per 1000 in those 65 years and older.

Case reports indicate that piroxicam can exacerbate reflux disease and occasionally lead to oesophageal ulceration and stricture (Kikendale, 1991). Piroxicam may also have deleterious effects on the small intestine, including stricture (Matsuhashi *et al.*, 1992), ulceration, perforation and diarrhoea (Kwo & Tremaine, 1995).

(b)   Blood pressure
In a meta-analysis of 50 randomized, placebo-controlled trials, treatment with NSAIDs raised supine mean blood pressure by 5 mm Hg (1.2–8.7) (Johnson *et al.*, 1994). Most NSAIDs appeared to have this effect, but the most marked increases were observed with piroxicam. Nonetheless, the numbers were too small to demonstrate statistically significant differences between different NSAIDs.

(c)   Reproductive and developmental effects
No data specifically related to the reproductive or developmental effects of piroxicam were available to the Working Group.

(d)   Other toxic manifestations
Piroxicam users report skin rashes and pruritus more often than users of other NSAIDs (Fries *et al.*, 1991).

7.1.2   Experimental animals

(a)   Gastrointestinal tract toxicity
The ulcerogenic dose or LD_{50} of orally administered piroxicam in starved rats was reportedly one-third to one-half that of indomethacin and fourfold greater than that of phenylbutazone. After rectal administration to rats, piroxicam had about one-half the ulcerogenic activity of that observed after oral administration (Schiantarelli & Cadel, 1981).

When piroxicam was given orally to fasted rats, the dose that induced gastric ulcers in 50% of rats was 6.2 mg/kg bw. The mean lesion score (a measure of ulceration intensity) was

9.5 $\pm$ 6.4 and 24.7 $\pm$ 10.5 for doses of 16 and 32 mg/kg bw piroxicam. No ulceration was seen at 2 mg/kg bw (Al-Ghamdi *et al.*, 1991).

In a study in which 62 dogs were given oral doses of 0.5–1.5 mg/kg bw piroxicam every 48 h, those receiving doses > 1 mg/kg bw had gastrointestinal irritation and ulceration after 7–120 days (median, 35 days) of treatment (Knapp *et al.*, 1992).

(b)   Effect on platelet function
Piroxicam inhibited collagen-induced platelet aggregation in dogs (Gaynor & Constantine, 1979).

(c)   Effect on articular cartilage and bone
Piroxicam administered to dogs at a dose of 0.3 mg/kg for eight weeks had no effect on articular cartilage structure (Mohr *et al.*, 1984). In a study of 12 rabbits given an oral dose of 10 mg/kg bw piroxicam per day for 12 weeks, a 3% decrease in tibial mineral content was seen, with 9% in controls, indicating that piroxicam may reduce the osteopenia caused by external fixation (Adolphson *et al.*, 1991).

(d)   Reproductive and developmental effects
Piroxicam has reportedly no dysmorphogenic, embryotoxic or teratogenic effects in rat or rabbit models when administered at concentrations of 2, 5 or 10 mg/kg bw (Perraud *et al.*, 1984). Also, no deleterious effect on mating or reproductive performance was observed when these doses were administered to animals before copulation.

Piroxicam does, however, affect parturition. Pregnant rats given piroxicam at 5 or 10 mg/kg bw on days 15–21 after insemination usually died. In surviving rats, labour was often prolonged, generally in relation to the dose and duration of piroxicam administered.

The numbers of live pups were reduced in rats treated with 5 or 10 mg/kg bw of piroxicam for at least five days, and the proportion of pups that were alive 24 h after birth was decreased as treatment was prolonged. Furthermore, lactation was impaired. Considerable maternal toxicity occurred 7–13 days after parturition in lactating female rats given 10 mg/kg bw of piroxicam (Perraud *et al.*, 1984).

These results cannot be extrapolated to pregnant or lactating women, since the standard daily dose of 20 mg piroxicam (equivalent to only about 0.3 mg/kg bw) is well below the threshold of 2 mg/kg bw at which any effect on gestation, labour or lactation was observed in rats (Brogden *et al.*, 1984).

(e)   Other toxic manifestations
Dogs given 1–1.5 mg/kg bw piroxicam orally every 48 h developed subclinical renal papillary necrosis (Knapp *et al.*, 1992). Intravenously administered piroxicam at cumulative doses up to 15 mg/kg bw had no significant effect on blood pressure or heart rate in experimental animals (Wiseman, 1978).

7.2   Genetic and related effects
7.2.1   Humans
Treatment with piroxicam at 20 mg/day for 14 days did not increase the frequency of sister chromatid exchange in peripheral blood lymphocytes (Kullich & Klein, 1986).

7.2.2   Experimental models
Piroxicam at 72 µg/ml increased the frequency of sister chromatid exchange in peripheral blood lymphocytes *in vitro* (Kullich *et al.*, 1990). It also enhanced the transformation of cultured rat tracheal cells (Steele *et al.*, 1990).

8. Summary of Data

8.1 Chemistry, occurrence and human exposure

Piroxicam, introduced in 1980, is a drug that has analgesic, anti-inflammatory and anti-pyretic properties. It has been widely and commonly used for the treatment of rheumatoid arthritis and osteoarthritis. Its use is in decline because of its gastrointestinal toxicity.

8.2 Metabolism and kinetics

Piroxicam is well absorbed after oral administration. Absorption is somewhat slower when the drug is administered rectally or with food. After initiation of therapy with the standard clinical dose of 20 mg/day, the plasma concentrations of piroxicam increase gradually and reach a steady state. This drug has a much longer half-life than other non-steroidal anti-inflammatory drugs.

Piroxicam is biotransformed in the liver to several metabolites. It is extensively bound to protein. It crosses the placenta and can be found in human milk.

8.3 Cancer-preventive effects
8.3.1 Humans

The only available data on the possible chemopreventive effects of piroxicam are from case series.

8.3.2 Experimental animals

The chemopreventive effects of piroxicam were studied in models of urinary bladder and lung carcinogenesis in mice and in models of colon, liver and mammary cancer in rats. In single studies in mice, piroxicam was preventive against urinary bladder and lung carcinogenesis. The preventive activity of piroxicam against adenomas in the intestine was demonstrated in mice predisposed to intestinal malignancy by a germ-line mutation in the *Apc* gene. Eight studies on colon cancer in rats indicate that piroxicam administered during the initiation and post-initiation phases of carcinogenesis reduces the incidence of both adenomas and adenocarcinomas. In rat models, piroxicam prevented liver carcinogenesis but had no preventive effect against mammary carcinogenesis.

8.3.3 Mechanism of action

The molecular mechanisms by which piroxicam exerts cancer preventive effects remain unclear; however, there is evidence that both prostaglandin-dependent and -independent events are involved, which result in suppression of cancer, regardless of whether piroxicam is administered early or many weeks after exposure to carcinogens.

8.4 Other beneficial effects

No data were available to the Working Group.

8.5 Carcinogenicity

No data were available to the Working Group.

8.6 Toxic effects
8.6.1 Humans

The spectrum of toxicity of piroxicam is similar to that of other aspirin-like non-steroidal anti-inflammatory agents, including gastrointestinal ulceration and bleeding, effects on blood pressure and skin rash.

8.6.2 Experimental animals

The most commonly observed toxic or adverse effect of piroxicam in experimental animals is ulceration and bleeding of the gastric and intestinal mucosa.

9. Recommendations for research

A central issue in relation to use of piroxicam as a cancer-preventive agent in humans is its toxic effects. Research on mitigating the toxicity of the drug while maintaining its cancer-preventive activity is recognized as a priority.

10. Evaluation[1]

10.1 Cancer-preventive activity
10.1.1 Humans
There is *inadequate evidence* in humans for the cancer-preventive activity of piroxicam.

10.1.2 Experimental animals
There is *sufficient evidence* for the cancer-preventive activity of piroxicam in experimental animals. This evaluation is based on models of cancers of the colon, urinary bladder, lung and liver.

10.2 Overall evaluation
Epidemiological studies in humans provide *inadequate evidence* for the cancer-preventive activity of piroxicam. In experimental animals, there is *sufficient evidence* that piroxicam prevents cancers at several sites. Because of the toxicity of piroxicam, however, it will probably have only limited use as a cancer-preventive agent in humans.

11. References

Abramson S.B., Leszczynska-Piziak, K.H. & Reibman, J. (1991) Non-steroidal anti-inflammatory drugs: Effects on a GTP-binding protein within the neutrophil plasma membrane. *Biochem. Pharmacol.*, 41, 567–573

Adolphson, P., Jonsson, U. & Dalen, N. (1991) Piroxicam-induced reduction in osteopenia after external fixation of rabbit tibia. *Acta orthoped. scand.*, 62, 363–366

Al-Ghamdi, M.S., Dissanayake, A.S., Cader, Z.A. & Jain, S. (1991) Tenoxicam-induced gastropathy in the rat: A comparison with piroxicam and diclofenac sodium and the inhibitory effects of ranitidine and sulcralfete. *J. int. med. Res.*, 19, 242–248

Ando, G.A. & Lombardino, J.G. (1983) Piroxicam — A literature review of new results from laboratory and clinical studies. *Eur. J. Rheumatol. Inflamm.*, 6, 3–23

Bayer, B., Kruth, H., Vaughn, M. & Breaven, M. (1979) Arrest of cultured cells in the G1 phase of the cell cyle by indomethacin. *J. Pharm. exp. Ther.*, 210, 106–111

Benveniste, C., Striberni, R. & Dayer, P. (1990) Indirect assessment of the enterohepatic recirculation of piroxicam and tenoxicam. *Eur. J. clin. Pharmacol.*, 38, 547–549

Blocкa, K.L.N., Richardson, C., Wallace, S.M., Ross, S.G. & Verbeeck, R.K. (1988) The effect of age on piroxicam disposition in rheumatoid arthritis. *J. Rheumatol.*, 15, 757–763

Boudinot, S.S., Funderburg, E.D. & Boudinot, F.D. (1993) Effects of age on the pharmacokinetics of piroxicam in rats. *J. pharm. Sci.*, 82, 254–257

Brogden, R.N., Heel, R.C., Speight, T.M. & Avery, G.S. (1981) Piroxicam: A review of its pharmacological properties and therapeutic efficacy. *Drugs*, 22, 165–187

Brogden, R.N., Heel, R.C., Speight, T.M. & Avery, G.S. (1984) Piroxicam: A reappraisal of its pharmacology and therapeutic efficacy. *Drugs*, 28, 292–323

Budavari, S., O'Neil, M.J., Smith, A., Heckelman, P.E. & Kinneary, J.F. (1996) *The Merck Index*, 12th Ed., Rahway, NJ, Merck & Co.

Caldwell, J.R. (1994) Comparison of the efficacy, safety, and pharmacokinetic profiles of extended-release ketoprofen and piroxicam in patients with rheumatoid arthritis. *Clin. Ther.*, 16, 225–235

Calin, A. (1988) Therapeutic focus: Piroxicam. *Br. J. clin. Pract.*, 42, 161–164

Campbell, A., Ferry, D.G. & Edwards, I.R. (1985) Pharmacokinetic projections for isoxicam and piroxicam in old and young subjects, *Br. J. Rheumatol.*, 24, 176–178

Darragh, A., Gordon, A.J., O'Bryne, H., Hobbs, D. & Casey, E. (1985) Single-dose and steady-state pharmacokinetics of piroxicam in elderly vs. young adults. *Eur. J. clin. Pharmacol.*, 28, 305–309

Dupont, D., Dayer, P., Balant, L., Gorgia, A. & Fabre, J. (1982) Inter- and intra-individual variations on the disposition of piroxicam. Pharmacokinetics in healthy men and the patient with renal insufficiency. *Pharm. Acta helv.*, 57, 20–26

---

[1] For definition of the italicized terms, see Preamble pp. 12–13

Earnest, D.L., Alberts, D.S., Hixson, L.J. & Meyskens, F.L. (1990) Dietary fiber or piroxicam as potential cancer prevention agents: Effects on rectal epithelial cell proliferation in humans at increased risk of colon cancer. In: Utsunomiya, J. & Lynch, H.T., eds, *Hereditary Colorectal Cancer*, Tokyo, Springer-Verlag, pp. 275–282

Earnest, D.L., Holubec, H., Wali, R.K., Jolley, C.S., Bissonette, M., Bhattacharyya, A.K., Roy, H., Khare, S. & Brasitus, T.A. (1994) Chemo-prevention of azoxymethane-induced colonic car-cinogenesis by supplemental dietary uroso-deoxycholic acid. *Cancer Res.*, **54**, 5071–5074

Edno, L., Bresolle, F., Combe, B. & Galtier, M. (1995) A reproducible and rapid HPLC assay for quantitation of piroxicam in plasma. *J. pharm. biomed. Anal.*, **13**, 785–789

Edwards, I.R., Ferry, D.G. & Campbell, A.J. (1985) Factors affecting the kinetics of 2 benzothiazine nonsteroidal anti-inflammatory medicines, pirox-icam and isoxicam. *Eur. J. clin. Pharmacol.*, **28**, 689–692

Emerit, I. & Cerutti, P.A. (1982) Tumor promoter phorbol 12-myristate 13-acetate induces a clasto-genic factor in human lymphocytes. *Proc. natl Acad. Sci. USA*, **79**, 7509–7513

Emerit, I., Levy, A. & Cerutti, P. (1983) Sup-pression of tumour promoter phorbol myristate acetate-induced chromosome breakage by antioxi-dants and inhibitors of arachidonic acid metabolism. *Mutat. Res.*, **110**, 327–335

Fernandez-Troconiz, J.I., Lopez-Bustamante, L.G. & Fos, D. (1991) Pharmacokinetics of piroxicam in rats. *Eur. J. Drug Metab. Pharmacokinet.*, **3**, 80–84

Ferry, D.G., Gazeley, L.R., Busby, W.J., Beasley, D.M., Edwards, I.R. & Campbell, A.J. (1990) Enhanced elimination of piroxicam by adminis-tration of activated charcoal and cholestyramine. *Eur J. clin. Pharmacol.*, **39**, 599–601

Fries, J.F., Williams, C.A. & Bloch, D.A. (1991) The relative toxicity of nonsteroidal antiinflammatory drugs. *Arthr. Rheum*, **34**, 1353–1360

Galbraith, E.A. & McKellar, Q.A. (1991) Pharma-cokinetics and pharmacodynamics of piroxicam in dogs. *Vet. Rec.*, **128**, 561–565

Garcia-Rodriguez, L.A., Walker, A.M. & Perez Gutthann, S. (1992) Nonsteroidal antiinflamma-tory drugs and gastrointestinal hospitalizations in Saskatchewan: A cohort study. *Epidemiology*, **3**, 337–342

Gaynor, B.J. & Constantine, J.W. (1979) Effect of piroxicam on platelet aggregation. *Experientia*, **35**, 797

Goodwin, J.S. (1984) Immunologic effects of non-steroidal antiinflammatory drugs. *Am. J. Med.*, **77**, 7–15

Gowen, G.F. (1996) Complete regression of villous adenomas of the colon using piroxicam, a nons-teroidal anti-inflammatory drug. *Dis. Colon Rectum*, **39**, 101–102

Guess, H.A., West, R., Strand, L.M., Helston, D., Lydick, E.G., Bergman, U. & Wolski, K. (1988) Fatal upper gastrointestinal hemorrhage or per-foration among users and nonusers of nons-teroidal anti-inflammatory drugs in Saskatchewan, Canada, 1983. *J. clin. Epidemiol.*, **41**, 35–45

Hanif, R., Pittas, A., Feng, Y., Koutsos, M.I., Qiao, L., Stiano-Coico, L., Shiff, S.I. & Riggs, B. (1996) Effects of nonsteroidal anti-inflammatory drugs on proliferation and on induction of apoptosis in colon cancer cells by a prostaglandin-independent pathway. *Biochem. Pharmacol.*, **52**, 237–245

Henry, D., Lim, L.L., Garcia Rodriguez, L.A., Perez Gutthann, S., Carson, J.L., Griffin, M., Savage, R., Logan, R., Monde, Y., Hawkey, C., Hill, S. & Fries, J.T. (1996) Variability in risk of gastrointestinal complications with individual non-steroidal anti-inflammatory drugs: Results of a collaborative meta-analysis. *Br. med. J.*, **312**, 1563–1566

Hial, V., De Mello, M.C.F., Horakova, Z. & Beaven, M.A. (1977) Antiproliferative activity of anti-inflammatory drugs in two mammalian cell cul-ture lines. *J. Pharmacol. exp. Ther.*, **202**, 446–454

Hixson, L.J., Earnest, D.L., Fennerty, M.B. & Sampliner, R.E. (1993) NSAID effect on sporadic colon polyps. *Am. J. Gastroenterol.*, **88**, 1652–1656

Hobbs, D.C. (1986) Piroxicam pharmacokinetics: Recent clinical results relating kinetics and plasma levels to age, sex, and adverse effects. *Am. J. Med.*, **81** (Suppl. 5B), 22–28

Hobbs, D.C. & Gordon, A.J. (1984) Absence of an effect of age on the pharmacokinetics of piroxi-cam. *R. Soc. Med. int. Congress Symp. Ser.*, **67**, 99–102

Hobbs, D.C. & Twomey, T.M. (1979) Piroxicam pharmacokinetics in man: Aspirin and antacid interaction studies. *J. clin. Pharmacol.*, 19, 270–281

Hobbs, D.C. & Twomey, T.M. (1981) Metabolism of piroxicam by laboratory animals. *Drug Metab. Disposition*, 9, 114–118

Hundal, O., Kvien, T.K., Glennas, A., Andrup, O., Karstensen, B., Thoen, J.E. & Rugstad, H.E. (1993) Total and free plasma and total synovial fluid piroxicam concentrations: Relationship to anti-inflammatory effect in patients with reactive arthritis and other arthritides. *Scand. J. Rheumatol.*, 22, 183–87

Ishizaki, T., Nomura, T. & Abe, T., (1979) Pharmacokinetics of piroxicam, a new non-steroidal anti-inflammatory agent, under fasting and postprandial states in man. *J. Pharmacokinet. Biopharmacol.*, 7, 369–381

Jacoby, R.F., Marshall, D.J., Newton, M.A., Novakovic, K., Tutsch, K., Cole, C.E., Lubet, R.A., Kelloff, G.J., Verma, A., Moser, A.R. & Dove, W.F. (1996) Chemoprevention of spontaneous instestinal adenomas in the *Apc*^Min mouse model by the nonsteroidal anti-inflammatory drug piroxicam. *Cancer Res.*, 56, 710–714

Jalbert, G. & Castonguay, A. (1992) Effects of NSAIDs on NNK-induced pulmonary and gastric tumorigenesis in A/J mice. *Cancer Lett.*, 66, 21–28

Johnson, A.G., Nguyen, T.V. & Day, R.O. (1994) Do nonsteroidal anti-inflammatory drugs affect blood pressure? A meta-analysis. *Ann. intern. Med.*, 121, 289–300

Kantor, H.S. & Hampton, M. (1978) Indomethacinin submicromolar concentrations inhibit cyclic AMP-dependent protein kinase. *Nature*, 276, 841–842

Kenzler, T.W. & Trush, M.A. (1984) Role of oxygen radicals in tumor promotion. *Environ. Mutag.*, 6, 593–616

Kikendale, J.W. (1991) Pill-induced esophageal injury. *Gastroenterol. Clin. North Am.*, 20, 835–846

Kitagawa, H. & Noguchi, M. (1994) Comparative effects of piroxicam and esculetin on incidence, proliferation, and cell kinetics of mammary carcinomas induced by 7,12-dimethylbenz[a]-anthracenene in rats on high- and low-fat diets. *Oncology*, 51, 401–410

Knapp, D.W., Richardson, R.C., Bottoms, G.D., Teclaw, R. & Chan, T.C.K. (1992) Phase I trial of piroxicam in 62 dogs bearing naturally occurring tumours. *Cancer Chemother. Pharmacol.*, 29, 214–218

Knapp, D.W., Chan, T.C.K., Kuczek, T. & Reagan, W.J. (1995) Evaluation of in vitro cytotoxicity of nonsteroidal anti-inflammatory drugs against canine tumour cells. *Am. J. vet. Res.*, 66, 801–805

Kulkarni, N., Zang, E., Kelloff, G. & Reddy, B.S. (1992) Effect of chemopreventative agents piroxicam and D,L-α-difluoromethylornithine on intermediate markers of colon cancer. *Carcinogenesis*, 13, 995–1000

Kullich, W. & Klein, G. (1986) Investigations of the influence of nonsteroidal antirheumatic drugs on the sister-chromatid exchange. *Mutat. Res.*, 174, 131–134

Kullich, W., Hermann, J. & Klein, G. (1990) [Cytogenetic studies of human lymphocytes under the influence of oxicams.] *Z. Rheumatol.*, 49, 77–81 (in German)

Kwo, P.Y. & Tremaine, W.J. (1995) Nonsteroidal anti-inflammatory drug induced enteropathy: Case discussion: A review of the literature. *Mayo Clin Proc.*, 70, 55–61

Langman, M.J.S., Weil, J., Wainwright, P., Lawson, D.H., Rawlins, M.D., Logan, R.F.A., Murphy, M., Vessey, M.P. & Colon-Jones, D.G. (1994) Risks of bleeding peptic ulcer associated with individual non-steroidal anti inflammatory drugs. *Lancet*, 343, 1075–1078

Laufen, H. & Leitold, M. (1986) The effect of activated charcoal on the bioavailability of piroxicam in man. *Int. J. clin. Pharmacol. Toxicol.*, 24, 48–52

Leemann, T.D., Transon, C., Bonnabry, P. & Dayer, P. (1993) A major role for cytochrome P-450_TB (CYP 2C subfamily) in the actions of non-steroidal anti-inflammatory drugs. *Drugs exp. clin. Res.*, 19, 189–195

Lombardino, J.G. & Wiseman, E.H. (1972) Sudoxicam and related N-heterocyclic carboxamides of 4-hydroxy-2H-1,2-benzothiazine–1,1-dioxide. Potent non-steroidal antiinflammatory agents. *J. med. Chem.*, 15, 848–489

Lombardino, J.G., Wiseman, E.H. & Chiaini, J. (1973) Potent antiinflammatory N-heterocyclic 3-carboxamides of 4-hydroxy-2-methyl-2H-1,2-benzothiazine-1,1 dioxide. J. med. Chem., 16, 493–496

Mäkelä, A.L., Olkkola, K.T., & Mattila, M.J. (1991) Steady-state pharmacokinetics of piroxicam in children with rheumatic diseases. Eur. J. clin. Pharmacol., 41, 79–81

Marnett, L.J. (1990) Prostaglandin synthase-mediated metabolism of carcinogens and a potential role for peroxyl radicals as reactive intermediates. Environ. Health Perspectives, 88, 5–12

Matsuhashi, N., Yamada, A., Hiraishi, M., Konishi, T., Minota, S., Saito, T., Sugano, K., Yozaki, Y., Mori, M. & Shiga, J. (1992) Multiple strictures of the small intestine after long-term non-steroidal anti-inflammatory drug therapy. Am. J. Gastroenterol., 87, 1183–1186

McLellan, E.A., Medline, A. & Bird, R.P. (1991) Sequential analysis of the growth and morphological characteristics of aberrant crypt foci: Putative preneoplastic lesions. Cancer Res., 51, 5270–5274

McManus, P., Primrose, J.G., Henry, D.A., Birkett, D.J., Lindner, J. & Day, R.O. (1996) Pattern of non-steroidal anti-inflammatory drug use in Australia 1990–1994. A report from the Drug Utilization Sub-committee of the Pharmaceutical Benefits Advisory Committee. Med. J. Aust., 164, 589–592

Mihalic, M., Hofman, H., Kajfez, F., Kuftinec, J., Blazevic, N. & Zinic, M. (1982) Physicochemical and analytical characteristics of piroxicam. Acta pharm. jugosl., 32, 13–20

Milligan, P.A. (1992) Determination of piroxicam and its major metabolites in the plasma, urine and bile of humans by high-performance liquid chromatography. J. Chromatogr. biomed. Appl., 114, 121–128

Mohr, W., Kirkpatrick, C.J., Wildfeuer, A. & Leitold, M. (1984) Effect of piroxicam on structure and function of joint cartilage. Inflammation, 8 (Suppl.), S139–S154

Moon, R.C., Kelloff, G.J., Detrisac, C.J., Steele, V.E., Thomas, C.F. & Sigman, C.C. (1993) Chemoprevention of OH-BBN-induced bladder cancer in mice by piroxicam. Carcinogenesis, 14, 1487–1489

Mukai, F.H. & Goldstein, B.D. (1976) Mutagenicity of malonaldehyde, a decomposition product of peroxidized polyunsaturated fatty acids. Science, 191, 868–869

Neupert, G. & Muller, P. (1975) Growth inhibition and morphological changes caused by indomethacin in fibroblasts in vitro. Exp. Pathol. Jena, 11, 1–9

Nigro, N.D., Bull, A.W. & Boyd, M.E. (1986) Inhibition of intestinal carcinogenesis in rats: Effect of difluoromethylornithine with piroxicam or fish oil. J. natl Cancer Inst., 77, 1309–1313

Noguchi, Y., Ishiko, J. & Ohtsuki, I. (1984) Comparative pharmacological profiles of piroxicam, indomethacin, phenylbutazone, diclofenac, ibuprofen and mefenamic acid. In: Richardson, R.G., ed., The Rheumatological Disease Process: Focus on Piroxicam, London, Royal Society of Medicine, pp. 69–75

Noguchi, M., Earashi, M., Minami, M., Miyazaki, I., Tanaka, M. & Sasaki, T. (1995) Effects of piroxicam and esculetin on the MDA-MB-231 human breast cancer cell line. Prostaglandins Leukotrienes Essential Fatty Acids, 53, 325–329

Olkkola, K.T., Brunetto, A.V. & Mattila, M.J., (1994) Pharmacokinetics of oxicam nonsteroidal anti-inflammatory agents. Clin. Pharmacokinet., 26, 107–120

Ostensen, M., Matheson, I. & Laufen, H. (1988) Piroxicam in breast milk after long-term treatment. Eur. J. clin. Pharmacol., 35, 567–569

Pereira, M.A., Barnes, L.H., Rassman, V.L., Kelloff, G.V. & Steele, V.E. (1994) Use of azoxymethane-induced foci of aberrant crypts in rat colon to identify potential cancer chemopreventive agents. Carcinogenesis, 15, 1049–1054

Pereira, M.A., Barnes, L.H., Steele, V.E., Kelloff, G.V. & Lubet, R.A. (1996) Piroxicam-induced regression of azoxymethane-induced aberrant crypt foci and prevention of colon cancer in rats. Carcinogenesis, 17, 373–376

Perraud, J., Stadler, J., Kessedijan, M.J. & Monro, A.M. (1984) Reproductive studies with the anti-inflammatory agent, piroxicam: Modification of classical protocols. Toxicology, 30, 59–63

Petry, T.W., Josephy, P.D., Pagano, D.A., Zeiger, E., Knecht, K.T. & Eling, T.E. (1989) Prostaglandin hydroperoxidase-dependent activation of heterocyclic aromatic amines. Carcinogenesis, 10, 2201–2207

Pollard, M. & Luckert, P.H (1984) Effects of piroxicam on primary intestinal tumors induced in
rats by N-methylnitrosourea. *Cancer Lett.*, **25**,
117–121

Pollard, M. & Luckert, P.H. (1989) Prevention and
treatment of primary intestinal tumors in rats by
piroxicam. *Cancer Res.*, **49**, 6471–6473

Pretlow, T.P., O'Riordan, M.A., Spancake, K.M. &
Pretlow, T.G. (1993) Two types of putative preneoplastic lesions identified in whole-mounts of
colon from F344 rats treated with carcinogen. *Am.
J. Pathol.*, **142**, 1695–1700

Rao, C.V., Tokumo, K., Rigotty, J., Zang, E., Kelloff,
G. & Reddy, B.S. (1991) Chemoprevention of
colon carcinogenesis by dietary administration of
piroxicam, α-difluoromethylornithine, 16α-fluo-
ro-5-androsten-17-one, and ellagic acid individually and in combination. *Cancer Res.*, **51**,
4528–4534

Reddy, B.S., Maruyama, H. & Kelloff, G. (1987)
Dose-related inhibition of colon carcinogenesis
by dietary piroxicam, a nonsteroidal antiinflammatory drug, during different stages of rat colon
tumour development. *Cancer Res.*, **47**, 5340–5346

Reddy, B.S., Nayini, J., Tokumo, K., Rigotty, J.,
Zang, E. & Kelloff, G. (1990) Chemoprevention of
colon carcinogenesis by concurrent administration
of piroxicam, a nonsteroidal antiinflammatory
drug with D,L-α-difluoromethylornithine, an
ornithine decarboxylase inhibitor, in diet. *Cancer
Res.*, **50**, 2562–2568

Reddy, B.S., Tokumo, K., Kulkarni, N., Aligia, C. &
Kelloff, G. (1992) Inhibition of colon carcinogenesis by prostaglandin synthesis inhibitors and
related compounds. *Carcinogenesis*, **13**, 1019–1023

Richardson, C.J., Blocka, K., Ross, S.G. & Verbeeck,
R.K. (1985) Effects of age and sex on piroxicam disposition. *Clin. pharmacol. Ther.*, **37**, 13–18

Richardson, C.J., Blocka, K.L. Ross, S.G. &
Verbeeck, P.K. (1987) Piroxicam and 5'-hydrox-
ypiroxicam kinetics following multiple dose
administration of piroxicam. *Eur. J. clin.
Pharmacol.*, **32**, 89–91

Rogers, H.J., Spector, R.G., Morrison, P.J. &
Bradbrook, I.D. (1981) Comparative steady-state
pharmacokinetic study of piroxicam and flurbiprofen in normal subjects. *Eur. J. Rheumatol.
Inflamm.*, **4**, 303–304

Rosenstein, E.D., Kunicka, J., Kramer, N. &
Goldstein, G. (1994) Modification of cytokine
production by piroxicam. *J. Rheumatol.*, **21**,
901–904

Roskos, L.K. & Boudinot, F.D. (1990) Effects of
dose and sex on the pharmacokinetics of piroxicam in the rat. *Biopharm. Drug Disposition*, **11**,
215–225

Roy, H.K., Bissonnette, M., Frawley, B.P., Wali,
R.K., Niedziela, S.M., Earnest, D. & Brasitus, T.A.,
(1995) Selective preservation of protein kinase C-
ζ in the chemoprevention of azoxymethane-
induced colonic tumors by piroxicam. *FEBS Lett.*,
366, 143–145

Rudy, A.C., Figueroa, N.L., Hall, S.D. & Brater D.C.
(1994) The pharmacokinetics of piroxicam in
elderly persons with and without renal impairment. *Br. J. clin Pharmacol.*, **37**, 1–5

Rugstad, H.E., Hundal, O., Holme, I., Herland,
O.B., Husby, G. & Giercksky K.E. (1986) Piroxicam
and naproxen plasma concentrations in patients
with osteoarthritis: Relation to age, sex, efficacy
and adverse events. *Clin. Rheumatol.*, **5**, 389–398

Schiantarelli, P. & Cadel, S. (1981) Piroxicam phar-
macologic activity and gastrointestinal damage by
oral and rectal route. Comparison with oral
indomethacin and phenylbutazone. *Arzneimittel.-
forsch.*, **31**, 87–91

Schiantarelli, P., Acerbi, D. & Bovis, G. (1981)
Some pharmacokinetic properties and bioavailability by oral and rectal route of piroxicam in rodents
and in man. *Arzneimittel.-forsch.*, **31**, 91–97

Shiff, S.J., Quao, L., Tsai, L. & Rigas, B. (1995)
Sulindac sulfide, an aspirin-like compound
inhibits proliferation, causes cell cycle quiescence
and induces apoptosis in HT-29 colon adenocarcinoma cells. *J. clin. Invest.*, **96**, 491–503

Shiff, S.J., Koutsos, M.I., Qiao, L. & Rigas, B. (1996)
Nonsteroidal antiinflammatory drugs inhibit the
proliferation of colon adenocarcinoma cells:
Effects on cell cyle and apoptosis. *Exp. Cell Res.*,
222, 179–188

Singh, J. Kulkarni, N., Kelloff, G. & Reddy, B.S.
(1994) Modulation of azoxymethane-induced
mutational activity of *ras* protooncogenes by
chemopreventative agents in colon carcinogenesis. *Carcinogenesis*, **15**, 1317–1323

Smalley, W.E., Griffin, M.R., Fought, R.L. & Ray, W.A. (1996) Excess costs for gastrointestinal disease among nonsteroidal anti-inflammatory drug users. *J. gen. intern. Med.*, **11**, 461–469

Smith, B.J., Curtis, J.F. & Eling, T.E. (1991) Bioactivation of xenobiotics by prostaglandin H synthase. *Chem.-biol. Interact.*, **79**, 245–264

Steele, V.E., Kelloff, G.J., Wilkinson, B.P. & Arnold, J.T. (1990) Inhibition of transformation in cultured rat tracheal epithelial cells by potential chemopreventive agents. *Cancer Res.*, **50**, 2068–2074

Tanaka, T., Kojima, T., Okumura, A., Sugie, S. & Mori, H. (1993) Inhibitory effect of the non-steroidal anti-inflammatory drugs, indomethacin and piroxicam on 2-acetylaminofluorene-induced hepatocarcinogenesis in male ACI/N rats. *Cancer Lett.*, **68**, 111–118

Tilstone, W.J., Lawson, D.H., Omara, F. & Cunningham, F. (1981) The steady-state pharmacokinetics of piroxicam: Effect of food and iron. *Eur. J. Rheumatol. Inflamm.*, **4**, 309–313

Tománková, H. & Sabartová, J. (1989) Determination of potential degradation products of piroxicam by HPTLC densiometry and HPLC. *Chromatographia*, **28**, 197–201

Trnavska, Z., Trnavsky, K. & Zlnay, D. (1984) Binding of piroxicam to synovial fluid and plasma proteins in patients with rheumatoid arthritis. *Eur. J. clin. Pharmacol.*, **26**, 457–461

Twomey, T.M., Bartolucci, S.R. & Hobbs, D.C. (1980) Analysis of piroxicam in plasma by high performance liquid chromatography. *J. Chromatogr.*, **183**, 104–108

Verbeeck, R.K., Richardson, C.J. & Blocka, K.L.N. (1986a) Clinical pharmacokinetics of piroxicam. *J. Rheumatol.*, **13**, 789–796

Verbeeck, R.K., Richardson, C.J. & Blocka, K.L.N. (1986b) Age and piroxicam disposition in rheumatoid arthritis (Abstract C2). *Clin. pharmacol. Ther.*, **29**, 233

Wali, R.K., Frawley, B.P., Hartmann, S., Roy, H.K., Khare, S., Scaglione-Seell, B.A., Earnest, D.L., Sitrin, M.D., Brasitus, T.A. & Bissonnette, M. (1995) Mechanism of action of chemoprotective ursodeoxycholate in the azoxymethane model of rat colonic carcinogenesis: Potential roles of proteinkinase C-α B$_{11}$ and ζ. *Cancer Res.*, **55**, 5257–5264

Wargovich, M.J., Chen, C.D., Harris, C., Yang, E. & Velasco, M. (1995) Inhibition of aberrant crypt growth by non-steroridal aniti-inflammatory agents and differentiation agents in the rat colon. *Int. J. Cancer*, **60**, 515–519

Weitberg, A.B. (1988) Effects of arachidonic acid and inhibitors of arachidonic acid metabolism on phagocyte-induced sister chromatid exchanges. *Clin. Genet.*, **34**, 288–292

Weitzman, S.A. & Stossel, T.P. (1981) Mutation caused by human phagocytes. *Science*, **212**, 546–547

Weitzman, S.A., Weitberg, A.B., Clark, E.P. & Stossel, T.P. (1985) Phagocytes as carcinogens: Malignant transformation produced by human neutrophils. *Science*, **227**, 1231–1233

Wessling, A., Boethius, G. & Sjoqvist, F. (1990) Prescription monitoring of drug dosages in the county of Jamtland and Sweden as a whole in 1976, 1982 and 1985. *Eur. J. clin. Pharmacol.*, **38**, 329–334

Whelton, A., Stout, R.L., Spilman, P.S. & Klassen, D.K. (1990) Renal effects of ibuprofen, piroxicam, and sulindac in patients with asymptomatic renal failure: A prospective, randomized, crossover comparison. *Ann. intern. Med.*, **112**, 568–576

Wiseman, E.H. (1978) *Review of Preclinical Studies with Piroxicam: Pharmacology, Pharmacokinetics and Toxicology* (Royal Society of Medicine International Congress Symposium Series No. 10), London, Royal Society of Medicine, pp. 11–13

Wiseman, E.H. & Hobbs, D.C. (1982) Review of pharmacokinetic studies with piroxicam. *Am. J. Med.*, **72**, 9–17

Wiseman, E.H., Lombardino, J.G., Holmes, C.L. & Perraud, J. (1982) Piroxicam. In: Goldberg, M.E., ed., *Pharmacological and Biochemical Properties of Drug Substances*, Vol. 3, Washington DC, American Pharmaceutical Association, pp. 324–346

Woolf, A.D., Rogers, H.J., Bradbrook, I.D. & Corbes, D. (1983) Pharmacokinetic observations on piroxicam in young adult, middle-aged and elderly patients. *Br. J. clin. Pharmacol.*, **16**, 433–437

Zhao, J., Leemann, T. & Dayer, P. (1992) In vitro oxidation of oxicam NSAIDs by a human liver cytochrome P450. *Life Sci.*, **51**, 575–581

Indomethacin

1. Chemical and Physical Characteristics

1.1 Name

Chemical Abstracts Services Registry Number
53-86-1

UPAC Systematic Chemical Name
1-(4-Chlorobenzoyl)-5-methoxy-2-methyl-1*H*-indole-3-acetic acid

Synonyms
1-(4-Chlorobenzoyl)-5-methoxy-2-methylindo-lo-3-acetic acid; 1-(*p*-chlorobenzoyl)-5-meth-oxy-2-methyl-3-indolylacetic acid; 1-(*p*-chloro-benzoyl)-5-methoxy-2-methylindole-3 acetic acid

1.2 Structural and molecular formulae and relative molecular mass

$C_{19}H_{16}ClNO_4$ Relative molecular mass: 357.81

1.3 Physical and chemical properties

From Budavari *et al.* (1996) and Reynolds and Prasad (1982), unless otherwise stated.

Description
White to yellow–tan, odourless crystalline powder

Melting-point
Indomethacin exhibits polymorphism, with a melting-point of ~155 °C for one form and ~162 °C for the other.

Solubility
Soluble in ether, acetone and castor oil; practically insoluble in water

Spectroscopy data
Absorbance spectrum in ethanol has maxima at 230, 260 and 319 nm

Stability
Stable in neutral or slightly acid media; decomposed by strong alkali.

Impurities
α–Substituted monoglyceryl esters of 4-chlorobenzoic acid and indomethacin are formed through chemical interaction of the drug with glycerin present in suppositories. Only trace or undetectable amounts of these and other impurities were recorded after analysis of bulk samples or after formulation as capsules (Curran *et al.*, 1980).

1.4 Technical products

Amuno, Argun, Artracin, Artrinovo, Artrivia, Bonidon, Catlep, Chibro-Amuno, Chrono-Indocid-75, Confortid, Dolcidium-PL, Dolovin, Durametacin, Elmetacin, Idomethine, Imbrilon, Inacid, Indacin, Indocid, Indocil, Indocin, Indocollyre, Indomecol, Indomed, Indomee, Indometacin, Indometacine, Indomethacine, Indomethine, Indomod, Indo-Phlogont, Indoptic, Indorektal, Indo-Rectalmin, Indo-Tablinen, Indoxen, Indren, Inflazon, Infrocin, Inteban SP, Lausit, Metacen, Metastril, Methazine, Metindal, Mezolin, Mikametan, Mobilan, Reumacide, Rheumacin LA, Sadoreum, Tannex, Vonum.

2. Occurrence, Production, Use, Analysis and Human Exposure

2.1 Occurrence

Indomethacin is not known to occur naturally.

2.2 Production

Indomethacin may be synthesized by several routes (Shen & Winter, 1977), which are generally modifications of the original procedure (Shen *et al.*, 1963) in which 5-methoxy-2-methylindole-3-acetic acid was used as the starting material. Technical details about its current commercial production were not available to the Working Group.

2.3 Use

The only known use of indomethacin is as a pharmaceutical agent. The drug is formulated as capsules or suppositories (Watanabe *et al.*, 1993). Experimental formulations of the drug are being investigated (Tsuji *et al.*, 1993). Indomethacin has analgesic, anti-inflammatory and anti-pyretic properties and is used extensively in the treatment of rheumatic disorders at doses of 25 mg and 50 mg two to four times daily up to 100–200 mg daily (Waller, 1983).

2.4 Analysis

In general, methods for the analysis of indomethacin are restricted to its determination in pharmaceutical preparations and in body fluids. Most of the methods involve high-performance liquid chromatography. Indomethacin can be determined in pharmaceutical preparations in the presence of other non-steroidal anti-inflammatory drugs (NSAIDs) (Rau *et al.*, 1991). Methods exist for its determination in plasma and urine (Hubert & Crommen, 1990; Singh *et al.*, 1991; Johnson & Ray, 1992).

2.5 Human exposure

Indomethacin is a commonly used NSAID (Griffin *et al.*, 1991; Langman *et al.*, 1994). Since its introduction in 1962, it has been used extensively for the treatment of acute and chronic arthritis and other inflammatory disorders. Although indomethacin is normally taken by mouth, it can be administered rectally in order to reduce the occurrence of gastrointestinal side-effects. This approach has been investigated in persons with familial adenomatous polyposis and remaining rectal segments (Hirata *et al.*, 1994; Hirota *et al.*, 1996). When it is used for the treatment of rheumatological disease, similar clinical benefits are seen with oral and rectal doses of indomethacin, although most patients prefer the oral route of administration (Huskisson *et al.*, 1970).

Indomethacin is currently available in five dosage formulations: a sterile solution containing 1 mg for intravenous administration, a conventional gelatin capsule, (25 or 50 mg) for oral administration, a 75-mg sustained release capsule; an oral suspension containing 25 mg indomethacin per 5 ml and a 50-mg suppository for rectal use (Billups & Billups, 1992).

3. Metabolism, Kinetics and Genetic Variation

3.1 Human studies

3.1.1 Metabolism

In adults, indomethacin undergoes extensive hepatic biodegradation by *O*-demethylation and *N*-deacylation reactions (Duggan *et al.*, 1972), and only a small amount is excreted in the urine unchanged (Helleberg, 1981) (Fig. 1). These metabolites lack anti-inflammatory activity (Shen, 1965).

Indomethacin is demethylated to form demethylindomethacin through the cytochrome P450 microsomal pathway (Duggan *et al.*, 1972). Leemann *et al.* (1993) showed in human liver microsomes, that a single cytochrome P450 monooxygenase plays a critical role in the elimination of indomethacin by the liver. Analysis of inhibition by indomethacin in comparison with other of NSAIDs suggested that a common isoenzyme, CYP2C9, catalyses oxidation of NSAIDS by human liver.

3.1.2 Pharmacokinetics

The pharmacokinetics of indomethacin in humans has been extensively studied and reviewed (Alvan *et al.*, 1975; Helleberg, 1981; Waller, 1983; Yeh, 1985).

(a) Absorption

Conventional indomethacin capsules are readily and completely absorbed after oral administration, with an estimated mean bioavailability of 85–122% (Duggan *et al.*, 1972; Alvan *et al.*, 1975; Kwan *et al.*, 1976; Yeh, 1985). Concomitant ingestion of foods may affect the absorption of indomethacin: total absorption is greater and the rate of absorption is generally quicker in fasting than in non-fasting subjects when delays of up to 4 h have been reported (Arnold & Brynger, 1970; Turakka & Airaksinen, 1974). Absorption of indomethacin from

Figure 1. 1-(p-Chlorobenzyl)-5-methoxy-2-methylindole-3-acetic acid (indomethacin) and its main metabolites

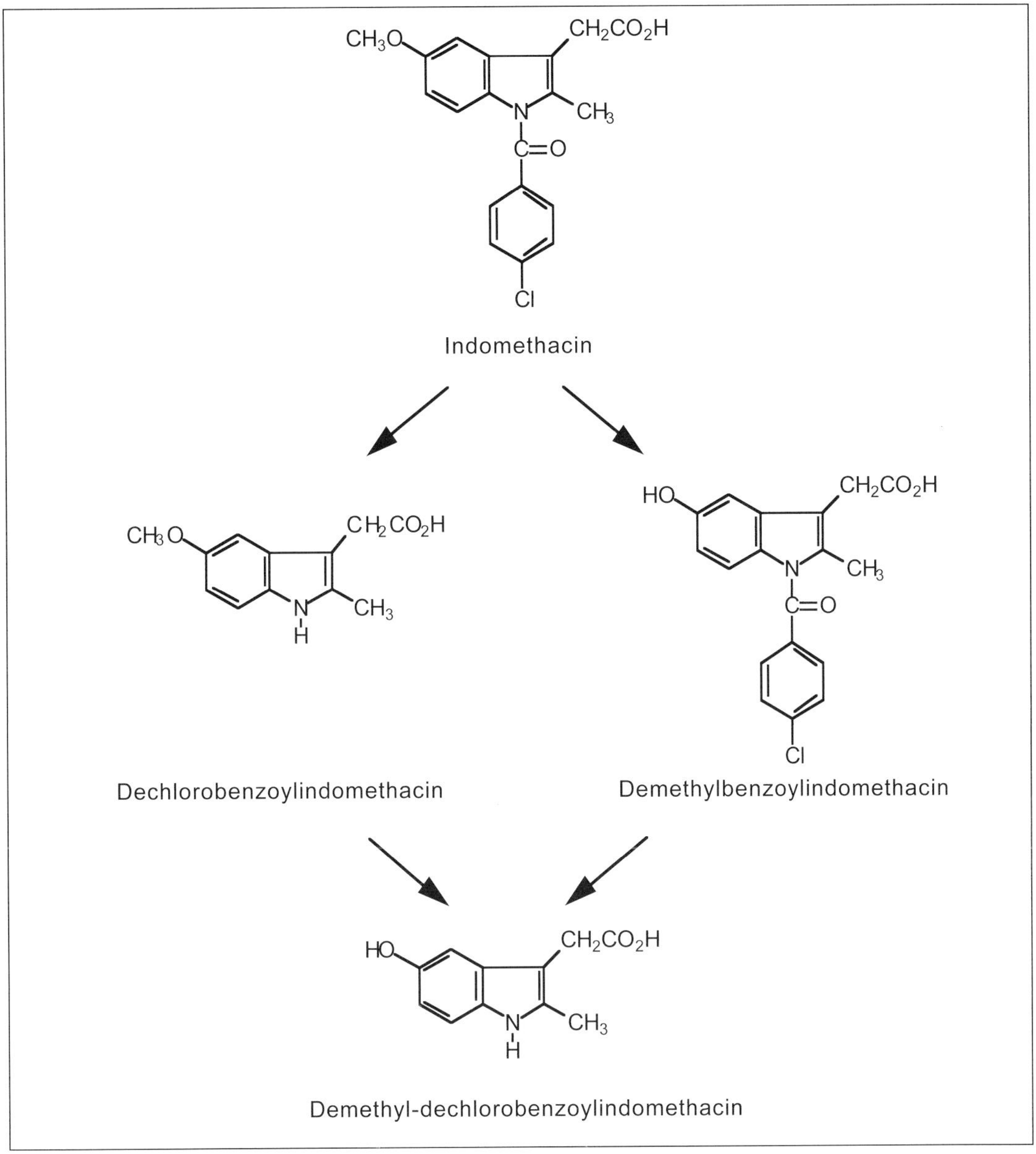

Indomethacin

Dechlorobenzoylindomethacin

Demethylbenzoylindomethacin

Demethyl-dechlorobenzoylindomethacin

50-mg gelatin capsules was nearly twice as long when taken with food than in fasting subjects (Rothermich, 1966; Emori *et al.*, 1976). Diets high in carbohydrates appear to delay absorption most, followed by high-protein and high-lipid diets (Wallusch *et al.*, 1978). The presence of antacids or antidiarrhoeal medications may also decrease the rate of absorption of orally administered indomethacin (Rothermich, 1966; Emori *et al.*, 1976). The overall bioavailability of indomethacin, is not however, influenced by the presence of food (Kwan *et al.*, 1976; Wallusch *et al.*, 1978), and similar values are reported in fasting and non-fasting subjects (Alvan *et al.*, 1975). Despite the possible effects on absorption, indomethacin and other NSAIDs are commonly taken with meals or antacids in order to lessen the gastric side-effects.

Comparisons of the bioavailability and pharmacokinetic profiles of sustained-release indomethacin and conventional capsules have been reported (Helleberg, 1981; Yeh *et al.*, 1982; Waller, 1983). The 75-mg sustained-release capsule contains 25 mg of an immediate-release fraction, and the remaining 50 mg are polymer-coated to ensure gradual release. The formulation is administered once or twice daily, as opposed to the less convenient three times daily dosing regime with conventional 25- or 50-mg capsules.

Use of the sustained-release formulation is associated with a slower rate of absorption and lower peak plasma concentrations, although the overall plasma concentration–time relationship is generally comparable to that of the conventional oral formulation. Waller (1983) reported peak plasma times of 2.0 ± 0.9 h with the sustained-release capsule and 1.0 ± 0.4 h with conventional capsules, and a 55% reduction in peak plasma concentrations. Schoog *et al.* (1981), however, in a cross-over study, found significant differences in the plasma concentration-time curves with 75-mg sustained-release and conventional capsules. The greatest differences were seen between 1 and 5 h after administration.

The peak plasma levels associated with rectal administration are generally lower than those with orally administered indomethacin capsules and are achieved earlier (Holt & Hawkins, 1965), although at least one author has disagreed on this point (Alvan *et al.*, 1975). Studies with volunteers showed that the maximal plasma concentrations of indomethacin after administration of suppositories (50–100 mg) were achieved within 60–80 min, with mean peak plasma concentrations of 1.5–2.8 µg/ml (Holt & Hawkins, 1965; Arnold & Brynger, 1970; Kwan *et al.*, 1976). The overall bioavailability of rectally delivered indomethacin is similar to that of orally administered ormulations, with values ranging from 80 to 100% (Alvan *et al.* 1975; Kwan *et al.*, 1976).

Circadian variation in the pharmacokinetics of indomethacin has been described (Clench *et al.*, 1981; Aronson *et al.*, 1993). In nine healthy volunteers, absorption of a single 100-mg oral dose of indomethacin was more rapid when it was taken at 7:00 or 11:00 h than at 15:00, 19:00 or 23:00 h (Clench *et al.*, 1981). Diurnal variations in the rate of gastric emptying may partially explain this effect, since the rate is significantly slower in the evening. Similarly, the transport mechanisms in the small bowel, where most indomethacin is absorbed, may be more efficient before midday. No diurnal variation was reported after rectal administration of a 100-mg suppository (Taggart *et al.*, 1987).

(b)   Distribution

Like most other acidic NSAIDs, indomethacin readily binds to human serum albumin and other plasma proteins (Hucker *et al.*, 1966; Hultmark *et al.*, 1975; Rane *et al.*, 1978; Zini *et al.*, 1979), with binding affinities similar to those of other NSAIDs (Hultmark *et al.*, 1975). The lack of binding to erythrocytes reported in earlier studies (McArthur *et al.*, 1971) was later disproved (Bruguerolle *et al.*, 1986), when a more sensitive detection technique was used. In this study, uptake of indomethacin by erythrocytes represented approximately 2.4% of the total blood indomethacin levels in both young and older volunteers.

The numbers of indomethacin-binding sites on human serum albumin have been calculated to be between four (Hultmark *et al.*, 1975) and 15 (Hvidberg *et al.*, 1972), with an association constant of 0.86×10^3 litre/mol (Hvidberg *et al.*, 1972), and the actual percentage of indomethacin bound to albumin has been reported to range from 92 to 99% (Mason & McQueen, 1974; Hultmark *et al.*, 1975). All of the studies showed consistent binding over the therapeutic dose range of indomethacin and at higher levels (Hucker *et al.*, 1966; Hvidberg *et al.*, 1972; Mason & McQueen, 1974; Hultmark *et al.*, 1975). At therapeutic doses, binding to albumin is independent of concentration (Rane *et al.*, 1978).

Binding of indomethacin is not altered in uraemic patients with chronic renal failure

(Sjoholm *et al.*, 1976); however, decreased protein binding has been observed in cancer patients with active disease, probably reflecting lower serum albumin levels in those patients (Raveendran *et al.*, 1992).

Indomethacin readily penetrates body tissues (Hucker *et al.*, 1966; Kohler *et al.*, 1981) and has been recovered in synovial fluid from rheumatoid arthritis patients (Caruso, 1971; Emori *et al.*, 1973) and in fatty tissue, muscle and bone (Kohler *et al.*, 1981). Indomethacin enters the synovial fluid slowly and exceeds plasma levels after 5 h (Emori *et al.*, 1973). Only trace amounts of indomethacin have been detected in saliva (Rothermich, 1971) and in brain tissue (Hucker *et al.*, 1966). Indomethacin readily crosses the human placenta (Traeger *et al.*, 1973; Moise *et al.*, 1990) and is distributed in fetal tissues (Parks *et al.*, 1977). Placental transfer is independent of gestational age (Moise *et al.*, 1990).

In women given indomethacin for pain relief, *post partum* negligible levels of indomethacin have been recovered from breast milk (Takyi, 1970; Lebedevs *et al.*, 1991). In one study, six of seven breast-fed infants had plasma indomethacin concentrations of < 20 µg/ml, below the detection limit of the assay, after maternal doses of 0.94–4.3 mg/kg bw per day (Lebedevs *et al.*, 1991). Since the average milk:plasma ratio of indomethacin in subjects with measurable levels was only 0.37, it was concluded that only small amounts of indomethacin could be ingested via breast milk.

(c)   Elimination

Most administered indomethacin is excreted in the urine either unchanged or in the form of conjugated and unconjugated metabolites which include demethylindomethacin, dechlorobenzoylindomethacin and demethyldechlorobenzoylindomethacin (Duggan *et al.*, 1972). After oral administration, these metabolites represent 19–42% of the dose recovered in faeces, whereas an average of nearly 60% appears in the urine as the parent drug and its glucuronide conjugates (Hucker *et al.*, 1966; Duggan *et al.*, 1972; Kwan *et al.*, 1976). In these studies, the amount of unchanged indomethacin in urine

was between less than 5% and up to 18%. No differences in the excretion pattern of indomethacin or its metabolites were found after oral, rectal or intravenous administration (Kwan *et al.*, 1976).

Indomethacin is also eliminated in bile, where it undergoes extensive enterohepatic recycling (Kwan *et al.*, 1978). Once discharged into the bile, indomethacin is subsequently hydrolysed and re-enters the circulation through the gastrointestinal tract (Hucker *et al.*, 1966). It has been estimated that 24–115% of a given dose is reabsorbed into the circulation by this mechanism (Kwan *et al.*, 1976). The sporadic nature of biliary clearance may be responsible for the wide fluctuations in plasma indomethacin levels and plasma half-lives reported in the literature. The lack of correlation between plasma indomethacin levels and clinical therapeutic effects further supports this theory. Biliary recycling and the presence of unchanged indomethacin in bile may con-tribute to the production of intestinal lesions in some patients.

A two-compartment, open kinetic model has been proposed to describe the pharmacokinetic profiles of individuals participating in single-dose studies and patients undergoing long-term therapy. Dissolution of indomethacin from the plasma follows a biexponential pattern, with an initial rapid phase lasting up to 8 h followed by a slower secondary phase lasting 2.6–11 h (Alvan *et al.*, 1975).

Linear pharmacokinetics have been demonstrated with oral doses of 25–75 mg, with typical peak plasma concentrations of 1.1–4.4 µg/ml within 30–60 min (Emori *et al.*, 1976). The half-life in plasma is extremely variable, ranging from 2 to 11 h, perhaps because of enterohepatic cycling (Flower *et al.*, 1985). Comparable measurements of the area under the curve of plasma concentration–time were observed in subjects given 25 mg indomethacin orally or intravenously (Alvan *et al.*, 1975). Marked variability in the peak plasma concentration between subjects and in the same subjects tested on three separate occasions were reported by Emori *et al.* (1976), while few differences in plasma levels have been noted by other investigators (Alvan *et al.*, 1975).

No evidence of altered elimination patterns after long-term treatment with indomethacin have been documented.

(d)   Effects of age

The total plasma clearance rates of indomethacin in adults are highly variable, ranging from 44 to 109 ml/h per kg bw (Alvan *et al.*, 1975); in premature infants, a substantially lower clearance rate of 7.6 ± 3.0 ml/h per kg bw has been reported after intravenous administration (Vert *et al.*, 1980). In children aged one year, the total clearance of indomethacin is substantially higher, at about 192 ml/h per kg bw (Olkkola *et al.*, 1989). Indomethacin has been widely used as a non-surgical treatment of patent ductus arteriosus in premature infants, at oral doses of 0.1–0.3 mg/kg bw. Plasma half-lives are considerably longer in premature newborns (11–90 h) than in adults, and wide variation is seen (Bhat *et al.*, 1979, 1980; Bianchetti *et al.*, 1980).

Some investigators have postulated that the plasma half-life is inversely correlated with gestational age (Evans *et al.*, 1979; Vert *et al.*, 1980). Decreased renal function or lower hepatic metabolism may explain the lower rate of elimination of indomethacin in premature infants. Alternatively, the differences related in half-life related to gestational age may correspond to maturation of drug metabolism systems (Evans *et al.*, 1981).

The pharmacokinetics of indomethacin in the elderly population has been described (Traeger *et al.*, 1973; Kunze *et al.*, 1974; McElnay *et al.*, 1992). No differences in absorption rate or peak plasma levels were seen between young volunteers and groups of healthy elderly subjects (McElnay *et al.*, 1992). One study, however, reported twofold higher levels in elderly patients than in young adults after a single 75-mg dose of indomethacin (Bruguerolle *et al.*, 1986), although the elimination rate of indomethacin was the same in the two groups. The clinical relevance of these data may be that untoward effects after indomethacin administration occur more frequently in patients over 60 years of age (Castleden & Pickles, 1988).

Age does not appear to influence the protein-binding capacity of indomethacin. After oral administration, more than 90% of a dose of indomethacin is bound to protein (Hultmark *et al.*, 1975) comparable values were found in premature newborns (Evans *et al.*, 1979), full-term infants (Friedman *et al.*, 1978) and the elderly (Bruguerolle *et al.*, 1986).

Some age-related alterations in excretion capacity have been noted. In one study, lower levels of unchanged indomethacin were recovered with increasing age, which were correlated with a reduction in renal function (Kunze *et al.*, 1974). The elimination kinetics in this group, were not affected, however. A 40% reduction in renal clearance of indomethacin was observed in a study of 12 healthy 36–50-year-old subjects in comparison with 15 healthy 19–34-year-old subjects (Wichlinski *et al.*, 1983). This study suggests that a reduction in renal clearance may accompany advancing age.

3.2   Experimental models

As in humans, biodegradation of indomethacin in most animal species involves deacylation and demethylation pathways (Harman *et al.*, 1964; Hucker *et al.*, 1966). While there is no evidence of demethylation reactions or metabolites in hamsters, both metabolic pathways have been shown in the rats, rabbits and guinea-pigs (Rowe & Carless, 1982). In monkeys, extensive metabolism of indomethacin into dechlorobenzoylindomethacin and excretion in the urine have been reported, whereas in rats indomethacin is metabolized principally into demethylindomethacin (Yesair *et al.*, 1970a).

Interspecies variations in the metabolism of drugs and in their binding affinities to plasma protein must be considered before data on the pharmacokinetics of indomethacin can be extrapolated. Marked differences in the absorption, plasma half-life, metabolism and excretion rate of indomethacin have been documented among animal species and in comparison with humans (Yesair *et al.*, 1970a).The plasma concentration is also influenced by the route of administration (Hucker *et al.*, 1966).

In an early study, higher plasma levels of ^{14}C-indomethacin were reported in dogs and rats than in rhesus monkeys or guinea-pigs after intravenous administration. The tissue distribution of the radiolabel was highest in guinea-pigs, which had a faster plasma clearance rate than the other species. The plasma half-lives of indomethacin were several hours in rats and minutes in monkeys and dogs (Hucker et al., 1966). In horses, a peak plasma level of about 125 ng/ml was seen within 1 h after a 250-mg oral dose of indomethacin (Phillips et al., 1980).

In horses given 100 mg indomethacin rectally, maximal urinary levels were observed 2 h later, with peak concentrations of 19–81 µg/ml (Delbeke et al., 1991). In rabbits, peak plasma levels appeared within 30–45 min after rectal administration of a 100-mg indomethacin suppository (Kuroda et al., 1983), comparable to the time in humans. In beagle dogs, gastric acidity influenced the absorption rate of a sustained-release indomethacin capsule: low gastric acid resulted in faster absorption, but bioavailability was reduced (Yamada et al., 1990).

As in humans, placental transfer of indomethacin has been documented. When given during late gestation, indomethacin readily crosses the placenta in rats (Sharpe et al., 1975), rabbits (Parks et al., 1977) and sheep (Levin et al., 1979; Anderson et al., 1980). In one study in rats, the maternal indomethacin plasma levels were 37–66 times higher than fetal levels when the drug was administered on days 11 and 12 of gestation, whereas only a three- to fourfold difference between maternal and fetal values was seen when it was given on day 21 (Klein et al., 1981). Progressive decreases in the maternal:fetal ratio of the concentration of indomethacin plasma with advancing gestational age have been confirmed in rats (Momma & Takao, 1987). In other animal models, such as the rabbit and sheep, fetal plasma levels exceeded maternal levels when the drug was given late in gestation (Parks et al., 1977; Harris & Van Petten, 1981).

Differences in the protein binding capacity of maternal and fetal blood may affect indomethacin transport throughout gestation. In rabbits, Parks et al. (1977) noted that the fetal levels of indomethacin increased as the maternal levels increased and there was always a substantial difference between the maternal and fetal concentrations, probably due to protein binding of indomethacin. Anderson et al. (1980)

found no difference in maternal and fetal plasma protein binding affinity in sheep. Evidence to support the theory that the plasma half-life of indomethacin is inversely correlated with gestational age was provided in a study in neonatal rats, in which an age-related increase in cytochrome P450 activity was reported (Clozel et al., 1986).

The increase in microsomal activity may be partially explained by an increased affinity of the enzyme for its substrate with age. An alternative theory is that the low affinity in the neonate is due to the presence of competitive inhibitors, as has been shown in neonatal rabbit liver (Evans et al., 1981).

The kidneys play a significant role in the elimination of indomethacin in some animal species, except dogs. In dogs, at least 80% of an administered dose of ^{14}C-indomethacin was excreted in the faeces as the parent compound, and large amounts were also present in bile. It was estimated that about 50% of the amount of indomethacin excreted in bile is reabsorbed by the intestines in dogs (Hucker et al., 1966). Enterohepatic recycling has been described in both rats (Hucker et al., 1966; Yesair et al., 1970a,b) and monkeys (Yesair et al., 1970a). Most excreted indomethacin is reabsorbed slowly by the intestine in rats (Hucker et al., 1966; Liss et al., 1968; Yesair et al., 1970b) and is thought to be involved in the occurrence of intestinal lesions in this species (Baer et al., 1974).

3.3 Genetic variation

No genetic variation in the pharmacokinetics of indomethacin has been described among different population groups.

4. Cancer-preventive Effects

4.1 Human studies
4.1.1 Studies of cancer occurrence

(a) Colorectal cancer
There are no studies that specifically address the risk for colorectal cancer after use of indomethacin alone. Studies that included separate estimates of NSAIDs other than aspirin and those in which aspirin and other NSAIDs were considered together are summarized in the chapter on aspirin.

(b)   Breast cancer

Indomethacin was included in a hypothesis-generating cohort study designed to screen 215 drugs for possible carcinogenicity, which covered more than 140 000 subscribers enrolled in July 1969 to August 1973 in a prepaid medical care programme in northern California (USA). Computer records of persons to whom at least one drug prescription had been dispensed were linked to cancer records from hospitals and the local cancer registry. The observed numbers of cancers were compared with expected numbers, standardized for age and sex, for the entire cohort. Three publications summarized the findings for follow-up periods of up to seven years (Friedman & Ury, 1980), nine years (Friedman & Ury, 1983) and 15 years (Selby *et al.*, 1989). Among 4867 persons who received indomethacin, there was a significant ($p < 0.01$) deficit of breast cancer (12 observed, 26 expected) in the seven-year follow-up. No negative or positive association with use of indomethacin was reported in the 15-year follow-up.

4.1.2   Studies of other relevant end-points

(a)   Sporadic adenomatous polyps in the colon

There are no controlled studies of the risk for sporadic adenomatous polyps of the colon and use of indomethacin alone. Studies of combined non-aspirin NSAIDs in this respect are summarized in the chapter on aspirin.

(b)   Adenomatous polyps in patients with familial adenomatous polyposis

Hirata *et al.* (1994) reported on two patients with familial adenomatous polyposis who had residual polyps in the rectal remnant after undergoing total colectomy and ileoproctoscopy. They were treated with 50-mg indomethacin suppositories once or twice daily and showed regression of polyps (both size and numbers) within three months. In one patient, polyps recurred after cessation of therapy and regressed again with reinstitution.

Eight patients with familial adenomatous polyposis who had undergone total colectomy with ileorectal anastomosis were given a 50-mg indomethacin suppository once or twice daily for four or eight weeks (Hirota *et al.*, 1996). In

six patients, the polyps regressed, but recurred on cessation of therapy.

(c)   Case studies of treatment for desmoid tumours

Waddell and Gerner (1980) reported three patients with refractory desmoid tumours who responded to indomethacin. Waddell *et al.* (1983) described two additional patients with desmoid tumours, one of whom responded to indomethacin. Klein *et al.* (1987) reported six patients treated with indomethacin for these tumours: one regressed completely, but no response was seen in the other five patients. Of four patients with desmoid tumours treated by Tsukada *et al.* (1992), one had complete remission of the tumour, but the others did not respond. Itoh *et al.* (1988) reported one patient with recurrent abdominal desmoid tumours who did not respond to indomethacin. Thus, of 16 patients reported, six responded to indomethacin.

4.2   Experimental models
4.2.1   Experimental animals

(a)   Colon

Studies on the prevention of colon carcinogenesis in rats treated with indomethacin are summarized in Table 1.

Eight-week-old male Donryu rats received intraperitoneal injections of 20 mg/kg bw methylazoxymethanol acetate once a week for six weeks. One group of rats received an intrarectal instillation of a 1-ml solution of indomethacin (macrogolum powder; 7.5 mg/kg bw) once a week on weeks 27, 28 and 29. One control group received instillations of 1.0 ml water (vehicle control), and another was untreated. Colon tumours were counted in week 30. The incidence of colon tumours in indomethacin-treated rats (15/30) was significantly lower than that in the vehicle control group (19/23) and in the untreated controls (26/30) ($p < 0.05$). Indomethacin treatment reduced the mean number of colon tumours per tumour-bearing rat (2.0) from that in the vehicle control group (3.5) and in untreated controls (3.3) ($p < 0.05$). Treatment also reduced the incidence of small intestine adenocarcinomas

Table 1. Prevention of colon tumourigenesis by indomethacin

Species, strain, sex	No. of animals/group	Carcinogen (dose)	Indomethacin Dose (route)	Treatment relative to carcinogen	Preventive efficacy	Reference
Rat, Donryu, male	30	MAM (20 mg/kg bw)	7.5 mg/kg bw (intrarectally)	After	Incidence, 42% ($p < 0.05$); multiplicity, 39%	Kudo et al. (1980)
Rat, Sprague-Dawley male	10	DMH (30 mg/kg bw)	20 mg/l (water)	3 d after 12 d after 35 d after	Multiplicity, 83% ($p < 0.01$) Multiplicity, 65% ($p < 0.01$) Multiplicity, 77% ($p < 0.01$)	Pollard & Luckert (1980)
			0.2 mg/kg bw (gavage)	After	Multiplicity, 48% (NS)	
Rat, Sprague-Dawley, male	7/8	NDMA-OAc (13 mg/kg bw)	20 mg/l (water)	After	Multiplicity, 90% ($p < 0.05$)	Pollard & Luckert (1981a)
Rat, Lobund Sprague-Dawley, male	9	DMH (30 mg/kg bw)	20 mg/l (water)	After	Incidence, 75% ($p < 0.01$); multiplicity, 83% ($p = 0.01$)	Pollard & Luckert (1981b)
	7	MAM (30 mg/kg bw)	20 mg/l (water)	After	Incidence, 81% ($p < 0.01$); multiplicity, 89% ($p < 0.01$)	
Rat, F344, female	29	MNU (2 mg/rat)	2.5 mg/kg (intraperitoneal)	After	Incidence, 55% ($p < 0.002$); multiplicity, 59% ($p < 0.02$)	Narisawa et al. (1981)
Rat, F344, female	30	MNU (2 mg/rat)	20 ppm (water)	After	Incidence, 75% ($p < 0.01$); multiplicity, 78% ($p < 0.01$)	Narisawa et al. (1982)
	30		10 ppm (water)	After	Incidence, 79% ($p < 0.01$); multiplicity, 80% ($p < 0.01$)	
Rat, F344, female	27 27 27	MNU (3 × 4 mg/rat)	10 ppm (water)	During 2–30 weeks 11 weeks after	Incidence, 58% ($p < 0.05$) Incidence 76% ($p < 0.01$) None	Narisawa et al. (1983)
Rat, Lobund Sprague-Dawley, male	10–27	DMH (2 × 30 mg/kg bw) MAM (30 mg/kg bw)	20 ppm (water)	After	Incidence, 81% Incidence, 79%	Pollard & Luckert (1983)

Table 1 (contd)

Species, strain, sex	No. of animals/group	Carcinogen (dose)	Indomethacin Dose (route)	Treatment relative to carcinogen	Preventive efficacy	Reference
Rat, Sprague-Dawley, male	30	DMH (20 mg/kg bw)	20 mg/L (water)	During and after	Incidence, 36% ($p < 0.005$)	Metzger et al. (1984)
Rat, Sprague-Dawley, male	50	NDMA-OAc (2 mg/kg bw)	10 ppm (water)	During After During and after	None Multiplicity, 32% ($p < 0.05$) Multiplicity, 55% ($p < 0.05$)	Narisawa et al. (1984a)
Rat, ACI/N, male	14	1-HA (1.5% in the diet)	16 ppm (water)	During and after	Incidence of colon adenoma + carcinoma, 100% ($p < 0.002$); of colon adenoma + adenocarcinoma, 100% ($p < 0.01$); of squamous cell papillomas of the forestomach, 72% ($p < 0.01$)	Tanaka et al. (1991)
Rat, F344, male	19–20	NDEA (100 mg/kg bw); MNU (20 mg/kg bw); NBHBA (500 ppm); DMH (40 mg/kg bw); NBHP (1000 ppm)	20 ppm (water)	After	Adenoma incidence, 100% Tumour incidence, 100% ($p < 0.05$)	Shibata et al. (1995)

MAM, methylazoxymethanol acetate; DMH, 1,2-dimethylhydrazine; NS, not significant; NDMA-OAc, N-nitrosodimethylacetoxyamine; F344, Fischer 344; MNU, N-methyl-N-nitrosourea; 1-HA, 1-hydroxyanthraquinone; NDEA, N-nitrosodiethylamine; NBHBA, N-nitrosobutyl(4-hydroxybutyl)amine; NBHP, N-nitrosobis-2-hydroxypropylamine to 4/30, from 10/23 in vehicle controls and 12/30 in untreated controls ($p < 0.05$) (Kudo et al., 1980).

Male Sprague-Dawley rats received five weekly intragastric administrations of 30 mg/kg bw 1,2-dimethylhydrazine as a solution of the hydrochloride in sterile saline, freshly prepared before administration. Three groups of 10 rats were given 20 mg/litre indomethacin in the drinking-water ad libitum starting 3, 12 or 35 days after the last dose of 1,2-dimethylhy-drazine, and three control groups were given tap-water that had been neither chlorinated nor acidified. The numbers of colon tumours were counted 20 weeks after the start of carcinogen treatment. Treatment with indomethacin reduced the number of tumours per rat from 5.3 to 0.9 ($p = 0.002$) when given three days after the carcinogen, from 2.6 to 0.9 ($p = 0.0065$) when given after 12 days and from 2.2 to 0.5 ($p = 0.007$) when given after 35 days. In the last group, the number of rats with tumours was reduced from 9/10 to 4/9 ($p = 0.0016$). Indomethacin treatment had no effect on body weight, and no lesion was observed in any other organ. In a second protocol, two groups of 10 rats received intragastric administrations of 1,2-dimethylhydrazine as above. Seven days after the fifth dose, one group received daily intragastric administrations of 0.25 mg/kg bw indomethacin obtained from commercial capsules (Indocin®), and the second group received an intragastric administration of the vehicle (1% cornstarch). Twenty weeks after the onset of treatment, a nonsignificant reduction in the number of tumours per rat, from 2.7 to 1.4, was seen ($p = 0.08$) (Pollard & Luckert, 1980).

Two groups of seven and eight male weanling Sprague-Dawley rats received a single intraperitoneal injection of 13 mg/kg bw N-nitrosomethyl(acetoxymethyl)amine. Two weeks later, the first group was given 20 mg/ml (3 mg/kg bw) indomethacin in the drinking-water for 18 weeks, at which time the experiment was terminated. The number of rats with tumours was reduced from 6/8 to 1/7 in the first experiment and from 8/10 to 0/5 in the second. [The statistical significance of these differences was not reported.] The number of

intestinal tumours per rat was reduced from 1.5 to 0.14 ($p < 0.05$). In a duplicate experiment with groups of five indomethacin-treated and 10 control rats, the number of tumours per rat was reduced from 1.4 to none (Pollard & Luckert, 1981a).

Weanling male Lobund strain Sprague-Dawley rats received a single dose of 30 mg/kg bw 1,2-dimethylhydrazine by gavage; 34 days later, indomethacin was given in the drinking-water (20 mg/l) and continued until the end of the experiment at 20 weeks. Indomethacin treatment reduced the incidence of colon tumours from 9/10 to 2/9 ($p < 0.01$) and the multiplicity of tumours from 1.30 to 0.22 ($p = 0.01$). Indomethacin also reduced the average body weight by 7% ($p < 0.05$). In a second experiment, rats were injected subcutaneously with methylazoxymethanol acetate (30 mg/kg bw) and 7 or 35 days later given indomethacin in the drinking-water (20 mg/l). The numbers of intestinal tumours in indomethacin-treated and untreated rats were determined at week 20. Treatment with indomethacin seven days after carcinogen treatment reduced the incidence from 7/9 to 1/7 ($p < 0.01$) and the multiplicity from 1.3 to 0.14 ($p < 0.01$). Treatment 35 days after carcinogen treatment reduced the incidence from 3/5 to 0/5 and the multiplicity from 1.4 to 0. No significant reduction in body-weight gain was seen with either protocol (Pollard & Luckert, 1981b).

Nine-week-old female Fischer 344 rats were given an intrarectal instillation of a 0.5-ml solution (2 mg) of 13.3 mg/kg bw N-methyl-N-nitrosourea three times a week in weeks 1–5. Groups of 29 and nine rats received intraperitoneal injections of 2.5 mg/kg bw indomethacin solution three times a week in weeks 11–25. Animals in the first group were killed at 25 weeks, and those in the second group were subjected to endoscopic examination and kept for an additional 10 weeks. A third group of nine rats was given indomethacin in weeks 26–35. The tumour incidences in the three groups were 9/29, 3/9 and 7/9, respectively, and the numbers of tumours per rat were 0.45, 0.33 and 1.0, respectively. Three control groups of 20, 30 and nine rats were treated with N-methyl-N-nitrosourea as above; one group then received intraperitoneal injections of 0.1 ml of the vehicle (methylcellulose); the other two groups were not treated. The tumour incidences in the three groups were 14/20, 20/30 and 6/9, respectively, and the numbers of tumours per rat were 1.1, 1.0 and 1.3 [p value not given]. Thus, indomethacin did not inhibit existing tumours when administered between 25 and 35 weeks (Narisawa *et al.*, 1981).

Three groups of 30 female Fischer 344 rats received intrarectal instillations of 2 mg N-methyl-N-nitrosourea in weeks 1–5. Two groups were given indomethacin at concentrations of 20 or 10 mg/l [20 or 10 ppm] in weeks 11–25 [consumption of water was not documented]; the third group was given tap-water. All rats were killed at week 26. Three rats given the high dose of indomethacin died before the end of treatment and a total of 8/90 rats died of pneumonia or lung abscess. In rats treated with 20 mg/l [20 ppm] of indomethacin, a reduction in the incidence of colon tumours was seen, from 18/27 to 4/24 ($p < 0.01$) and a reduction in the multiplicity from 1.04 to 0.23 tumours per rat ($p > 0.01$). With a dose of 10 mg/l [10 ppm] indomethacin, the reduction in incidence was from 18/27 to 4/28 ($p < 0.01$) and the reduction in multiplicity from 1.04 to 0.21 ($p < 0.01$) (Narisawa *et al.*, 1982).

Colonic tumours were induced in female Fischer 344 rats by intrarectal administration of 4 mg per rat of a freshly prepared 0.5-ml solution of N-methyl-N-nitrosourea on days 3, 5 and 7. Indomethacin was given at a concentration of 0.001% [10 ppm] in drinking-water for various periods. The incidence of tumours in control rats killed at week 31 was 12/27. Administration of indomethacin on days 1–7 reduced the incidence to 5/27 ($p < 0.05$), and administration in weeks 2–30 to week 30 reduced the incidence to 3/28 ($p < 0.01$). The reduction in the incidence (6/28) of colon tumours when indomethacin was given in weeks 11–30 was not significant. The incidence of colon tumours in rats given indomethacin in weeks 2–30 and killed on week 41 (10/22) was significantly higher ($p < 0.01$) than in rats receiving identical treatment with indomethacin but killed in week 31 (Narisawa *et al.*, 1983).

Groups of 10–27 male weanling Lobund Sprague-Dawley rats received two intragastric administrations of 30 mg/kg bw 1,2-dimethyl-hydrazine hydrochloride at seven-day intervals or a single subcutaneous injection of 30 mg/kg bw methylazoxymethanol acetate. Treatment with 20 mg/l indomethacin in the drinking-water (estimated intake, 2.5 mg/kg bw per day) was initiated 14 or 63 days after 1,2-dimethyl-hydrazine treatment and 14 or 77 days after methylazoxymethanol acetate treatment. The development of intestinal tumours was prevented or retarded significantly with indomethacin in comparison with that of control animals. In the rats treated with 1,2-dimethyl-hydrazine, the incidence of colon tumours was reduced from 20/25 to 4/27 ($p < 0.05$) after 14 days and from 12/12 to 10/13 ($p < 0.05$) after 63 days. In those treated with methylazoxy-methanol acetate, the incidence of colon tumours was reduced from 16/17 to 3/15 ($p < 0.05$) after 14 days and from 10/10 to 9/10 after 77 days (Pollard & Luckert, 1983).

Two groups of 30 male Sprague-Dawley rats, with an average weight of 120 g, were given subcutaneous injections of 20 mg/kg bw 1,2-dimethylhydrazine hydrochloride once a week for 20 weeks. One group of rats was given 20 mg/l [20 ppm] indomethacin in drinking water during the initiation and post-initiation phases. The rats were killed 32 weeks after the start of carcinogen treatment. Indomethacin had no significant effect on food intake or water consumption, and the average body weights of the two groups were similar. The incidence of colonic tumours was reduced from 88 to 56% ($p < 0.005$). The numbers of metastases to lymph nodes were comparable (Metzger *et al.*, 1984).

Male Sprague-Dawley rats, eight weeks old, were given Altromin-1320 chow and an intrarectal instillation of 2 mg/kg bw N-nitroso-dimethyl(acetoxymethyl)amine once a week in weeks 1–10. Three groups of 50 rats were given 0.001% [10 ppm] indomethacin in the drinking-water in weeks 1–10, 11–20 and 1–20. Two control groups were given 0.1% ethanol in water or water only. Indomethacin given after the carcinogen treatment reduced the multiplicity of colon tumours from 4.7 to

3.2 ($p < 0.05$); when it was given during and after the carcinogen it reduced the multiplicity from 4.7 to 2.1 ($p < 0.05$) (Narisawa *et al.*, 1984).

Six-week-old male ACI/N rats were fed a diet containing 1.5% 1-hydroxy-anthraquinone [purity and diet consumption unspecified] for 48 weeks. A second group was given 1-hydroxy-anthraquinone as above plus 16 ppm indomethacin in the drinking-water for 48 weeks [water intake unspecified]. A control group received basal diet and tap-water only. Treatment with 1-hydroxyanthraquinone decreased body weight by 7% ($p < 0.02$) and increased the relative liver weight by 15% ($p < 0.001$). The number of rats with adenomas or adenocarcinomas in the colon (12/27) was reduced to 0 by co-administration of indomethacin ($p < 0.01$), and the number of squamous-cell papillomas of the forestomach was reduced from 14/27 to 2/14 ($p < 0.01$) (Tanaka *et al.*, 1991).

(b)   Oesophagus

These studies are summarized in Table 2. In a first experiment, groups of 24 and 45 three-month-old C57BL male mice were given N-nitrosodiethylamine [purity unspecified] at concentration of 0.04 µl/ml [37.7 ppm] and indomethacin at a concentration of 16 mg/l [16 ppm] in the drinking-water daily for two weeks and then three times a week for 18 weeks [water intake not monitored]. The number of

oesophageal tumours per centimetre was reduced from 6.04 to 3.74 ($p < 0.001$). In a second experiment, groups of eight and 16 mice were given the same treatments daily for 30 days and then twice a week for 16 weeks. The number of oesophageal tumours per centimetre was reduced from 4.10 to 2.66 ($p < 0.01$). In a third experiment, 16 mice were given the carcinogen daily for 30 days and then twice a week for four months, and 19 mice received indomethacin in the drinking-water four months after the beginning of carcinogen treatment. Both groups were killed eight months after that date. The number of tumours per centimetre was reduced from 6.10 to 4.74 ($p < 0.01$) (Rubio, 1984). [The Working Group noted that body weights and gastrointestinal toxicity were not documented.]

Groups of 18–61 female C57BL mice, three months of age, were given N-nitrosodiethylamine [purity unspecified] in the drinking-water at a concentration of 0.4 mg/l [0.4 ppm] daily for three months. The first group was killed at the end of treatment and the second group three months after the end of treatment; the third group was given indomethacin at a concentration of 1.6 mg/l [1.6 ppm] for three months from the end of carcinogen treatment. Indomethacin treatment reduced the number of tumours per centimetre of oesophageal mucosa from 5.01 to 2.85 ($p < 0.01$). In a second experiment, two

Table 2. Prevention of oesophageal tumourigenesis by indomethacin

Species, strain, sex	No. of animals/ group	Carcinogen (dose)	Indomethacin Dose (route)	Treatment relative to carcinogen	Preventive efficacy	Reference
Mouse, C57BL, male	24 + 45	NDEA (37.7 ppm)	16 ppm	During	38%; $p < 0.001$	Rubio (1984)
	8 + 16		(drinking-water)	During	35%; $p < 0.01$	
	16 + 19			During and after	22%; $p < 0.01$	
Mouse, C57BL, female	18–61	NDEA (0.4 ppm)	1.6 ppm	After	43%; $p < 0.01$	Rubio (1986)
	18 + 19		(drinking-water)	After	21%; p 0.05	
					32%; $p < 0.01$	
	35 + 39			After	32% $p < 0.01$	
Rat, LIO, male	35 + 58	NSEE (50 mg mg bw)	25 ppm (diet)	After	63%; $p < 0.05$	Bespalov *et al.* (1989)

NDEA, N-nitrosodiethylamine; NSEE, N-nitrososarcosine ethyl ester groups of 19 and 18 mice were given the same concentration of N-nitrosodiethylamine in the drinking-water for three months. The first group was killed six months after treatment and the second was given indomethacin in the drinking-water for six months starting at the end of carcinogen treatment, after which they were killed. Indomethacin treatment reduced the tumour index from 4.79 to 3.78 ($p < 0.05$). In a third experiment, three groups of 39, 35 and 36 mice were given the carcinogen treatment for four months. The first group was killed at the end of treatment and the second three months after treatment; the third group was given 1.6 mg/l [1.6 ppm] indomethacin for three months after carcinogen treatment. A reduction in the tumour index from 5.23 to 3.55 ($p < 0.01$) was observed with indomethacin treatment (Rubio, 1986). [The Working Group noted that body weights and gastrointestinal toxicity were not reported.]

A group of male outbred LIO rats, weighing 120–130 g, received N-nitrososarcosine ethyl ester [purity unspecified] by gavage at a dose of 50 mg/kg bw, five times per week for 16 weeks. After this treatment, a control group of 58 rats was given basal diet, and a second group of 35 rats received a diet containing 25 mg/kg [25 ppm] indomethacin [intake not documented]. All rats were killed 32 weeks after the beginning of carcinogen treatment, and tumours of the oesophagus were examined macroscopically and histologically. Three rats died with a perforating gastric ulcer. Indomethacin treatment reduced the incidence of oesophageal tumours from 89.7 to 65.7% ($p < 0.05$), and their multiplicity from 4.3 ± 0.6 to 1.6 ± 0.4. The incidence of forestomach tumours was also decreased, from 41.4 to 14.3% ($p < 0.05$), and their multiplicity from 0.9 ± 0.1 to 0.4 ± 0.3 (Bespalov et al., 1989).

(c) Mammary gland

These studies are summarized in Table 3. Female Sprague-Dawley rats, 50 days of age, received a single intragastric administration of 5 mg 7,12-dimethylbenz[a]anthracene (DMBA). Three days later, 32 rats were given a low-fat diet (5% corn oil) and 34 rats a high-fat diet (18% corn oil), with or without indomethacin. Indo-

methacin was added to the diet at a concentration of 0.004% (w/w) [40 ppm] [food intake unspecified]. This treatment did not change the body weights significantly. In rats fed the low-fat diet, the reductions in the incidence, multiplicity and size of mammary tumours were not significant. In rats fed the high-fat diet, indomethacin had no significant effect on the incidence or multiplicity of mammary tumours, but the mean tumour size was reduced from 4.08 to 1.46 g ($p < 0.01$) (Carter et al., 1983).

Female Sprague-Dawley rats, 50 days old, received intragastric administrations of 16 mg/rat DMBA in 1 ml sesame oil. Four groups of 25 rats were given indomethacin at 25 or 50 mg/kg diet [25 or 50 ppm] from weeks -2 to +1 or from week +1 for 150 days. When administered from weeks –2 to +1, indomethacin delayed the appearance of mammary tumours by 10–20 days. After 150 days of indomethacin treatment, the total number of tumours per rat was reduced from 8.66 to 5.79 with 50 ppm ($p < 0.01$) and to 5.94 with 25 ppm ($p < 0.01$). When administered at 50 ppm from weeks +1 to the end, indomethacin reduced the multiplicity of mammary carcinomas from 6.40 to 3.71 ($p < 0.01$), that of benign tumours from 2.26 to 0.40 ($p < 0.01$) and that of all tumours from 8.66 to 4.11 ($p < 0.01$). Administration of the lower dose of indomethacin during the same period changed none of the three parameters. The experiment was repeated with a dose of 8 mg DMBA per rat. The results of the two experiments were comparable (McCormick et al., 1985).

Virgin female Sprague-Dawley rats, 36 days old, received an intragastric administration of 10 mg DMBA in 1 ml of sesame oil. Indomethacin was mixed into the diet at a concentration of 50 mg/kg diet [50 ppm], which was given either from weeks –2 to +1 or weeks +1 to the end of the experiment at 27 weeks. Treatment had no effect on body weights. Administration of indomethacin from weeks –2 to +1 did not reduce the multiplicity of mammary cancers or of all tumours, but administration from weeks +1 to the end of experiment reduced mammary carcinoma multiplicity from 3.46 to 2.56 ($p < 0.05$) and total tumour multiplicity from 3.65 to 1.88 ($p < 0.01$) (McCormick & Wilson, 1986).

Table 3. Prevention of mammary tumourigenesis by indomethacin

Species, strain, sex	No. of animals/ group	Carcinogen (dose)	Indomethacin Dose (route)	Treatment relative to carcinogen	Preventive efficacy	Reference
Rat, Sprague-Dawley, female	32–34	DMBA (5 mg/rat)	40 ppm (diet)	After	None	Carter et al. (1983)
Rat, Sprague-Dawley, female	25	DMBA (16 mg/rat)	25 or 50 ppm (diet)	Before and during After	Benign tumours, multiplicity, 81% ($p < 0.01$) Carcinomas, multiplicity, 42% ($p < 0.01$)	McCormick et al. (1985)
Rat, Sprague-Dawley, female	25	DMBA (10 mg/rat)	50 ppm (diet)	Before and during After	None Carcinoma multiplicity, 26%; $p < 0.05$	McCormick & Wilson (1986)
Rat, Sprague-Dawley, female	28–29	DMBA (10 mg/rat)	40 ppm (diet)	After	None	Abou-El-Ela et al. (1989)
Rat, Sprague-Dawley, female	32–33	DMBA (5 mg/rat)	50 ppm (diet)	After	High fat: tumour incidence, 63% ($p < 0.01$) Low fat: none	Noguchi et al. (1991)
Rat, LIO, female	21	MNU (12 mg/rat)	25 ppm (diet)	After	Tumour incidence, 37%; $p < 0.05$	Bespalov et al. (1992)

DMBA, 7,12-dimethylbenz[a]anthracene; MNU, N-methyl-N-nitrosourea

Virgin female Sprague-Dawley rats, 50 days old, received a single intragastric administration of 10 mg DMBA. Three weeks later, groups of 28–29 rats were placed on high-fat diets (20% corn oil) and 0.004% (w/w) [40 ppm] indomethacin until the end of the experiment at 16 weeks. Indomethacin had no significant effect on body weight or food intake and did not reduce the incidence, latency or number of mammary tumours per tumour-bearing rat (Abou-El-Ela et al., 1989).

Four groups of 32 or 33 virgin female Sprague-Dawley rats received an intragastric administration of 5 mg DMBA. Seven days later, two groups were given a high-fat diet (20% corn oil), and the two other groups received a low-fat diet (0.5% corn oil). One group on each diet was given 0.005% (w/w) [50 ppm] indomethacin seven days after DMBA up to the end of the experiment, 20 weeks after DMBA administration. Indomethacin treatment reduced the number of rats with tumours from 26/32 to 10/33 in the high-fat group ($p < 0.01$) but increased the number of tumour-bearing rats from 9/33 to 11/32 in the group on the low-fat diet. Indomethacin reduced the multiplicity of mammary tumours in the high-fat groups from 2.3 to 0.9 ($p < 0.001$) but had no preventive effect in rats fed the low-fat diet (Noguchi et al., 1991).

Female LIO (outbred) albino rats, weighing 200–230 g, were given one dose of 1 mg N-methyl-N-nitrosourea in 0.1 ml saline solution into each of the 12 mammary glands (total dose, 12 mg/rat). A control group of 25 rats then received basal diet, and 21 rats were given indomethacin at 25 mg/kg in the diet [25 ppm] for six months, when all animals were killed [feed intake unspecified]. Most of the mammary tumours were adenocarcinomas. Indomethacin reduced the incidence of mammary tumours from 19/25 to 10/21 ($p < 0.05$) but did not affect their multiplicity (1.36 and 1.14, respectively) (Bespalov et al., 1992).

(d)   Tongue

Two groups of 17 and 13 six-week-old male ACI/N rats, weighing 120 g, were given 4-nitroquinoline-1-oxide at 10 ppm in the drinking-water for 12 weeks. One group was switched to tap-water and the second to 10 ppm indomethacin for 24 weeks [water consumption unspecified]. No difference between the two groups in body weight or relative liver weight was seen. The incidence of all tumours (squamous-cell papilloma or carcinoma) was reduced from 12/17 to 3/13 ($p < 0.02$) and the incidence of carcinoma from 12/17 to 2/13 ($p < 0.005$) (Tanaka et al., 1989); see also Table 4).

(e)   Oral cavity

Two groups of five female and five male Syrian golden hamsters, eight weeks of age, received applications of a 0.5% solution of DMBA in mineral oil three times a week on the left buccal pouch. One of the groups simultaneously received a 0.5% solution of indomethacin (1 mg/animal) in the mouth daily until killing. A group of five male and five female animals was left untreated. One female and one male from each treated group were killed in weeks 8, 10, 12, 13 and 14. No morphological changes were seen in untreated hamsters. Indomethacin treatment reduced the multiplicity of tumours from 6.4 to 2.8 ($p < 0.05$) (Perkins & Shklar, 1982). [The Working Group noted the small number of animals per group.]

Three groups of 10–11 male Syrian golden hamsters, three to four months old, were treated with either mineral oil, a 0.5% solution of DMBA in mineral oil, DMBA in mineral oil plus an indomethacin suspension or mineral oil plus the indomethacin suspension. DMBA was applied to the right buccal pouch three times a week for 14.5 weeks; four drops of a suspension of indomethacin (1 mg/animal) was administered orally daily. All hamsters were killed 16.5 weeks after the beginning of treatment. Indomethacin had no effect on the incidence of all oral tumours or of carcinomas or on the latency or multiplicity of tumours (Gould et al., 1985).

Two groups of six to 12 male Syrian hamsters, four to six weeks old, received applications of a 0.5% solution of DMBA in liquid paraffin on both cheek pouches three times a week for 10 weeks. During weeks 12–22 (time of terminal kill), one group of hamsters received a daily oral dose of 1 mg/animal (0.1 ml solution) sodium indomethacin trihydrate; the second group was not treated. The total number of

Table 4. Prevention of tumorigenesis in other organs by indomethacin

Sex, species, strain	No. of animals/ group	Carcinogen (dose)	Organ	Indomethacin Dose (route)	Treatment relative to carcinogen	Preventive efficacy	Reference
Rat, ACI/N, male	13	4-NQO (10 ppm)	Tongue	10 ppm (water)	After	Incidence: total tumour, 67% ($p < 0.002$); carcinoma, 78% ($p < 0.005$)	Tanaka et al. (1989)
Hamster, Syrian golden, male and female	10	DMBA (unspecified)	Oral cavity	1 mg (oral)	During	Multiplicity, 56% ($p < 0.02$)	Perkins & Shklar (1992)
Hamster, Syrian golden, male	10–11	DMBA (unspecified)	Oral cavity	1 mg (oral)	During	0	Gould et al. (1985)
Hamster, Syrian golden, male	6–12	DMBA (unspecified)	Oral cavity	1 mg (oral)	During	0	Franklin & Craig (1987)
Rat, ACI/N, male	10	AAF (200 ppm)	Liver	10 ppm (water)	Before, during and after	Incidence: adenoma, 86% ($p < 0.01$); carcinoma, 100% ($p < 0.001$); multiplicity, 97% ($p < 0.001$)	Tanaka et al. (1993)
Hamster, Syrian golden, female	20–30	BOP (10 mg/kg)	Pancreas	20 ppm (water)	After	Multiplicity, 51% ($p < 0.05$)	Takahashi et al. (1990)
Mouse, BDF, male	78–80	OH-BBN (8 doses of 7.5 mg/mouse)	Urinary bladder	7.5 ppm (diet)	Before, during and after	Incidence, 79% ($p < 0.05$)	Grubbs et al. (1993)
	78–84			15.0 mg/kg (diet)	Before, during and after	Incidence, 100% ($p < 0.01$)	
Mouse, Swiss, female	26	3-Methylcholanthrene	Cervix	40 ppm (diet)	Before, during and after	Incidence, 71% ($p < 0.01$)	Rao & Hussain (1988)

Table 4. (contd)

Sex, species, strain	No. of animals/ group	Carcinogen (dose)	Organ	Indomethacin Dose (route)	Treatment relative to carcinogen	Preventive efficacy	Reference
Mouse, albino outbred, female	30–61	DMBA (8 doses of 25 µg)	Vagina and cervix	20 mg/l (water)	After	Carcinoma incidence, 40.5% ($p < 0.05$)	Bespalov et al. (1992)
Mouse, Balb/c, male	6	BaP (100 µg/rat)	Skin	8.4 µg/mouse (topically)	Before and during	Tumour weight reduced by 46%	Andrews et al. (1991)
	6	DMBA unspecified	Skin			None	
Mouse, hr/hr, female	20	UV radiation	Skin	1.8 mg/kg (water)	During	0	Haedersdal et al. (1995)
Rat, LIO, male and female	25	ENU (75 mg/kg bw)	Brain, kidney	20 mg/l (water) postnatally	After	Incidence: brain, 35% ($p < 0.05$); kidney, 29% ($p > 0.05$)	Alexandrov et al. (1996)

4-NQO, 4-nitroquinoline-1-oxide; 2-AAF, 2-acetylaminofluorene; OH-BBN, N-nitrosobutyl(4-hydroxybutyl)amine; DMBA, 7,12-dimethylbenz[a]anthracene; BaP, benzo[a]pyrene; BOP, N-nitrosobis(2-oxopropyl)amine; UV, ultraviolet; ENU, N-ethyl-N-nitrosourea small and large tumours of the oral cavity in the two groups was similar (Franklin & Craig, 1987).

(f)   Liver

Two groups of 10 five-week-old male inbred ACI/N rats were fed a diet containing 200 ppm 2-acetylaminofluorene in weeks 0–6 and basal diet in weeks 17–36. One group was given 10 ppm indomethacin in the drinking-water starting one week before carcinogen treatment to week 17. The experiment was terminated in week 36. Treatment with 2-acetylaminofluorene increased the liver weight from 3.47 to 4.75 g/100 g bw ($p < 0.001$); and administration of indomethacin reduced the weight to 3.69 g/100 g bw ($p < 0.05$). Indomethacin treatment also reduced the incidence of hepatic adenomas from 7/10 to 1/10 ($p < 0.01$) and that of hepatic carcinomas from 8/10 to 0/10 ($p < 0.001$). The number of all hepatic neoplasms per rat was reduced from 4.00 to 0.10 ($p < 0.001$) (Tanaka *et al.*, 1993; see also Table 4).

(g)   Pancreas

Outbred female Syrian golden hamsters, five weeks old, received five weekly doses of 10 mg/kg bw *N*-nitrosobis(2-oxopropyl)amine subcutaneously. One group of 20 hamsters was given 20 ppm indomethacin in weeks 6–32 (after which they were killed), and a control group of 30 hamsters was given tap-water. Indomethacin treatment had no effect on body-weight gain but induced a nonsignificant reduction in the incidence of pancreatic tumours, from 20/28 to 10/19, and a significant reduction in the multiplicity of pancreatic adenocarcinomas, from 1.29 to 0.63 ($p < 0.05$) (Takahashi *et al.*, 1990).

(h)   Urinary bladder

Groups of 78, 80 and 84 male C57BL x DBA/2F$_1$ mice, 49 days of age, received 7.5 mg *N*-nitrosobutyl(4-hydroxybutyl)amine [purity unspecified] dissolved in 0.1 ml/l ethanol:water (20:80) by intragastric administration once a week for eight weeks. The first group of mice was given the carcinogen alone, and the second and third groups received diets containing indomethacin at 7.5 and 15 mg/kg diet [7.5 and 15 ppm] starting one week before carcinogen treatment and

continuing until the end of the experiment at 180 days; the higher concentration was determined to be the maximal nontoxic dose. Indomethacin reduced the incidence of urinary bladder tumours from 14 to 4% ($p < 0.05$) when given at 7.5 ppm and to 0 ($p < 0.01$) when given at 15 ppm. The incidence of all bladder tumours, including papillomas, was reduced from 24 to 5% ($p < 0.05$) and 0 ($p < 0.01$), respectively (Grubbs *et al.*, 1993; see also Table 4).

(i)   Cervix and vagina:

These studies are summarized in Table 4. Random-bred, 10–12-week-old virgin Swiss mice were treated with 3-methylcholanthrene [purity unspecified] by the insertion of sterile, double cotton threads impregnated with beeswax containing approximately 600 μg 3-methylcholanthrene into the uterine cervix [levels of exposure unspecified]. Four groups of 25 mice were given 0, 10, 20 or 40 mg/kg of diet [0, 10, 20 or 40 ppm] indomethacin starting two weeks before carcinogen treatment up to 16 weeks, when all animals were killed. Control groups of 15 mice received beeswax-impregnated threads and the same diets as described above [dietary intake not documented]. Indomethacin treatment did not reduce body-weight gain. No cervical tumours were observed in the mice treated with beeswax-impregnated thread. In 3-methylcholanthrene-treated mice, indomethacin at 40 ppm reduced the cervical tumour incidence from 21/23 to 6/23 ($p < 0.01$). The reduction at lower doses of indomethacin was not significant (Rao & Hussain, 1988). [The Working Group noted that the linearity of the preventive efficacy in relation to the doses of indomethacin was not documented.]

Groups of 30 outbred albino (SHR) virgin female mice, 12 weeks old received polymer sponge tampons impregnated with a 0.1% triethylene glycol solution of DMBA intravaginally. The average dose of DMBA was 25 μg per application. The tampons were changed twice weekly for eight weeks, for a total of 16 applications. Nine weeks after the start of DMBA treatment, 61 mice received no further treatment and 30 received indomethacin in the drinking-water at 20 mg/l [20 ppm; water consumption unspecified] for a further 28 weeks. All surviving mice were killed 36 weeks after the start of the experiment, but 30–60% died with progressing tumours of the vagina and cervix before that time. All tumours were examined histologically. The total incidence of vaginal and cervical (papillomas plus carcinomas) was similar in the two groups (63–72%), but the ratio of carcinomas to papillomas was lower in mice given DMBA followed by indomethacin (12 carcinomas and 7 papillomas) than in mice given DMBA alone (41 carcinomas and 3 papillomas; carcinoma:papilloma ratio, 14). Significantly more control than indomethacin-treated mice died before the end of the experiment (61% and 37%, respectively; $p < 0.05$) (Bespalov et al., 1992).

(j) Skin
Two groups of six male Balb/c mice, aged six to eight weeks, received two weekly applications of 20 μl benzo[a]pyrene [purity unspecified] dissolved in 0.5% acetone (total dose, 100 μg per rat). One group was given 8.4 μg indomethacin dissolved in acetone at a concentration of 0.42 mg/ml 20 min before the benzo[a]pyrene application on the same area of the shaved dorsal trunk. Treatment lasted for six months. Indomethacin pretreatment increased the time of tumour onset from 19.8 to 24.8 weeks ($p < 0.05$) but reduced the mean weight of tumours from 0.57 to 0.31 g. Two other groups received weekly applications of DMBA dissolved in lanolin plus liquid paraffin [dose of DMBA unspecified], and one group was treated weekly with 16.8 μg indomethacin 20 min before DMBA application, as described above. No difference in tumour onset or weight was seen between the two groups (Andrews et al., 1991; see also Table 4).

Two groups of 20 female hr/hr C3H/Tif mice, 14–15 weeks of age, were exposed to ultraviolet radiation at a daily dose of 12.6 kJ/m^2 for 8 min/day on four days per week. Indomethacin was given in the drinking-water [concentration unspecified] at an intake estimated to be 1.8 mg/kg bw per day. Mice were treated until they were killed by tumours. Indomethacin delayed the time of appearance of the first tumours ($p < 0.001$) but increased the mortality rate ($p < 0.0005$) (Haedersdal et al., 1995).

(k) Transplacental carcinogenesis
Groups of 6–10 LIO outbred albino rats, three to four months of age, were injected intravenously on day 21 of gestation with 75 mg/kg bw N-ethyl-N-nitrosourea in saline; there were 12-16 pregnant controls. Two groups of 42 and 25 pups of each sex were treated with water alone or with 20 mg/l [20 ppm] indomethacin in the drinking-water throughout postnatal life. The daily intake of indomethacin was estimated to be 1.6 mg/kg bw. The incidence of brain tumours was reduced from 36/42 to 14/25 ($p < 0.05$) and their multiplicity was decreased from 1.95 to 0.92 ($p < 0.05$). The multiplicity of kidney tumours was reduced from 0.45 to 0.32 ($p < 0.05$). There was no significant difference in body weights between the groups [exact data not provided] (Alexandrov et al., 1996; see also Table 4).

(l) Multi-organ carcinogenesis
Groups of 19–20 male Fischer 344 rats, six weeks of age, were treated sequentially with five carcinogens, as follows: a single intraperitoneal injection of 100 mg/kg bw N-nitrosodiethylamine on day 1; intraperitoneal injections of 20 mg/kg bw N-methyl-N-nitrosourea on days 3, 9 and 12; administration of N-nitrosobutyl(4-hydroxybutyl)amine in the drinking-water (0.05%) [500 ppm] during weeks 1 and 2; subcutaneous injections of 40 mg/kg bw 1,2-dimethylhydrazine on days 17, 20, 23 and 26; administration of N-nitrosobis-2-hydroxypropylamine in the drinking-water (0.1%) [1000 ppm] during weeks 3 and 4. Groups of rats were given indomethacin in the drinking-water [20 ppm] and basal diet in weeks 6–28. Indomethacin did not reduce body-weight gain or food or water consumption. The incidences and multiplicities of lung adenomas were significantly decreased in indomethacin-treated rats. Indomethacin treatment did not reduce the incidence or multiplicity of urinary bladder papillomas but did decrease the development of preneoplastic lesions. The incidence of adenomas of the large intestine and the number of rats bearing tumours were decreased in the indomethacin-treated group in comparison with control. Only the decrease in tumour incidence was statistically significant ($p < 0.05$) controls (Shibata et al., 1995; see also Table 1).

4.2.2 In-vitro models

(a) Cultured mammalian cells

Non-regressing, premalignant, nodule-like alveolar lesions can be induced in cultured mouse mammary organs by DMBA. Female Balb/c mice were pretreated with oestradiol and progesterone for nine days to stimulate hormones, and then their mammary glands were excised and cultured for 10 days with insulin, prolactin, aldosterone and hydrocortisone to promote growth. During this period, the cultures were exposed to 2 μg/ml DMBA for 72–96 h. After the promotion period, all of the hormones except insulin were withdrawn to induce regression of the lobular alveolar structures. Half of the mammary glands were also treated with indomethacin at doses of (10^{-9} to 10^{-5} mol/l during the first 10 days of culture. The average incidence of mammary gland lesions in the DMBA-treated group was 63%; indomethacin inhibited the formation of DMBA-induced lesions, the most effective dose of 10^{-6} mol/l causing 77% inhibition (Mehta et al., 1991).

Inhibition of TPA-induced early antigen of Epstein-Barr virus in lymphoblastoid Raji cells has been used to screen for anti-tumour promoters. Indomethacin inhibited the induction in a dose-related manner; the effective concentration resulting in 50% inhibition was 13 μg/ml (Saito et al., 1986).

Indomethacin was a competitive inhibitor of dihydrodiol dehydrogenase in isolated hepatocytes from uninduced Sprague-Dawley rats. Preincubation of cells with 30 μmol/l indomethacin before addition of (±)-trans-7,8-dihydroxy-7,8-dihydrobenzo[a]pyrene prevented the formation of benzo[a]pyrene-7,8-dione, which may be an activated metabolite of the carcinogen benzo[a]pyrene. (Flowers-Geary et al., 1995).

(b) Antimutagenicity in short-term tests

The antimutagenicity effects of indomethacin are summarized in Table 5 and are displayed graphically as an activity profile in Figure 2.

Indomethacin reduced aflatoxin-induced mutagenicity in Saccharomyces cerevisiae (Niggli et al., 1986) and clastogenicity in human lymphocytes (Amstad et al., 1984). It inhibited arachidonic acid-induced sister chromatid exchange in Chinese hamster ovary cells co-cultured with human leukocytes (Weitberg, 1988). Indomethacin inhibited the induction of sister chromatid exchange by arachidonic acid in combination with benzo[a]pyrene or DMBA in a human tumour-derived cell line and inhibited sister chromatid exchange induction by the last two compounds in a rat tumour-derived cell line (Abe, 1986). Indomethacin completely inhibited the mutagenicity of 7,8-dihydroxy-7,8-dihydrobenzo[a]pyrene in V79 cells pretreated with arachidonic acid (Sevanian & Peterson, 1989). In Salmonella typhimurium strain TA98, indomethacin reduced the mutagenicity of N-acetylbenzidine, but it enhanced benzidine-induced mutagenicity. It inhibited DNA binding induced by benzidine or benzidine analogues in a microsomal activation system initiated by arachidonic acid but had no effect when the activation system was initiated by hydrogen peroxide (Petry et al., 1988). It partially inhibited benzidine- or diethylstilboestrol-induced sister chromatid exchange in cell lines derived from rat and human hepatomas (Buenaventura et al., 1984; Grady et al., 1986), and it inhibited sister chromatid exchange induced by diethylstilboestrol in mouse cells (Hillbertz-Nilsson & Forsberg, 1989). It also reduced the frequency of chromium chloride-induced chromosomal aberrations in human lymphocytes (Friedman et al., 1987). It inhibited DNA single-strand breaks induced by the tumour promoter, fecapentane-12, but it did not inhibit hydrogen peroxide-induced breaks (Plummer et al., 1995). Pretreatment of rats with indomethacin prevented hydralazine hydrochloride-induced unscheduled DNA synthesis in hepatocytes in vitro (Martelli et al., 1995). Indomethacin did not inhibit mitomycin C-induced sister chromatid exchange in human lymphocytes (Ekmekci et al., 1995). It inhibited DNA binding induced by phenylhydroquinone in vitro (Pathak & Roy, 1993), and it inhibited the effects of the tumour promoter, TPA, including chromosomal aberrations in human lymphocytes and sister chromatid exchange in Chinese hamster ovary cells co-cultured with human leukocytes (Emerit & Cerutti, 1982; Weitberg, 1988). Indomethacin enhanced the frequency of styrene- and styrene

Table 5. Antimutagenic effects of indomethacin

Mutagen	Dose of mutagen (µg/ml)	Test code[a]	% Inhibition[b] (% enhancement)	Dose range (µg/ml) Low	Dose range (µg/ml) High	Reference
Aflatoxin B1	0.09	CHL	38	10.0	10.0	Amstad et al. (1984)
Aflatoxin B1	78.0	SCG	55	0.1	0.7	Niggli et al. (1986)
Arachidonic acid	24.3	SIC	86	10.7	10.7	Weitberg (1988)
Benzo[a]pyrene + arachidonic acid	25.2	SHT	(9)	18.0	36.0	Abe (1986)
Benzo[a]pyrene	25.2	SHT	40	36.0	36.0	Abe (1986)
Benzo[a]pyrene	126	SIC	0	18.0	36.0	Abe (1986)
Benzo[a]pyrene	50.4	SIT	0	18.0	36.0	Abe (1986)
Benzo[a]pyrene	75.6	SIT	69	36.0	36.0	Abe (1986)
B[a]P-diol	0.5	G9H	100	7.2	7.2	Sevanian & Peterson (1989)
B[a]P-diol	1.0	G9H	100	7.2	7.2	Sevanian & Peterson (1989)
B[a]P-diol	1.5	G9H	100	7.2	7.2	Sevanian & Peterson (1989)
Benzidine + arachidonic acid	4.6	BID	99	7.2	7.2	Petry et al. (1988)
Benzidine	0.028	SA9	(42)	3.6	36.0	Petry et al. (1988)
Benzidine	5.0	SHT	80	3.6	3.6	Grady et al. (1986)
Benzidine	7.5	SHT	75	3.6	3.6	Grady et al. (1986)
Benzidine	10.0	SHT	56	3.6	3.6	Grady et al. (1986)
Benzidine	1.0	SIT	25	3.6	3.6	Grady et al. (1986)
Benzidine	5.0	SIT	100	3.6	3.6	Grady et al. (1986)
Benzidine	7.5	SIT	100	3.6	3.6	Grady et al. (1986)
Benzidine	10.0	SIT	80	3.6	3.6	Grady et al. (1986)
Dichlorobenzidine	6.3	BID	55	7.2	7.2	Petry et al. (1988)
N-Acetylbenzidine	5.6	BID	76	7.2	7.2	Petry et al. (1988)
N-Acetylbenzidine	0.034	SA9	37	3.6	36.0	Petry et al. (1988)
Tetramethylbenzidine	6.0	BID	93	7.2	7.2	Petry et al. (1988)
Chromium chloride	2.5	CHL	57	10.7	21.0	Friedman et al. (1987)
Dianisidine	6.1	BID	99	7.2	7.2	Petry et al. (1988)
Diethylstilboestrol	0.027	SHT	100	3.6	3.7	Buenaventura et al. (1984)
Diethylstilboestrol	0.27	SIM	65	0.4	3.6	Hillbertz-Nilsson & Forsberg (1989)
Diethylstilboestrol	2.7	SIT	100	3.6	3.6	Buenaventura et al. (1984); Shamon et al. (1994)
DMBA	5.1	SHT	5	17.9	36.0	Abe (1986)
DMBA + arachidonic acid	5.1	SHT	54	35.8	36.0	Abe (1986)
DMBA	128	SIC	5	17.9	36.0	Abe 1986)
DMBA	51	SIT	4	17.9	36.	Abe (1986)
	51	SIT	64	35.8	36.0	Abe (1986)
Fecapentane-12	12.5	DIH	100	35.8	36.0	Plummer et al. (1995)
Fecapentane-12	25.0	DIH	100	35.8	36.0	Plummer et al. (1995)
Hydrogen peroxide	3.4	DIH	(17)	35.80	36.0	Plummer et al. (1995)
Hydrogen peroxide	6.8	DIH	10	35.80	36.0	Plummer et al. (1995)
Hydralazine	110	URP	73	5.0	5.0	Martelli et al. (1995)
Hydralazine	200	URP	55	5.0	5.0	Martelli et al. (1995)
Mitomycin C	0.03	SHL	21	0.0	0.0	Ekmekci et al. (1995)
Phenyl hydroquinone	186	BID	92	179	179	Pathak & Roy (1993)
TPA	0.1	CHL	79	10.0	10.0	Emerit & Cerutti (1982)
TPA	0.1	SIC	88	10.7	10.7	Weitberg (1988)
Styrene	52.0	SHL	(52)	26.9	53.7	Lee & Norppa (1995)
Styrene	104	SHL	(63)	26.9	53.7	Lee & Norppa (1995)
Styrene oxide	6	SHL	(181)	26.9	53.7	Lee & Norppa (1995)
Styrene oxide	12.0	SHL	(51)	26.9	53.7	Lee & Norppa (1995)

B[a]P-diol, 7,8-dihydroxy-7,8-dihydrobenz[a]pyrene; DMBA, 7,12-dimethylbenz[a]anthracene; TPA, 12-O-tetradecanoylphorbol 13-acetate

[a] The test codes are defined in Appendix 2

[b] A positive value is the percentage inhibition of the effect induced by the mutagen in the test; a negative value (in parentheses) is the percentage enhancement of the effect.

Figure 2. Antimutagenicity profile of indomethacin

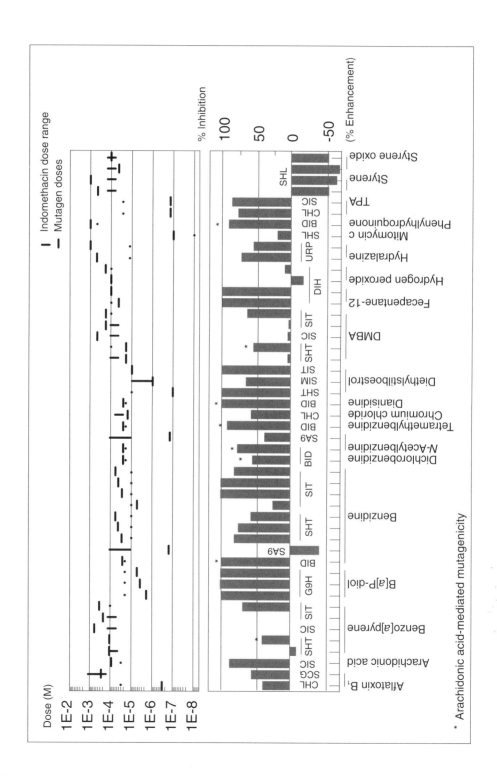

oxide-induced sister chromatid exchange in human lymphocytes (Lee & Norppa, 1995).

Indomethacin at 100 μmol/l inhibited DMBAinduced forward mutation to 8-azaguanine resistance in *S. typhimurium* strain TM677 by 69% (Shamon *et al.*, 1994). Transformed foci can be induced in Balbc3T3 cells in a two-stage assay, with initiation by 3-methylcholanthrene (0.5 μg/ml) and promotion by TPA 0.1 μg/ml). Indomethacin inhibited the induction of transformed foci in a dose-dependent manner, causing 81% inhibition at a concentration of 20 μg/ml (Semba & Inui, 1990).

Indomethacin reversed the inhibition of gap-junction intercellular communication in liver cells from male Wistar rats induced by the hepatic tumour promoter phenobarbital, 1,1,1-trichloro-2,2-(*p*-chlorophenyl)ethane (DDT) or γ-hexachlorocyclohexane (lindane). Treatment with 2 mmol/l phenobarbital inhibited intercellular communication by 30%, as measured by microinjection of fluorescent Lucifer Yellow dye after a 5-h incubation. Indomethacin did not reverse the inhibition of communication induced by DDT or lindane (Leibold & Schwartz, 1993)

4.3   Mechanisms of chemoprevention
4.3.1   Inhibition of carcinogen activation
In 1971, Vane reported that indomethacin inhibits prostaglandin production by interfering with the cyclooxygenase(COX)[1]-catalysed oxygenation of arachidonic acid. For a full description of this mechanism, see the General Remarks. An additional important mechanism by which indomethacin may prevent cancer is inhibition of carcinogen activation (Szarka *et al.*, 1994).

There is indirect evidence that COX catalyses conversion of the benzene metabolite, hydroquinone, into reactive oxygen products that accumulate in bone marrow and damage DNA. Indomethacin inhibits activation of hydroquinone,. thereby preventing DNA damage and further myelotoxicity (Schlosser *et al.*, 1990). Another mutagen similarly activated and formed during protein pyrolysis is 3-methylimidazo[4,5-*f*]quinoline (IQ). Once formed, IQ and its methylated derivatives are potent mutagens (Wild & Degen, 1987; Petry *et al.*, 1989).

Indomethacin and other NSAIDs which prevent bioactivation of these molecules may prevent cancer through this mechanism (Earnest *et al.*, 1992).

4.3.2   Effects on cell proliferation and apoptosis
Early investigations demonstrated that indomethacin and other NSAIDs interfere with a diverse range of biological processes related to cell growth including reductions in glycolysis (Cooney & Dawson, 1977), uncoupling of oxidative phosphorylation (Whitehouse, 1964), decreased mucopolysaccharide formation (Kalbhen *et al.*, 1967) and interference with calcium ion uptake and other calcium-mediated processes (Northover, 1977). Enzyme pathways found subsequently to be inhibited by indomethacin include phospholipase A_2 (Kaplan *et al.*, 1978; Lobo & Hoult, 1994), 15-lipoxygenase (Siegel *et al.*, 1980), myeloperoxidase (Shacter *et al.*, 1991) and glutathione *S*-transferase (Wu & Mathews, 1983).

A direct inhibitory effect of indomethacin on cellular proliferation is indicated by the results of studies of cell cultures, showing that indomethacin inhibits cell multiplication and progression of the cell cycle from G_1 to S phase (Bayer & Beaven, 1979; Bayer *et al.*, 1979). Several recent reports support the concept that indomethacin prevents tumour cell growth through alterations in the cell cycle and induction of apoptosis leading to cell death (Lu *et al.*, 1995; Shiff *et al*, 1996). In one study, indomethacin reduced the levels of two key cyclin-dependent kinases, p33 and p34, in HT-29 colon cells, both of which are crucial to cell cycle progression. Indomethacin induced apoptosis in these cells and increased the proportion of cells in the G_0/G_1 phases, which correlated with its ability to suppress cell proliferation (Shiff *et al.*, 1996). A similar mechanism has not yet been demonstrated in human colon tissue.

Indomethacin may also protect against cancer by altering the activity of enzymes other than cyclooxygenase. These effects include inhibition of enzymes such as cyclic AMP protein kinase and phosphodiesterase, both of which may be critical to cancer initiation and promotion (Kantor & Hampton, 1978;

[1] Used as a synonym for prostaglandin endoperoxide synthase (PGH synthase)

Abramson & Weissmann, 1989). Likewise, indomethacin may exert cancer preventive effects in the colon by preventing induction of ornithine decarboxylase, the first and rate-limiting enzyme in polyamine biosynthesis (Narisawa *et al.*, 1985, 1987). Data showing an association between ornithine decarboxylase activity, tumour promotion and cell proliferation in various organs including the colon and skin have been reported (Pegg & McCann, 1982; Slaga, 1983). More importantly, in patients with adenomatous polyps, ornithine decarboxylase activity is markedly elevated (Luk & Baylin, 1984). Suppression of ornithine decarboxylase by indomethacin in mouse skin with concomitant prevention of skin carcinogenesis by the tumour promoter TPA (Furstenberger & Marks, 1978, 1980; Verma *et al.*, 1980) further supports the theory that this enzyme is involved in carcinogenesis.

Although not direct chemopreventive mechanisms, other growth regulatory effects exerted by indomethacin, such as inhibition of angiogenesis (Gullino, 1981; Ziche *et al.*, 1982; Peterson, 1986), may be relevant. The results of a recent study conducted in murine 3T3 fibroblasts suggest that the ability of indomethacin to block angiogenesis may be related to its inhibitory effect on hyaluronic acid production (August *et al.*, 1994). Hyaluronic acid has been recovered from the stroma of several malignant tumours (Knudson *et al.*, 1984), including human breast tumours (Bertrand *et al.*, 1992; Shuster *et al.*, 1993), and is believed to play a role in cell migration. Interruption of hyaluronic acid synthesis, therefore, may be yet another potential target of the action of indomethacin.

Nitric oxide stimulates COX-2 activity in a concentration-dependent manner (Salvemini *et al.*, 1993). At pharmacological, micromolar doses, indomethacin had no effect on nitric oxide synthase activity or mRNA expression, in contrast to aspirin, which inhibited the enzyme through a post-translational modification mechanism at millimolar concentrations (Amin *et al.*, 1995).

4.3.3 Immune surveillance

Another mechanism that may be relevant to the chemopreventive action of indomethacin is immunomodulation (Honn *et al.*, 1981; Plescia, 1982; Goodwin & Ceuppens, 1985; Hwang, 1989). Of the arachidonic acid metabolites, only prostaglandin E_2 has a defined function in regulating both humoral and cellular immune responses (Goodwin, 1981, 1984). Elevated tissue levels of prostaglandin E_2 have been shown to suppress immune surveillance by inhibiting T-cell proliferation, natural killer cell cytotoxicity and lymphokine production (Taffet & Russell, 1981; Goodwin & Ceuppens, 1983). Apparently, prostaglandin E_2 exerts its activity by interfering with the production and activity of interleukin 2, a potent lymphokine needed for T-cell proliferation. Drugs such as indomethacin, which block cyclooxygenase activity and prostaglandin production, stimulate the immune response both *in vitro* and *in vivo* (Han *et al.*, 1983; Goodwin, 1984).

An alternative mechanism implicating the immune system involves the ability of indomethacin to restore expression of major histocompatability antigens (HLA) in human colon cancer cells (Arvind *et al.*, 1996). In human colon tumours and in histologically normal mucosa distant from colon adenomas, expression of class I and II HLA antigens is either reduced or lost. Loss of HLA antigen expression allows cancer cells to escape immune surveillance (McDougall *et al.*, 1990; Tsioulias *et al.*, 1992, 1993). Indomethacin induced expression of the class II antigen, HLA-DR, in a time- and dose-dependent manner and increased the steady-state levels of HLA-DR mRNA (Arvind *et al.*, 1996).

The capacity of indomethacin to stimulate the lipoxygenase pathway, particularly 15-lipoxygenase (Vanderhoek *et al.*, 1984), and influence the immune system through production of leukotrienes and other metabolites is an alternative mechanism worthy of further study. Additional experiments conducted with specific COX-2 inhibitors will assist in delineating the role of this enzyme in chemoprevention.

5.   Other Beneficial Effects

Rogers *et al.* (1993) randomized 44 patients with a clinical diagnosis of Alzeimer's disease to indomethacin (100–150 mg/day) or a matching placebo in a double-blind study of six months' duration. Only 14 of 24 (58%) of those randomized to indomethacin and 14 of 20 (70%) of those randomized to placebo completed the trial and were available for measurements. More subjects on indomethacin stopped their treatment, primarily because of gastrointestinal side-effects. Patients on indomethacin who completed the study showed a 1.3% improvement in standardized tests, whereas those on placebo showed a 8.4% decline; at least a 4% decline was seen in only 2 of 14 patients on indomethacin and 12 of 14 patients on placebo.

The remainder of the studies on Alzheimer disease (McGeer *et al.*, 1996), which were observational in nature, were based on a variety of conditions used as surrogates for NSAID use, including history of arthritis and analgesic use. These are summarized in the chapter on aspirin.

6.   Carcinogenicity

6.1   Humans
No data were available to the Working Group.

6.2   Experimental animals
Groups of six-week-old female Sprague-Dawley rats received indomethacin in the drinking-water at a concentration of 10 mg/l [10 ppm] for 92 weeks. The cumulative dose of indomethacin was estimated to be 200 mg per rat. Control rats were given drinking-water only. A significant increase in moderate (10/48; $p < 0.05$) and severe (5/48; $p < 0.05$) hyperplasia of the urinary tract was observed in comparison with the control group (5/49 and 1/49, respectively). The number of rats with mammary adenocarcinomas was higher in those given indomethacin (5/48) than in the untreated control group (1/49; $p < 0.01$). The authors reported a higher incidence of benign mammary gland tumours in the treated (19/48) than in untreated rats (11/49; $p < 0.01$) (Holmäng *et al.*, 1995).

Groups of 50 28-day-old (adolescent) and 97-day-old (adult) male Sprague-Dawley rats received a single application of 25 mg/kg bw indomethacin dissolved in 1 ml acetone on the shaved dorsal skin. A second group received the same dose of indomethacin and acetone plus 21.3 mg/animal of a carrier substance (Amuno®). Control groups received either 1 ml acetone or the carrier only. The animals were observed until natural death. Adolescent rats treated with indomethacin with or without carrier had a lower average body weight than control rats ($p < 0.05$). More malignant tumours were observed in the indomethacin-treated adolescent rats with or without carrier than in their respective controls ($p < 0.02$). In contrast, treatment of adult rats with indomethacin with or without carrier had no effect of the incidence of malignant tumours. Leydig-cell tumours of the testis (distinguished from hyperplasia) were more frequent in indomethacin-treated rats than in either adolescent ($p = 0.005$) or adult ($p = 0.03$) controls. Malignant intestinal tumours were observed in 3/50 adolescent rats treated with indomethacin and in 8/50 also given the carrier but not in control rats (0/50). The increase was not significant. No difference was seen in the adult treated rats (Goerttler *et al.*, 1992). [The Working Group noted that a single dose of indomethacin was used and that the route of administration was inappropriate for carcinogen evaluation.]

Two groups of six-week-old female Sprague-Dawley rats were fed a semisynthetic pelleted diet containing 0.2% N-[4-(5-nitro-2-furyl)-2-thiazolyl]formamide for seven weeks. They were then fed the basal diet up to week 92. One group was given indomethacin in the drinking-water at a concentration of 1 mg/l for 92 weeks starting one week before the carcinogen treatment, for an estimated cumulative dose of 200 mg per rat. The controls were fed synthetic diet for 92 weeks. There was no significant difference in body weight between treated and untreated rats. Indomethacin treatment increased the incidence of urothelial tumours from 4/50 to 10/48 ($p < 0.05$) (Holmäng *et al.*, 1995).

Weanling female Fischer 344 rats were fed standard diet and water *ad libitum* [type of diet and consumption not specified] and given subcutaneous injections of 1,2-dimethyl-hydrazine [purity unspecified] at 40 mg/rat once a week for 10 weeks. After laparotomy, 42 rats were found to be free of visible metastases and 16 rats had grossly apparent metastases in regional nodes, the peritoneum, the omentum and the liver. One-half of the animals with no metastases were given indomethacin in drinking-water at a concentration of 20 μg/ml [20 ppm] until they died or became moribund; the remaining 21 rats were given drug-free water. Indomethacin treatment reduced the median survival from 69 to 29 days ($p < 0.01$) and increased the number of rats with grossly evident metastases from three to nine ($p = 0.035$). When eight rats with metastases were treated with indomethacin as described above, there was no significant effect on mean survival (Danzi *et al.*, 1984). [The Working Group noted that assignment of rats with and without metastases on the basis of staging laparotomy could be subject to considerable variation.]

7.   Other Toxic Effects

7.1   Adverse effects
7.1.1   Humans
See also General Remarks and the chapter on sulindac.

(a)   Gastrointestinal tract toxicity
In the meta-analysis of Henry *et al.* (1996), described in the chapter on aspirin, the risks for serious upper gastrointestinal complications after use of indomethacin were statistically indistinguishable from those of most other NSAIDs. Within individual studies, however, indomethacin was consistently associated with a higher risk for such complications, and in a ranking analysis it ranked 5 (with 1 the most and 12 the least toxic) of 12 NSAIDs analysed. The pooled relative risk estimate from a meta-analysis of five studies that included indomethacin was 3.0 (95% CI, 2.2–4.2) for low-dose indomethacin users and 7.0 (95% C1, 4.4–11) for high-dose users in comparison with non-users. Given baseline risks for ulcer disease of 0.5 per 1000 per year in younger adults (Garcia Rodriguez *et al.*, 1992) and 4 per 1000 in older adults (Smalley *et al.*, 1996), the rates of serious ulcer complications among indomethacin users can be estimated to be 2 per 1000 in younger adults and 10–20 per 1000 in those 65 years and older.

(b)   Reproductive and developmental effects
In non-randomized trials of short courses (one to three days) of indomethacin at doses of 100–400 mg/day for the prevention of pre-term labour, no increase in the risk for congenital anomalies, premature closure of the ductus arteriosus or pulmonary hypertension was observed (Ostensen, 1994). Of 57 infants delivered at or before 30 weeks who had been exposed to indomethacin prenatally, 62% had persistent ductus arteriosus, compared with 44% of unexposed infants matched with exposed infants on gestational age and sex (Norton *et al.*, 1993). This difference was statistically significant. More of the indomethacin-exposed infants with persistent ductus arteriosus required surgical ligation than affected infants who had not been exposed.

There have been case reports of perinatal death associated with severe oligohydramnios in the infants of mothers who used indomethacin (Itskovitz *et al.*, 1980; Veersema *et al.*, 1983). Of 37 fetuses exposed to indomethacin for treatment of pre-term labour, 70% were diagnosed with oligohydramnios, in comparison with 3% of fetuses whose mothers had been treated with agents other than NSAIDs (Hendricks *et al.*, 1990).

In two studies, indomethacin treatment of mothers for pre-term labour was associated with necrotizing enterocolitis in the neonate (Norton *et al.*, 1993; Major *et al.*, 1994).

An unspecified defect was identified from hospital discharge records in one infant among the offspring of 50 women who were members of a health care cooperative in Seattle (USA) and who filled a prescription for indomethacin during the first trimester (Aselton *et al.*, 1985).

(c)   Other toxic manifestations
Indomethacin users report a variety of signs and symptoms more frequently than users of other NSAIDs These include vertigo and headache (Fries *et al.*, 1991).

7.1.2 Experimental animals

Many of the toxic effects of indomethacin in non-human species may result from its action as a prostaglandin synthesis inhibitor. As in humans, the primary site of acute toxicity in various species is the gastrointestinal tract. Drug-induced adverse effects have also been reported in the tissues of the kidney, liver, heart and bone, and significant adverse reproductive and developmental effects have been found.

(a)   Acute and short-term toxicity

Indomethacin was toxic to several species when administered at low levels. The LD$_{50}$ values were as follows: mouse, 5.7 mg/kg bw day orally for five days (Julou et al., 1969); and rat, 2.4 mg/kg bw per day orally for 14 days (Awouters et al., 1975) and 13 mg/kg bw intraperitoneally for seven days (Klaassen, 1976). No defined symptoms of toxicity were reported (Klaassen, 1976). When slightly higher levels of 5–10 mg/kg bw per day orally were administered to male and female rats for up to 21 days, 77–100% of the animals died within four to 10 days. Surviving female rats had a lower weight gain (Gaetani et al., 1972).

Marked growth inhibition, measured as decreased body-weight gain, and decreased food and water consumption were seen in rats treated with indomethacin at 2.5–5 mg/kg per day orally on five days per week for up to 26 weeks. All female and 40% of male rats treated at 5 mg/kg bw per day died within 24 weeks. Overt signs of toxicity included bloody faeces, emaciation, hypoactivity, piloerection, urinary incontinence, loss of grooming activity and anorexia. None of the surviving rats exhibited any abnormal appearance or behaviour, and no significant changes were seen on haematology, blood chemistry, urinalysis, organ weight analysis or pathology (Nomura et al., 1978).

All male and female rats given indomethacin 1–3 mg/kg bw per day orally on six days per week for 30 days or 3 mg/kg bw per day orally for six to 12 weeks survived and remained in good health. Two of six rats at 6 mg/kg bw per day died after 10 and 13 days (Nomura et al., 1978; Anthony et al., 1994).

(b)   Gastrointestinal tract toxicity

Instillation of indomethacin at 12 mg/kg per day directly into the stomach of male and female marmosets resulted in the death of all animals within 20 days. Diarrhoea was observed in animals of each sex treated with the drug at this level of 6 mg/kg per day orally for up to four weeks (Oberto et al., 1990).

Gastrointestinal damage induced by indomethacin has been reported in rats, mice, rabbits, guinea-pigs, dogs and marmosets. Typical lesions include gastric inflammation, mucosal and submucosal haemorrhages, ulceration, perforations and adhesions of the small bowel and peritonitis. The extent of toxicity appears to vary with the excretion of intact drug into the bile and the length of its contact in the small intestine, due to enterohepatic circulation of the drug (Hucker et al., 1966; Yesair et al., 1970a; Duggan et al., 1973, 1975; Klaassen, 1976; Cronen et al., 1982).

In rats, a species considered to be highly susceptible to the ulcerogenic effect of indomethacin (Wilhelmi, 1974), low oral doses rapidly induced marked gastric and duodenal damage when administered as either a single acute dose or over several weeks. Unspecified gastrointestinal lesions were observed within 24–48 h of a single oral dose of 16 mg/kg bw in female rats (Fracasso et al., 1987), while oral doses as low as 6–10 mg/kg bw produced small haemorrhages, small to large (> 2 mm) ulcers and slight to marked hyperaemia (30–100% incidence) within two to five days of treatment (Shriver et al., 1977; Laufer et al., 1994). Multiple oral doses of 6–9 mg/kg bw per day for up to four days or 3 mg/kg per day for up to 11 days resulted in similar lesions, small bowel perforation and adhesions in male rats (Shriver et al., 1977; Laufer et al., 1994). Oral doses of 5 mg/kg bw per day on five days per week for up to 26 weeks produced fibrinous peritonitis, due to perforated ulcers, in the ileum in 40% of male and 100% of female rats that died during the experimental period (Nomura et al., 1978). Few lesions were reported in rats after single or multiple daily oral doses of 1–3 mg/kg for up to four days (Shriver et al., 1977).

Non-ulcerated lesions in the rat caecum, consisting of prominent mucosal folds showing submucosal fibrosis with fibrous obliteration and thickening of the muscularis mucosae, were induced by indomethacin administered in a regimen designed to mimic a course of human treatment. Anthony *et al.* (1994) treated rats for 30 weeks with consecutive doses of 3 mg/kg bw per day for 12 weeks, 4.5 mg/kg bw per day for one week, 6 mg/kg bw per day for one week, no drug for six weeks, 4.5 mg/kg bw per day for two weeks and control diet for eight weeks. These diaphragm-like caecal lesions, similar to lesions observed in the ileum of some patients treated for long periods with NSAIDs (Lang *et al.*, 1988), appear to arise from healed caecal ulcers.

Gastrointestinal ulceration was also reported in mice and guinea-pigs treated twice with indomethacin at doses of 2.5–10 mg/kg bw and 50–100 mg/kg bw orally, respectively (Wilhelmi, 1974). Regions of focal necrosis and subepithelial oedema were noted in rabbits treated intraluminally into the stomach with a solution delivering 100 mg/kg bw of drug for 15 min (Wallace *et al.*, 1991). In dogs, ulceration and inflammation were reported in the small and large intestines after treatment with 2.5 mg/kg bw per day indomethacin orally for up to three years (Stewart *et al.*, 1980). Subacute diffuse inflammation of the gastrointestinal submucosa and serosa with peritoneal involvement, necrosis or ulceration of the mucosa and haemorrhages were also reported in male and female marmosets (*Callithrix jacchus*) treated with indomethacin at 6–12 mg/kg bw per day for up to four weeks (Oberto *et al.*, 1990).

Gastrointestinal damage seems to stem from the ability of indomethacin to suppress prostaglandin synthesis. In this region, prostaglandins are involved in modulation of gastric acid and mucus production, intestinal bicarbonate secretion, regulation of mucosal blood flow and the inflammatory process. Thus, development of indomethacin-induced gastrointestinal lesions may be prevented until weaning in suckling rat pups by prostaglandins, which are known to be present in milk (Bedrick & Holtzapple, 1986). Lesions may develop as a result of drug-induced ischaemia in the mesenteric tissues, an effect demonstrated in dogs, in regions corresponding to drug-induced ulceration (Cronen *et al.*, 1982).

Exacerbation of indomethacin-induced gastrointestinal damage was reported in rats and dogs by an experimentally induced increase in gastric acid production or a decrease in duodenal alkaline secretion. Duodenal lesions (up to a 100% incidence), some penetrating to the muscularis mucosae, and a few lesions in the stomach were precipitated in dogs subsequently injected with gastric acid-inducing histamine (40–80 μg/kg bw intramuscularly, four times per hour for 6 h) beginning 12 h after a single oral dose of 70 mg indomethacin. Alone, this dose produced no ulcers in either the stomach or duodenum within 18 h (Takeuchi *et al.*, 1988). A similar increase in gastric damage was produced in rats (Elliot *et al.*, 1996).

In 630 Wistar rats receiving 12–14 mg/kg bw indomethacin by gavage, there was significantly more intestinal ulceration (two- to fourfold) in those receiving a regular diet than in those on fat-free diets, independent of feeding schedule, sex or castration. Fasting also reduced the intestinal toxicity observed in animals fed a regular diet by two- to fivefold (Del Soldato & Meli, 1977).

(c)   Nephrotoxicity

The primary renal lesions induced by indomethacin in animals and frequently in human patients are papillary necrosis and interstitial inflammation (Jackson & Lawrence, 1978). Drug-induced alterations in renal function and architecture were observed in rats, dogs and marmosets, which may be the result of either tissue phospholipid accumulation, inhibition of prostaglandin synthesis or a combination of the two. Renal damage induced by other agents may also be enhanced by indomethacin.

Papillary necrosis was observed in rats after a single dose of 75 mg/kg bw (Arnold *et al.*, 1974). Renal papillary necrosis associated with either short- or long-term treatment with indomethacin may be the result of selective phospholipid accumulation in renal tissue, the papillae being the most sensitive. In rats treated subcutaneously with 10 or 50 mg/kg bw per day for three days, indomethacin caused a marked increase in all papillary phospholipids (sphingomyelin, phosphatidylcholine, phosphatidylinositol, phosphatidylserine and phosphatidylethanolamine), with an increase in sphingomyelin and phosphatidylethanolamine in the cortex and no observed effect in the medulla. Alterations in renal papillary phospholipid concentrations were observed even at doses as low as 1 mg/kg per day for up to four weeks, but no significant changes were observed in the medulla or cortex (Fernández-Tomé & Sterin Speziale, 1994). This result agrees with other reports of phospholipid accumulation preceding cellular necrosis (Mingeot-Leclercq et al., 1988).

Other renal effects of indomethacin include degenerative changes in the renal parenchyma after oral administration of 5–10 mg/kg bw per day to male and female rats for up to 21 consecutive days (Gaetani et al., 1972), and dose-related subacute interstitial inflammation of the renal cortex in female and male marmosets treated with 2–12 mg/kg bw per day for up to four weeks (Oberto et al., 1990). Although no renal lesions were seen on histological examination of rats treated orally with 2 mg/kg bw for up to four months (Kleinknecht et al., 1983), indomethacin accelerated the destruction of renal glomeruli in puromycin aminonucleoside-induced nephrosis.

Intravenous administration of 4 mg/kg bw indomethacin to anaesthetized dogs produced a very rapid, sharp decrease in renal blood flow and a decrease in water and sodium excretion (Tost et al., 1995). These effects may be related to inhibition of prostaglandin synthesis, as prostaglandins are involved in the regulation of renal blood pressure (Flower et al., 1985); however, this effect was not observed in alert dogs or rats, suggesting an interaction with anaesthesia (Swain et al., 1975).

(d)   Cardiovascular toxicity

Indomethacin caused premature constriction of the ductus arteriosus in the offspring of rats (Momma & Takao, 1989), rabbits (Sharpe et al., 1975) and sheep (Levin et al., 1979) when given near the end of gestation. In pregnant rats treated orally with 2.5–10 mg/kg bw on gestational day 21 or 22, fetal ductal constriction appeared within 6 h of maternal treatment and

lasted for up to 36 h. Hampering of fetal cardiac function by retardation of significant blood flow through the ductus arteriosus can result in fetal acidaemia, hypoxaemia, pulmonary arterial hypertension, altered morphological development of the pulmonary vascular bed, right ventricular hypertrophy, diminished ventricular cavity, left ventricular dilatation, degenerative changes in the papillary muscles of the tricuspid valve, fetal death within 24 h of maternal treatment and respiratory difficulties in the neonate (Momma & Takao, 1989).

Intraventricular injection of 4 mg/kg bw indomethacin to cats diminished the coronary circulation and, to a lesser degree, reduced myocardial oxygen consumption (Stepaniuk & Stoliarchuk, 1985).

Indomethacin impairs scar formation after experimental myocardial infarct in dogs and enhances murine myocarditis due to coxsackie virus B_4 (Hammerman et al., 1983; Khatib et al., 1992).

(e)   Hepatotoxicity

Degenerative changes in the liver, including vacuolar changes and fatty liver, were reported in male and female rats treated with 5–10 mg/kg bw per day for up to 21 days (Gaetani et al., 1972). Alterations in a variety of hepatic microsomal drug-metabolizing enzymes were observed in rats dosed with indomethacin (Burke et al., 1983), as noted above.

(f)   Effects on bone formation

Bone formation during the healing of fractures or induction of heterotopic bone is retarded or completely inhibited by indomethacin. This effect, observed experimentally in rats and rabbits, may be elicited in the early phase of bone induction by a reduction in the inflammatory response, causing less favourable circumstances for bone formation (Rö et al., 1976; Sudmann & Bang, 1979; Allen et al., 1980).

(g)   Haematological effects

Indomethacin induced changes in blood and blood chemistry, including iron-deficiency (microcytic) anaemia, hypoalbuminaemia, leukocytosis, thrombocytosis and decreased total serum proteins, in rats treated with 3–6 mg/kg bw per day in the diet for up to 12 weeks or 5 mg/kg bw per day orally for up to 21 days (Gaetani *et al.*, 1972; Anthony *et al.*, 1994). No drug-induced alterations in haematological or blood chemical parameters were observed after treatment of male and female rats orally with 1–3 mg/kg bw per day on six days per week for 30 days (Nomura *et al.*, 1978).

Slight hypotrophy of the bone marrow, thymus and testis and slight thyroid hypertrophy were seen after oral administration of 5–10 mg/kg bw per day indomethacin to male and female rats for up to 21 days (Gaetani *et al.*, 1972).

(h)   Reproductive and development effects

Indomethacin induced reductions in fetal and decidual tissue weights, fetal malformations, fetal death and prolonged gestation and parturition. The developmental toxicity of indomethacin was recently reviewed (Lione & Scialli, 1995).

Effects on fertility. Indomethacin reduced fertility in male mice treated with 146 µg/day for seven days and rats treated with 0.8 mg/kg bw orally daily for 28 days or 2 mg/kg bw intraperitoneally for seven days. It had anti-mating effects in female rats treated with 0.8-4 mg/kg bw orally, daily from pro-estrous for a period of six cycles before mating (Marley & Smith, 1974; Yegnanarayan & Joglekar, 1978; Löscher & Blazaki, 1986). Significant increases in the number of abnormal sperm were observed in mice treated with 12–36 mg/kg bw per day orally or 12–24 mg/kg bw per day intraperitoneally for 2–30 days (Shobha Devi & Polasa, 1987).

Effects on ovulation. Indomethacin has been reported to suppress ovulation in rats, mice, rabbits, cows, and two species of monkey. The doses sufficient to completely block induced ovulation were reported to be 7 mg/kg bw subcutaneously or 7.5–8 mg per animal intraperitoneally in rats, (Armstrong & Grinwich, 1972; Orczyk & Behrman, 1972; Yegnanarayan & Joglekar, 1978), 200 µg subcutaneously in mice (Saksena *et al.*, 1974), 3 mg/kg bw orally for two days before induction of ovulation in rabbits (O'Grady *et al.*, 1972; Yegnanarayan & Joglekar, 1978) or two injections of 15 mg/kg bw intramuscularly in cynomolgus monkeys

(*Macaca fascicularis*) (Jaszczak, 1975). Induced ovulation was also suppressed in rhesus monkeys (*Macaca mulatta*) (Wallach *et al.*, 1975). In cows, injection of 20 mg of the drug directly into the preovulatory ovarian follicle completely blocked ovulation; however, it was ineffective when given as 5 g intramuscularly five times over 24 h or by intrauterine infusion of 1440 mg total dose per uterine horn (De Silva & Reeves, 1985).

Effects on gestation. Pregnancy disruption resulting from indomethacin treatment, reported in many species may result from reductions in implantation, suppressed placental development or adverse fetal effects. Prostaglandin inhibition may prevent implantation, resulting in lowered ova retention due to tubal disturbances or reduced uterine vascular permeability. Inhibition or delay of implantation was reported after treatment early in gestation in mice (150 µg/day subcutaneously on gestation days 1–4 or a single injection of 225 µg on day 2; Lau *et al.*, 1973), in rats (4 mg/kg bw orally daily on days 1–7, 3 mg/kg subcutaneously on days 3 and 4, or 400 µg into the uterine horns on day 4; Yegnanarayan & Joglekar, 1978; Gupta *et al.*, 1981; Phillips & Poyser, 1981), in rabbits (8–20 mg/kg bw intravenously every 12 h from 2 days before mating to nine days after mating, and similar doses administered on gestation days 4–7; El-Banna *et al.*, 1976; Hoffman, 1978), and in hamsters (0.1 mg/kg bw subcutaneously to pregnant females on gestation day 4; Evans & Kennedy, 1978). Other implantation-related effects include reductions in litter size in hamsters and marked reductions in the number of decidual implantation sites, fetal, placental and decidual tissue weights, and fetal viability. Increased fetal resorptions in rabbits (an apparent anti-implantation effect if it occurs early in gestation) were also observed (Hoos & Hoffman, 1983).

Inhibition of placental development was suggested to be the basis of pregnancy failure in mature gilts given 10 mg/kg bw per day indomethacin in the diet on days 10–25 of gestation (Kraeling *et al.*, 1985).

Post-implantation effects. Maternal treatment with indomethacin in the post-implantation period (mid-gestation) resulted in increased numbers of intrauterine deaths and fetal resorptions in mice (5 mg/kg subcutaneously on gestation days 8–15 or 15 mg/kg bw subcutaneously on days 8–10 or 13–15, Persaud & Moore, 1974); apparent abortion and no successful deliveries at term in rats (4 mg/kg bw orally daily on days 10–16 of pregnancy; Yegnanarayan & Joglekar, 1978) and a reduction in the viability of implanted fetuses in rabbits (8 mg/kg bw subcutaneously twice daily on gestation days 9–12; Hoffman, 1978).

Maternal treatment near term resulted in increased numbers of fetal deaths in rats (0.1 and 1.0 mg/kg bw twice daily on days 18–21 of gestation; Aiken, 1972), in rabbits (2.5–10 mg/kg bw per day subcutaneously on gestation days 26–29; Harris, 1980) and in ewes (0.5–1 mg/kg bw intravenously or 75 mg orally three times daily for four days on gestation days 123–139; Levin et al., 1979). Some of the stillbirths in rats were attributed to placental separation (Aiken, 1972).

Teratogenicity. Indomethacin appears to be teratogenic in mice but not rats. Mouse fetuses were born with eventration of the abdominal viscera, meromelia and defective limb posture when pregnant mice were treated subcutaneously with either 5 mg/kg bw on days 8–15 or 15 mg/kg bw on gestation days 13–15 (Persaud & Moore, 1974). Evidence that indomethacin induces cleft palate in mice was provided both *in vitro* and *in vivo* (Montenegro & Palomino, 1989, 1990). Indomethacin was not teratogenic in rats when administered to dams on gestation days 10–11 at 4 mg/kg bw orally three times (Klein et al., 1981).

Prolongation of gestation. Delay in the onset of parturition, previously a therapeutic indication for use of indomethacin in humans, has also been reported in laboratory animals, including hamsters, rabbits and rhesus monkeys. Parturition onset was delayed in pregnant and pseudopregnant hamsters (300 or 600 µg twice daily on days 14–16 of pregnancy or 1 mg daily from day 5 of pseudopregnancy), although the treatment did not affect the duration of parturition (Lau et al., 1975). In rabbits, prolongation of the

gestation period was route- and time-dependent: 8–10 mg/kg per day in the drinking water from day 20 until delivery prolonged gestation, while subcutaneous administration of similar levels near the end of gestation (days 29–31) did not suppress plasma prostaglandin levels and did not prolong gestation (Challis et al., 1975). With doses similar to those used in human therapy, Novy et al. (1974) reported up to 20 days' prolongation of gestation in rhesus monkeys treated with 100 mg/day on days 150–165 of gestation and 200 mg/day on days 166–187 of gestation. These results were confirmed at lower doses (10–15 mg/kg bw per day on days 150–165 of gestation and 21–28 mg/kg bw per day from day 166 of gestation until delivery) (Manaugh & Novy, 1976).

Administration of indomethacin at the end of gestation appeared to provoke both maternal and fetal adverse events at parturition in rats, rabbits and rhesus monkeys. The maternal events included protracted parturition, haemorrhage and gastric ulcers in rats treated with 0.1 or 1.0 mg/kg bw twice daily on days 18–21 of gestation (Aiken, 1972). Fetal events including signs of prolonged intrauterine stress (staining of the fetal skin, umbilical cord and placental membranes with meconium and a virtual absence of amniotic fluid) were noted in rhesus monkey fetuses at delivery. Four of eight fetuses died, two probably from prolonged labour-induced stress or hypoxia. No gross morphological abnormalities were seen in either the fetuses or the placentas (Manaugh & Novy, 1976). Fetal lung maturation was inhibited at birth after treatment of pregnant rabbits at 10 mg/kg bw per day intramuscularly for three days before delivery (Bustos et al., 1978). Persistent fetal circulation syndrome was reported in neonatal rats in a study in which pregnant rats were treated with 2–4 mg/kg bw per day orally from gestation day 17 to delivery (Harker et al., 1981). The appearance of medial hypertrophy and newly muscularized arterioles, combined with immature, thick saccular walls, produced a decreased surface for oxygen exchange and increased pulmonary vascular resistance.

Prolongation of the length of the oestrus cycle was reportedly induced by indomethacin in guinea-pigs injected subcutaneously with 10 mg/kg bw twice daily for 12 days beginning on day 7 of the cycle or implanted with 33 mg per uterine horn, providing a slow-release dose of 0.2–0.6 mg/day. Oestrus cycles were lengthened by three days in the animals treated with 20 mg/kg bw per day, while cycles of up to 75 days were observed in the implanted animals. Two animals treated with 20 mg/kg bw per day died with gastrointestinal perforations after 11 days of treatment. The authors suggested that the drug blocked the formation of luteolysin in the uterus, prolonging the life of the corpus lutea (Horton & Poyser, 1973). No effect on the length of the oestrus cycle was noted in female rats treated with 0.8–4 mg/kg bw per day orally from pro-oestrus for six cycles before mating (Yegnanarayan & Joglekar, 1978). The authors suggested that the doses used in the studies could not result in the high intrauterine concentrations required to inhibit corpus luteum regression.

7.2 Genetic and related effects
7.2.1 Humans
No data were available to the Working Group.

7.2.2 Experimental models
The genetic and related effects of indomethacin are listed in Table 6.

Indomethacin induced DNA damage in *Bacillus subtilis* (Kuboyama & Fujii, 1992). It did not induce mutation in *Escherichia coli* or *Drosophila melanogaster* (King *et al.*, 1979), but it induced mutation in *Salmonella typhimurium* tester strain TA100 in the presence of exogenous metabolic activation (Kuboyama & Fujii, 1992). It did not induce chromosomal aberrations or aneuploidy (Ishidate *et al.*, 1988) in hamster cells *in vitro*. Indomethacin induced chromosomal aberrations and sperm abnormalities in mice *in vivo* (Shobha Devi & Polasa, 1987). Conflicting results were reported for micronucleus induction in mice (Shobha Devi & Polasa, 1987; King *et al.*, 1979). It did not induce sister chromatid exchange in human lymphocytes *in vivo* (Kullich & Klein, 1986).

Table 6. Genetic and related effects of indomethacin

End-point	Test code	Test system	Results[a] –	+	Dose[b] (LED or HID)	Reference
D	BSD	*B. subtilis rec*, differential toxicity	+	0	100	Kuboyama & Fujii (1992)
G	SA5	*S. typhimurium* TA1535, reverse mutation	–	–	1790	King *et al.* (1979)
G	SA7	*S. typhimurium* TA 1537, reverse mutation	–	–	1790	King *et al.* (1979)
G	SA8	*S. typhimurium* TA 1538, reverse mutation	–	–	1790	King *et al.* (1979)
G	SA9	*S. typhimurium* TA 98, reverse mutation	–	–	1790	King *et al.* (1979)
G	SA9	*S. typhimurium* TA98, reverse mutation	–	–	27	Kuboyama & Fujii (1992)
G	SA0	*S. typhimurium* TA100, reverse mutation	–		1790	King *et al.* (1979)
G	SA0	*S. typhimurium* TA100, reverse mutation	–	+	27	Kuboyama & Fujii (1992)
G	ECK	*E. coli* K12, forward or reverse mutation	–	0	10 740	King *et al.* (1979)
G	DMX	*D. melanogaster*, sex-linked receessive recessive lethal mutation	–	0	895	King *et al.* (1979)
C	CIC	Chromosomal aberration, Chinese hamste r cells *in vitro*	–	0	250	Ishidate *et al.* (1988)
C	SLH	Sister chromatid exchange, human lymphocytes *in vitro*	–	0	1.1	Kullich & Klein (1986)
A	AIA	Aneuploidy, human cells *in vitro*	–	0	250	Ishidate *et al.* (1988)
C	CVA	Chromosomal aberation, mouse spermatocytes *in vivo*	+	0	12	Shobha Devi & Polasa (1987)
M	MVM	Micronucleus formation, mice *in vivo*	(+)	0	24	Shobha Devi & Polasa (1987)
M	MVM	Micronucleus formation, mice *in vivo*	+	0	179	King *et al.* (1979)
P	SPM	Sperm morphology, mice *in vivo*	+	0	12	Shobha Devi & Polasa (1987)

Definitions of the abbreviations and terms used are given in Appendix 1.
[a] In the absence (–) and presence (+) of an exogenous metabolic activation system; + positive, (+) weakly positive; – negative; 0, not determined
[b] Lowest effective dose (LED) or highest ineffective dose (HID) expressed as µg/ml for in-vitro studies and as mg/kg body weight per day for in-vivo studies

8. Summary of Data

8.1 Chemistry, occurrence and human exposure

Indomethacin has been used for over 30 years as an analgesic and anti-inflammatory agent. It is used in the treatment of a variety of musculoskeletal conditions, notably rheumatoid and osteoarthritis. It is conventionally prescribed at doses of 25–100 mg three or four times daily.

8.2 Metabolism and kinetic properties

Conventional oral administration results in a high level of bioavailability, although foods taken concomitantly may delay and/or reduce absorption. Indomethacin is strongly bound to serum albumin. After its distribution, indomethacin undergoes glucuronide conjugation, O-demethylation and N-deacylation. Less than 10% of an oral dose is recovered as the unchanged parent compound in urine; indomethacin is also eliminated in bile and undergoes extensive enterohepatic recirculation.

8.3 Cancer-preventive effects
8.3.1 Humans

No studies have been reported that specifically address protection by indomethacin against cancer. Case reports of the use of indomethacin in patients with familial adenomatous polyposis showed regression of polyps in about one-half of the patients.

8.3.2 Experimental animals

The chemopreventive efficacy of indomethacin was assessed in mouse, rat and hamster models. In seven studies in mice, the effects of indomethacin were studied on carcinogenesis in the oesophagus, urinary bladder, cervix and skin. Indomethacin was effective in all of the studies, but appeared to be less effective during late stages of carcinogenesis and in the skin.

The cancer-preventive efficacy of indomethacin was investigated in 20 studies in rats in models of cancers of the oesophagus, colon, urinary bladder, tongue, liver, mammary gland, nervous system and kidney. It was effective in all 12 studies in which the colon was the target organ, but inconsistent results were obtained in models of mammary gland carcinogenesis: it

was effective in three studies and ineffective in another three. In single studies in rats, indomethacin had chemopreventive effects in models of cancers of the urinary bladder, liver and tongue.

The efficacy of indomethacin in inhibiting oral cavity tumorigenesis in hamsters remains controversial. No conclusive reduction was seen in pancreatic tumorigenesis in hamsters.

Indomethacin had antimutagenic activity in a variety of test systems.

8.3.3 Mechanism of action

While the anti-inflammatory action of indomethacin is directly linked to its ability to inhibit the cyclooxygenases, the precise molecular mechanism(s) whereby indomethacin and other non-steroidal anti-inflammatory drugs exert their chemopreventive effects remain unclear. Mechanisms secondary to prostaglandin reduction, such as enhanced immune surveillance and stimulation of T-cell proliferation, may be involved. Furthermore, indomethacin may exert a protective effect against cancer by influencing receptors or affecting enzymes other than cyclooxygenases.

8.4 Other beneficial effects

One small clinical trial in which many patients could not be followed up suggests that indomethacin slows the progression of Alzheimer's disease.

8.5 Carcinogenicity
8.5.1 Humans

No data were available to the Working Group.

8.5.2 Experimental animals

Indomethacin given to rats in the drinking-water for life induced hyperplasia of the urinary tract. In a further study in rats, the incidence of urinary bladder tumours induced by N-[4-(5-nitro-2-furyl)-2-thiazolyl]formamide was enhanced by concomitant treatment with indomethacin.

8.6 Toxic effects
8.6.1 Humans

Indomethacin has a wide variety of adverse effects, the most clinically important of which are ulcers and bleeding in the upper gastrointestinal tract. Indomethacin increases the risk for these complications in a dose-dependent manner. Indomethacin decreases renal function and increases blood pressure, sometimes causes rash and headache and rarely results in hepatotoxicity and aseptic meningitis.

8.6.2 Experimental animals

Many of the toxic effects of indomethacin in experimental animals may be due to inhibition of prostaglandin synthesis. As in humans, the primary site of acute toxicity is the gastrointestinal tract, although adverse effects have also been reported in kidney, liver, heart and bone.

Toxic effects on male fertility, female mating behaviour, ovulation and gestation, teratogenicity and effects on fetal circulatory development have been reported in isolated studies in experimental animals.

In one study in mice treated *in vivo*, indomethacin induced chromosomal aberrations in spermatocytes and micronuclei in bone marrow.

9. Recommendations for Research

Toxicity would be a major drawback to developing indomethacin as a chemopreventive agent in humans. The preventive efficacy of indomethacin has been assessed extensively in animal models, and no further experimental investigation is needed, unless specific mechanisms of action are addressed.

10. Evaluation[1]

10.1 Cancer-preventive activity

10.1.1 Humans

There is *inadequate evidence* that indomethacin has cancer-preventive activity in humans.

10.1.2 Experimental models

There is *sufficient evidence* that indomethacin has cancer-preventive activity in experimental animals. This evaluation is based on models of cancers of the colon and oesophagus.

10.2 Overall evaluation

Epidemiological studies in humans provide *inadequate evidence* for the cancer-preventive activity of indomethacin, although some data suggest that it prevents the progression of adenomatous polyps in patients with familial adenomatous polyposis. In experimental animals, there is *sufficient evidence* that indomethacin prevents colon cancer. The adverse effects of indomethacin include dose-dependent bleeding and ulceration in the upper gastrointestinal tract and hepatic and renal toxicity.

Despite the availability of extensive data from studies of experimental models, indomethacin cannot be regarded as a chemopreventive agent in humans, because of inadequate epidemiological data.

11. References

Abe, S. (1986) Effects of arachidonic acid and indomethacin on sister-chromatid exchange induction by polycyclic aromatic hydrocarbons in mammalian cell lines. *Mutat. Res.*, **173**, 55–60

Abou-El-Ela, S.H., Prasse, K.W., Farrell, R.L., Carroll, R.W., Wade, A.E. & Bunce, O.R. (1989) Effects of D,L-2-difluoromethylornithine and indomethacin on mammary tumor promotion in rats fed high n-3 and/or n-6 fat diets. *Cancer Res.*, **49**, 1434–1440

Abramson, S.B. & Weissmann, G. (1989) The mechanisms of action of nonsteroidal antiinflammatory drugs. *Arthritis Rheum.*, **32**, 1–9

Aiken, J.W. (1972) Aspirin and indomethacin prolong parturition in rats: Evidence that prostaglandins contribute to expulsion of foetus. *Nature*, **240**, 21–25

Alexandrov, V.A., Bespalov, V.G., Petrov, A.S., Troyan, D.N. & Lichks, M.Y. (1996) Study of post-natal effect of chemopreventive agents on ethylnitrosoura-induced transplacental carcinogenesis in rats. III Inhibitory action of indomethacin, voltaren, theophylline and e-amniocaproic acid. *Carcinogenesis*, **17**, 1935–1939

Allen, H.L., Wase, A. & Bear, W.T. (1980) Indomethacin and aspirin: Effect of nonsteroidal anti-inflammatory agents on the rate of fracture repair in the rat. *Acta orthopaed. scand.*, **51**, 595–600

Alvan, G., Orme, M., Bertilsson, L., Ekstrand, R. & Palmer, L. (1975) Pharmacokinetics of indomethacin. *Clin. pharmacol. Ther.*, **18**, 364–373

---

[1] For definitions of the italicized terms, see the Preamble, pp. 12–13

Amin, A.R., Vyas, P., Attur, M., Leszczynska-Piziak, J., Patel, I.R., Weissmann, G. & Abramson, S.B. (1995) The mode of action of aspirin-like drugs: Effect on inducible nitric oxide synthase. *Proc. natl Acad. Sci. USA.*, **92**, 7926–7930

Amstad, P., Levy, A., Emerit, I. & Cerutti, P. (1984) Evidence for membrane-mediated chromosomal damage by aflatoxin B1 in human lymphocytes. *Carcinogenesis*, **5**, 719–723

Anderson, D.F., Phernetton, T.M. & Rankin, J.H.G. (1980) The measurement of placental drug clearance in near-term sheep: Indomethacin. *J. pharmacol. exp. Ther.*, **213**, 100–104

Andrews, F.J., Halliday, G.M. & Muller, H.K. (1991) A role of prostaglandins in the suppression of cutaneous cellular immunity and tumour development in benzo(a)pyrene- but not 7,12-dimethyl-benz(a)anthracene-treated mice. *Clin. exp. Immunol.*, **85**, 9–13

Anthony, A., Dhillon, A.P., Sim, R., Nygard, G., Pounder, R.E. & Wakefield, A.J. (1994) Ulceration, fibrosis and diaphragm-like lesions in the caecum of rats treated with indomethacin. *Aliment. Pharmacol. Ther.*, **8**, 417–424

Armstrong, D.T. & Grinwich, D.L. (1972) Blockade of spontaneous and LH-induced ovulation in rats by indomethacin, an inhibitor of prostaglandin biosynthesis. *Prostaglandins*, **1**, 21–28

Arnold, E. & Brynger, H. (1970) [Serum concentrations after administration of indomethacin capsules and suppositories. *Opusc. Med*, **15**, 333–336 (in Swedish)

Arnold, L., Collins, C. & Starmer, G.A. (1974) Renal and gastric lesions after phenylbutazone and indomethacin in the rat. *Pathology*, **6**, 303–313

Aronson, J.K., Chappell, M.J., Godfrey, K.R. & Yew, M.K. (1993) Modelling circadian variation in the pharmacokinetics of non-steroidal anti-inflammatory drugs. *Eur. J. clin. Pharmacol.*, **45**, 357–361

Arvind, P., Qiao, L., Papavassiliou, E.D., Goldin, E., Koutsos, M. & Rigas, B. (1996) Aspirin and aspirin-like drugs induce HLA-DR expression in HT29 colon cancer cells. *Int. J. Oncol.*, **8**, 1207–1211

Aselton, P., Jick, H., Milunsky, A., Hunter, J.R. & Stergachis, A (1985) First-trimester drug use and congenital disorders. *Obstet. Gynecol.*, **65**, 451–455

August, E.M., Nguyen, T., Malinowski, N.M. & Cysyk, R.L. (1994) Non-steroidal anti-inflammatory drugs and tumor progression: Inhibition of fibroblast hyaluronic acid production by indomethacin and mefenamic acid. *Cancer Lett.*, **82**, 49–54

Awouters, F., Niemegeers, C.J.E., Lenaerts, F.M. & Janssen, P.A.J. (1975) The effects of suprofen in rats with mycobacterium butyricum-induced arthritis. *Arzneimittel.-forsch.*, **25**, 1526–1537

Baer, J.E., Hucker, H.B. & Duggan, D.E. (1974) Bioavailability of indomethacin in man. *Ann. clin. Res.*, **6**, 44–47

Bayer, B.M. & Beaven, M.A. (1979) Evidence that indomethacin reversibly inhibits cell growth in the G1 phase of the cell cycle. *Biochem. Pharmacol.*, **28**, 441–443

Bayer, B.M., Kruth, H.S., Vaughan, M. & Beaven, M.A. (1979) Arrest of cultured cells in the G1 phase of the cell cycle by indomethacin. *J. Pharmacol. exp. Ther.*, **210**, 106–111

Bedrick, A.D. & Holtzapple, P.G. (1986) Indomethacin fails to induce ulceration in the gastrointestinal tract of newborn and suckling rats. *Pediatr. Res.*, **20**, 598–601

Bertrand, P., Girard, N., Delpech, B., Duval, C., d'Anjou, J. & Dauce, J.P. (1992) Hyaluronan (hyaluronic acid) and hyaluronectin in the extracellular matrix of human breast carcinomas: Comparison between invasive and non-invasive areas. *Int. J. Cancer*, **52**, 1–6

Bespalov V.G., Troyan D.N., Petrov A.S. & Alexandrov V.A. (1989) Inhibition of the esophagus tumor development by anti-inflammatory non-steroidal and steroidal drugs indomethacin and dexamethasone. *Pharmacol. Toxicol.*, **52**, 67–70

Bespalov, V.G., Lidak, M.Y., Petrov, A.S., Troyan, D.N. & Alexandrov, V.A. (1992) Study of anticarcinogenic effect of ortophen and indomethacin in rats and mice with induced tumours of different organs. *Exp. Oncol.*, **14**, 36–40

Bhat, R., Vidyasagar, D., Vadapalli, M., Whallcy, C., Fisher, E., Hastreiter, A. & Evans, M. (1979) Disposition of indomethacin in preterm infants. *J. Pediatr.*, **95**, 313–316

Bhat, R., Vidyasagar, D., Fisher, E., Hastreiter, A., Ramirez, J.L., Burns, L. & Evans, M. (1980) Pharmacokinetics of oral and intravenous indomethacin in preterm infants. *Dev. Pharmacol.*, **1**, 101–110

Billups, N.F. & Billups, S.M. eds (1992) *American Drug Index*, 36th Ed., St Louis, MO, Facts and Comparisons, p. 307

Bruguerolle, B., Barbeau, G., Belanger, P.M. & Labrecque, G. (1986) Pharmacokinetics of a sustained-release product of indomethacin in the elderly. *Gerontology.*, **32**, 277–285

Budavari, S., O'Neil, M.J., Smith, A., Heckelman, P.E. & Kinneary, J.F., eds (1996) *Merck Index*, 12th Ed., Rahway, NJ, Merck & Co., p. 4995

Buenaventura, S.K., Jacobson-Kram, D., Dearfield, K.L. & Williams, J.R. (1984) Induction of sister chromatid exchange by diethylstilbestrol in metabolically competent hepatoma cell lines but not in fibroblasts. *Cancer Res.*, **44**, 3851–3855

Burke, M.D., Falzon, M. & Milton A.S. (1983) Decreased hepatic microsomal cytochrome P450 due to indomethacin: Protective roles of 16,16-dimethyl-prostaglandin F2 alpha and inducing agents. *Biochem. Pharmacol.*, **32**, 389-397

Bustos, R., Ballejo, G., Giussi, G., Rosas, R. and Isa, J.C. (1978) Inhibition of fetal lung maturation by indomethacin in pregnant rabbits. *J. Perinat. Med.*, **6**, 240–245

Carter, C.A., Milholland, R.J., Shea, W. & Ip. M.M. (1983) Effect of the prostaglandin synthetase inhibitor indomethacin on 7,12-dimethylbenz(*a*)-anthracene-induced mammary tumorigenesis in rats fed different levels of fat. *Cancer Res.*, **43**, 3559–3562

Caruso, I. (1971) [Distribution of indomethacin in blood and synovial fluid of patients with rheumatoid arthritis.] *Arzneimittel.-forsch.*, **21**, 1824–1826 (in German)

Castleden, C.M. & Pickles, H. (1988) Suspected adverse drug reactions in elderly patients reported to the Committee on Safety of Medicines. *Br. J. clin. Pharmacol.*, **26**, 347–353

Challis, J.R.G., Davies, I.J. & Ryan, K.J. (1975) The effects of dexamethasone and indomethacin on the outcome of pregnancy in the rabbit. *J. Endocrinol.*, **64**, 363–370

Clench, J., Reinberg, A., Dziewanowska, Z., Ghata, J. & Smolensky, M. (1981) Circadian changes in the bioavailability and effects of indomethacin in healthy subjects. *Eur. J. clin. Pharmacol.*, **20**, 359–369

Clozel, M., Beharry, K. & Aranda, J.V. (1986) Indomethacin metabolism in liver microsomes during postnatal development in the rat. *Biol. Neonate*, **50**, 83–90

Cooney, G.J. & Dawson, A.G. (1977) Effects of indomethacin on the metabolism of glucose by isolated rat kidney tubules. *Biochem. Pharmacol.*, **26**, 2463–2468

Cronen, P.W., Nagaraj, H.S., Janik, J.S., Groff, D.B., Passmore, J.C. & Hock, C.E. (1982) Effect of indomethacin on mesenteric circulation in mongrel dogs. *J. pediatr. Surg.*, **17**, 474–478

Curran, N.M., Lovering, E.G., McErlane, K.M. &

Watson, J.R. (1980) Impurities in drugs IV: Indomethacin. *J. pharm. Sci.*, **69**, 187–189

Danzi, M., Ferulano, G.P., Abate, S. & Califano, G. (1984) Enhancement of colonic cancer by indomethacin treatment in dimethylhydrazine pretreated rats. *Carcinogenesis.*, **5**, 287–289

Delbeke, F.T., Debackere, M. & Vynckier, L. (1991) Disposition of human drug preparations in the horse. I. Rectally administered indomethacin. *J. Vet. Pharmacol. Ther.*, **14**, 145–149

Del Soldato, P. & Meli, A. (1977) Factors influencing indomethacin toxicity in the rat. *Farmaco. Sci*, **32**, 845–852

De Silva, M. & Reeves, J.J. (1985) Indomethacin inhibition of ovulation in the cow. *J. Reprod. Fertil.*, **75**, 547–549

Duggan, D.E., Hogans, A.F., Kwan, K.C. & McMahon, F.G. (1972) The metabolism of indomethacin in man. *J. Pharmacol. exp. Ther.*, **181**, 563-575

Duggan, D.E., Hogans, A.F. & Kwan, K.C. (1973) Species differences in total biliary secretion of indomethacin (Abstract 3334). *Fed. Proc.*, **32**, 809

Duggan, D.E., Hooke, K.F., Noll, R.M. & Kwan, K.C. (1975) Enterohepatic circulation of indomethacin and its role in intestinal irritation. *Biochem. Pharmacol.*, **24**, 1749–1754

Earnest, D.L., Hixson, L.J. & Alberts, D.S. (1992) Piroxicam and other cyclooxygenase inhibitors: Potential for cancer chemoprevention. *J. cell. Biochem.*, **161**, 156–166

Ekmekci, A., Sayli, A., Donmez, H. & Bal, F. (1995) In vitro effects of prostaglandin E1 and indomethacin on mitomycin C-induced sister-chromatid exchanges in mitogen-stimulated human lymphocytes. *Mutat. Res.*, **328**, 49–53

El-Banna, A.A., Sacher, B. & Schilling, E. (1976) Effect of indomethacin on egg transport and pregnancy in the rabbit. *J. Reprod. Fertil.*, **46**, 375–378

Elliott, S.L., Ferris, R.J., Giraud, A.S., Cook, G.A., Skeljo, M.V. & Yeomans, N.D. (1996) Indomethacin damage to the gastric mucosa is markedly dependent on luminal pH. *Clin. exp. Pharm. Physiol.*, **23**, 432–434

Emerit, I. & Cerutti, P.A. (1982) Tumor promoter phorbol 12-myristate 13-acetate induces a clastogenic factor in human lymphocytes. *Proc. natl. Acad. Sci. USA.*, **79**, 7509–7513

Emori, H.W., Champion, G.D., Bluestone, R. & Paulus, H.E. (1973) Simultaneous pharmacokinetics of indomethacin in serum and synovial fluid. *Ann. rheum. Dis.*, **32**, 433–435

Emori, H.W., Paulus, H., Bluestone, R., Champion, G.D. & Pearson, C. (1976) Indomethacin serum concentrations in man. Effects of dosage, food, and antacid. *Ann. rheum. Dis.*, **35**, 333–338

Evans, C.A. & Kennedy, T.G. (1978) The importance of prostaglandin synthesis for the initiation of blastocyst implantation in the hamster. *J. Reprod. Fertil.*, **54**, 255–261

Evans, M.A., Bhat, R., Vidyasagar, D., Vadapalli, M., Fisher, E. & Hastreiter, A. (1979) Gestational age and indomethacin elimination in the neonate. *Clin. pharmol. Ther.*, 26, 746–751

Evans, M.A., Papazafiratou, C., Bhat, R.,& Vidyasagar, D. (1981) Indomethacin metabolism in isolated neonatal and fetal rabbit hepatocytes. *Pediatr. Res.*, **15**, 1406–1410

Fernández Tomé, M.C. & Sterin Speziale N.B. (1994) Short and long term treatment with indomethacin causes renal phospholipid alteration : a possible explanation for indomethacin nephrotoxicity. *Pharmacology*, **48**, 341–348

Flower, R.J., Moncada, S. & Vane, J.R. (1985) Analgesic-antipyretics and anti-inflammatory agents. Drugs employed in the treatment of gout. In: Gilman, A.G., Goodman, L.S., Rall, T.W. & Murad, F., eds, *The Pharmacological Basis of Therapeutics*. 7th Ed., New York, Macmillan Publishing Co., pp. 674–715

Flowers-Geary, L., Harvey, R.G. & Penning, T.M. (1995) Identification of benzo[*a*]pyrene-7,8-dione as an authentic metabolite of (±)-*trans*-7,8-dihydroxy-7,8-dihydrobenzo[*a*]pyrene in isolated rat hepatocytes. *Carcinogenesis*, **16**, 2707–2715

Fracasso, M.E., Cuzzolin, L., Del Soldato, P., Leone, R., Velo, G.P. & Benoni, G. (1987) Multisystem toxicity of indomethacin: Effects on kidney, liver and intestine in the rat. *Agents Actions*, **22**, 310–313

Franklin, C.D. & Craig, G.T. (1987) The effect of indomethacin on tumor regression in DMBA-induced epithelial neoplasia of hamster cheek pouch mucosa. *Oral Surg.*, **63**, 335–339

Friedman, G.D. & Ury, H.K. (1980) Initial screening for carcinogenicity of commonly used drugs. *J. natl Cancer Inst.*, **65**, 723–733

Friedman, J., Shabtai, F., Levy, L.S. & Djaldetti, M. (1987) Chromium chloride induces chromosomal aberrations in human lymphocytes via indirect action, *Mutat. Res.*, **191**, 207–210

Friedman, Z., Whitman, V., Maisels, M.J., Berman, W., Jr. Marks, K.H. & Vesell, E.S. (1978) Indomethacin disposition and indomethacin-induced platelet dysfunction in premature infants. *J. clin. Pharmacol.*, **18**, 272–279

Friedman, G.D. & Ury, H.K. (1983) Screening for possibile drug carcinogenicity: Second report of findings. *J. natl Cancer Inst.*, **71**, 1165–1175

Fries, J.F., Williams, C.A. & Bloch D.A. (1991) The relative toxicity of nonsteroidal antiinflammatory drugs. *Arthritis Rheum.*, **34**, 1353–1360

Furstenberger, G. & Marks, F. (1978) Indomethacin inhibition of cell proliferation induced by the phorbol ester TPA is reversed by prostaglandin E2 in mouse epidermis *in vivo*. *Biochem. biophys. Res. Commun.*, **84**, 1103–1111

Furstenberger, G. & Marks, F. (1980) Early prostaglandin E synthesis is an obligatory event in the induction of cell proliferation in mouse epidermis *in vivo* by the phorbol ester TPA. *Biochem. biophys. Res. Commun.*, **92**, 749–756

Gaetani, M., Debeus, R., Vidi, A. & Coppi, G. (1972) Toxicological investigations of 4-prenyl-1,2-diphenyl-3,5-pyrazolidinedione (DA 2370). A comparative study of short-term toxicity of DA 2370 and other non-steroidal anti-inflammatory drugs (phenylbutazone, mefenemic acid, indometacin and benzydamine) in the rat. *Arzneimittel.-forsch.*, **22**, 226–234

Garcia Rodriguez, L.A., Walker, A.M. & Gutthann, S.P. (1992) Nonsteroidal antiinflammatory drugs and gastrointestinal hospitalizations in Saskatchewan: A cohort study. *Epidemiology*, **3**, 337–342

Goerttler, K., Edler, L. & Loehrke, H. (1992) Long term tumorigeniciy of a single application of indomethacin or Amuno® in adolescent and in adult male Sprague Dawley rats. *Exp. Toxicol. Pathol.*, **44**, 361–370.

Goodwin, J.S. (1981) Prostaglandins and host defense in cancer. *Med. Clin. North Am.*, **65**, 829–844

Goodwin, J.S. (1984) Immunologic effects of nonsteroidal anti-inflammatory drugs. *Am. J. Med.*, **77**, 7–15

Goodwin, J.S. & Ceuppens, J. (1983) Regulation of the immune response by prostaglandins. *J. clin. Immunol.*, **3**, 295–315

Goodwin, J.S. & Ceuppens, J.L. (1985) Prostaglandins, cellular immunity and cancer. *Prostaglandins Leukotrienes Cancer*, **4**, 1–34

Gould, A.R., Miller, R.L., Grant, F.T. & Perry, D.A. (1985) Indomethacin and 7,12-dimethylbenz(a)-anthracene-induced carcinogenesis in the hamster buccal pouch. *J. Oral Pathol.*, **14**, 398–404

Grady, M.K., Jacobson-Kram, D., Dearfield, K.L. & Williams, J.R. (1986) Induction of sister chromatid exchanges by benzidine in rat and human hepatoma cell lines and inhibition by indomethacin. *Cell Biol. Toxicol.*, **2**, 223–230

Griffin, M.R., Piper, J.M., Daugherty, J.R., Snowden, M. & Ray, W.A. (1991) Nonsteroidal anti-inflammatory drug use and increased risk for peptic ulcer disease in elderly persons. *Ann intern. Med.*, **114**, 257–263

Grubbs, C.J., Juliana, M.M., Eto, I., Casebolt, T., Whitaker, L.M., Canfield, G.J., Manczak, M., Steele, V.E. & Kelloff, G.J. (1993) Chemoprevention by indomethacin of n-butyl-n-(4-hydroxybutyl)-nitrosamine-induced urinary bladder tumors. *Anticancer Res.*, **13**, 33–36

Gullino, P.M. (1981) Angiogenesis and neoplasia. *New Engl. J. Med.*, **305**, 884–885

Gupta, U., Malhotra, N., Varma, S.K. & Chaudhury, R.R. (1981) Effect of intrauterine administration of antiprostaglandin drugs on implantation in the rat. *Contraception*, **24**, 283–288

Haedersdal, M., Poulsen, T. & Wulf, H.C. (1995) Effects of systemic indomethacin on photocarcinogenesis in hairless mice. *J. Cancer Res. clin. Oncol.*, **121**, 257–261

Hammerman, H., Kloner, R.A., Schoen, F.J., Brown, E.J., Jr, Hale, S. & Braunwald, E. (1983) Indomethacin-induced scar thinning after experimental myocardial infarction. *Circulation*, **67**, 1290–1295

Han, T., Nemoto, T., Ledesma, E.J. & Bruno, S. (1983) Enhancement of T lymphocyte proliferative response to mitogens by indomethacin in breast and colorectal cancer patients. *Int. J. Immunopharmacol.*, **5**, 11–15

Harker, L.C., Kirkpatrick, S.E., Friedman, W.F. & Bloor, C.M. (1981) Effects of indomethacin on fetal rat lungs: A possible cause of persistent fetal circulation (PFC). *Pediatr. Res.*, **15**, 147–151

Harman, R.E., Meisinger, M.A.P., Davis, G.E. & Kuehl, F.A., Jr (1964) The metabolites of indomethacin, a new anti-inflammatory drug. *J. Pharmacol. exp. Ther.*, **143**, 215–220

Harris, W.H. (1980) The effects of repeated doses of indomethacin on fetal rabbit mortality and on the patency of the ductus arteriosus. *Can. J. Physiol. Pharmacol.*, **58**, 212–216

Harris, W.H. & Van Petten, G.R. (1981) Placental transfer of indomethacin in the rabbit and sheep. *Can. J. Physiol. Pharmacol.*, **59**, 342–346

Helleberg, L. (1981) Clinical pharmacokinetics of indomethacin. *Clin. Pharmacokinet.*, **6**, 245–258

Hendricks, S.K., Smith, J.R., Jr, Moore D.E. & Brown, Z.A. (1990) Oligohydramnios associated with prostaglandin synthetase inhibitors in preterm labour. *Br J Obstet Gynaecol.*, **97**, 312–316

Henry, D., Lim, L.-Y., Garcia Rodriguez, L.A., Perez Gutthan, S., Carson, J.L., Griffin, M., Savage, R., Logan, R., Moride Y., Hawkey, C., Hill, S., Fries, J.R. (1996) Variability in risk of major upper gastrointestinal complications with individual NSAIDs. Results of a collaborative meta-analysis. *Br. med. J.*, **312**, 1563–1566

Hillbertz-Nilsson, K. & Forsberg, J.G. (1989) Genotoxic effects of estrogens in epithelial cells from the neonatal mouse uterine cervix: Modifications by metabolic modifiers. *Teratog. Carcinog. Mutag.*, **9**, 97–110

Hirata, K., Itoh, H. & Ohsato, K. (1994) Regression of rectal polyps by indomethacin suppository in familial adenomatous polyposis. Report of two cases. *Dis. Colon Rectum*, **37**, 943–946

Hirota, C., Lida, M., Aoyagi, K., Matsumoto, T., Tada, S., Yao, T. & Fujishima, M. (1996) Effect of indomethacin suppositories on rectal polyposis in patients with familial adenomatous polyposis. *Cancer*, **78**, 1660–1665

Hoffman, L.H. (1978) Antifertility effects of indomethacin during early pregnancy in the rabbit. *Biol. Reprod.*, **18**, 148–153

Holmäng, S., Cano, M., Grenabo, L. , Hedelin, H. & Johansson, S.L. (1995) Effect of indomethacin on N-4-(5-nitro-2-furyl)-2-thiazolyl]formamide-induced urinary tract carcinogenesis. *Carcinogenesis*, **16**, 1493–1498

Holt, L.P.J. & Hawkins, C.F. (1965) Indomethacin: Studies of absorption and of the use of indomethacin suppositories. *Br. med. J.*, **i**, 1354–1356

Honn, K.V., Bockman, R.S. & Marnett, L.J. (1981) Prostaglandins and cancer: A review of tumor initiation through tumor metastasis. *Prostaglandins*, **21**, 833–864

Hoos, P.C. & Hoffman, L.H. (1983) Effect of histamine receptor antagonists and indomethacin on implantation in the rabbit. *Biol. Reprod.*, **29**, 833–840

Horton, E.W. & Poyser, N.L. (1973) Elongation of oestrous cycle in the guinea-pig following subcutaneous or intra-uterine administration of indomethacin. *Br. J. Pharmacol.*, **49**, 98–105

Hubert, P. & Crommen, J. (1990) Automatic determination of indomethacin in human plasma using liquid–solid extraction on disposable cartridges in combination with HPLC. *J. liq. Chromatogr.*, **13**, 3891–3907

Hucker, H.B., Zacchei, A.G., Cox, S.V., Brodie, D.A. & Cantwell, N.H.R. (1966) Studies on the absorption, distribution and excretion of indomethacin in various species. *J. clin. Pharmacol. exp. Ther.*, **153**, 237–249

Hultmark, D., Borg, K.O., Elofsson, R. & Palmer, L. (1975) Interaction between salicylic acid and indomethacin in binding to human serum albumin. *Acta pharmacol. suec.*, **12**, 259–276

Huskisson, E.C., Taylor, R.T., Burston, D., Chuter, P.J. & Hart, F.D. (1970) Evening indomethacin in the treatment of rheumatoid arthritis. *Ann. rheum. Dis.*, **29**, 393–396

Hvidberg, E., Lausen, H.H. & Jansen, J.A. (1972) Indomethacin: Plasma concentrations and protein binding in man. *Eur. J. clin. Pharmacol.*, **4**, 119–124

Hwang, D. (1989) Essential fatty acids and immune response. *FASEB J.*, **3**, 2052–2061

Ishidate, M., Jr., Harnois, M.C. & Sofuni, T. (1988) A comparative analysis of data on the clastogenicity of 951 chemical substances tested in mammalian cell cultures. *Mutat. Res.*, **195**, 151–213

Itoh, H., Ikeda, S., Oohata, Y., Iida, M., Inoue, T. & Onitsuka H. (1988) Treatment of desmoid tumors in Gardner's syndrome. *Dis. Colon Rectum*, **31**, 459–461

Itskovitz, J., Abramovici H. & Brandes, J.M. (1980) Oligohydramnion, meconium and perinatal death concurrent with indomethacin treatment in human pregnancy. *J. reprod. Med.*, **24**, 137–140

Jackson, B. & Lawrence, J.R. (1978) Renal papillary necrosis associated with indomethacin and phenylbutazone treated rheumatoid arthritis. *Aust. N.Z. J. Med.*, **8**, 165-167

Jaszczak, S.E. (1983) Anovulatory luteal cycles in primates. *Contraception*, **27**, 505–514

Johnson, A.G. & Ray, J.E. (1992) Improved high-performance liquid-chromatographic method for the determination of indomethacin in plasma. *Ther. Drug Monit.*, **14**, 61–65

Julou, P.L., Guyonnet, J.C., Ducrot, R., Bardone, M.C., Detaille, J.Y. & Laffargue, B. (1969) General pharmacological properties of metiazinic acid (16 091 R.P.). *Arzneimittel.-forsch.*, **19**, 1198–1206

Kalbhen, D.A., Karzel, K. & Domenjoz, R. (1967) The inhibitory effects of some antiphlogistic drugs on the glucosamine incorporation into mucopolysaccharides synthesized by fibroblast cultures. *Med. Pharmacol. exp.*, **16**, 185–189

Kantor, H.S. & Hampton, M. (1978) Indomethacin in submicromolar concentrations inhibits cyclic AMP-dependent protein kinase. *Nature*, **276**, 841–842

Kaplan, L., Weiss, J. & Elsbach, P. (1978) Low concentrations of indomethacin inhibit phospholipase A2 of rabbit polymorphonuclear leukocytes. *Proc. natl Acad. Sci. USA*, **75**, 2955–2958

Khatib, R., Reyes, M.P., Khatib, G., Smith, F., Rezkella, S. & Kloner, R.A. (1992) Focal ventricular thinning caused by indomethacin in the late phase of coxsackievirus B4 murine myocarditis. *Am. J. med. Sci.*, **303**, 95–98

King, M.T., Beikirch, H., Eckhardt, K., Gocke, E. & Wild, D. (1979) Mutagenicity studies with X-ray-contrast media, analgesics, antipyretics, antirheumatics and some other pharmaceutical drugs in bacterial, Drosophila and mammalian test systems. *Mutat. Res.*, **66**, 33–43

Klaassen, C.D. (1976) Studies on the mechanism of spironolactone protection against indomethacin toxicity. *Toxicol. appl. Pharmacol.*, **38**, 127–135

Klein, K.L., Scott, W.J., Clark, K.E. & Wilson, J.G. (1981) Indomethacin – Placental transfer, cytotoxicity, and teratology in the rat. *Am. J. Obstet. Gynecol.*, **141**, 448–452

Klein, W.A., Miller, H.H., Anderson, M. & DeCosse J.J. (1987) The use of indomethacin, sulindac, and tamoxifen for the treatment of desmoid tumors associated with familial polyposis. *Cancer.*, **60**, 2863–2868

Kleinknecht, C., Laouari, D., Gubler, M.-C. & Gros, F. (1983) Adverse effects of indomethacin in experimental chronic nephrosis. *Int. J. pediatr. Nephrol.*, **4**, 83–86

Knudson, W., Biswas, C. & Toole, B.P. (1984) Interactions between human tumor cells and fibroblasts stimulate hyaluronate synthesis. *Proc. natl Acad. Sci. USA*, **81**, 6767–671

Kohler, G., Dell, H.-D. & Kamp, R. (1981) Tissue concentrations of non-steroidal anti-inflammatory agents in chronic polyarthritis patients. *Z. Rheumatol.*, **40**, 97–99

Kraeling, R.R., Rampacek, G.B. & Fiorello, N.A. (1985) Inhibition of pregnancy with indomethacin in mature gilts and prepuberal gilts induced to ovulate. *Biol. Reprod.*, **32**, 105–110

Kuboyama, N., & Fujii, A. (1992) Mutagenicity of analgesics, their derivatives, and anti-inflammatory drugs with S-9 mix of several animal species. *J. Nihon Univ. Sch. Dent.*, **34**, 183–195

Kudo, T., Narisawa, T. & Abo, S. (1980) Antitumor activity of indomethacin on methylazoxymethanol-induced large bowel tumors in rats. *Gann*, **34**, 260–264

Kullich, W., & Klein, G. (1986) Investigations of the influence of nonsteroidal antirheumatic drugs on the rates of sister-chromatid exchange. *Mutat. Res.* **174**, 131–134

Kunze, V.M., Stein, G., Kunze, E. & Traeger, A. (1974) [The pharmacokinetics of indomethacin relating to age, bile duct obstruction, reduced kidney function and incompatibility symptoms.] *Dtsch. Gesundheitsw.*, **29**, 351–354 (in German)

Kuroda, T., Yokoyama, T., Umeda, T., Matsuzawa, A., Kuroda, K. & Asada, S. (1983) Studies on sustained-release dosage forms. II. Pharmacokinetics after rectal administration of indomethacin suppositories in rabbits. *Chem. Pharm. Bull.*, **31**, 3319–3325

Kwan, K.C., Breault, G.O., Umbenhauer, E.R., McMahon, F.G. & Duggan, D.E. (1976) Kinetics of indomethacin absorption, elimination, and entero-hepatic circulation in man. *J. Pharmacokinet. Biopharm.*, **4**, 255–280

Kwan, K.C., Breault, G.O., Davis, R.L., Lei, B.W., Czerwinski, A.W., Besselaar, G.H. & Duggan, D.E. (1978) Effects of concomitant aspirin administration on the pharmacokinetics of indomethacin in man. *J. Pharmacokinet. Biopharm.*, **6**, 451–476

Lang, J., Price, A.B., Levi, A.J., Burke, M., Gumpel, J.M. & Bjarnason, I. (1988) Diaphragm disease: Pathology of disease of the small intestine induced by non-steroidal anti- inflammatory drugs. *J. clin. Pathol.*, **41**, 516–526

Langman, M.J.S, Weil, J., Wainwright, P., Lawson, D.H., Rawlins, M.D., Logan, R.F., Murphy, M., Vessey, M.P. & Colin Jones, D.G. (1994). Risks of bleeding peptic ulcer associated with individual non-steroidal anti-inflammatory drugs. *Lancet.*, **343**, 1075–1078

Lau, I.F., Saksena, S.K. & Chang, M.C. (1973) Pregnancy blockade by indomethacin, an inhibitor of prostaglandin synthesis: Its reversal by prostaglandins and progesterone in mice. *Prostaglandins.*, **4**, 795–803

Lau, I.F., Saksena, S.K. & Chang, M.C. (1975) Effect of indomethacin and prostaglandin F2 on parturition in the hamster. *Prostaglandins*, **10**, 1011–1018

Laufer, S., Tries, S., Augustin, J., Elsasser, R., Algate, D.R., Atterson, P.R. & Munt, P.L. (1994) Gastrointestinal tolerance of [2,2-dimethyl-6-(4-chlorophenyl-7-phenyl-2,3-dihydro-1H-pyrrolizine-5-yl]acetic acid in the rat. *Arzneimittel.-forsch.*, **44**, 1329–1333

Lebedevs, T.H., Wojnar-Horton, R.E., Yapp, P., Roberts, M.J., Dusci, L.J., Hackett, L.P. & Ilett, K.F. (1991) Excretion of indomethacin in breast milk. *Br. J. clin. Pharmacol.*, **32**, 751–754

Lee, S.-H. & Norppa, H. (1995) Effects of indomethacin and arachidonic acid on sister chromatid exchange induction by styrene and styrene-7,8-oxide. *Mutat. Res.*, **348**, 93–99

Leemann,T.D., Transon, C., Bonnabry, P., & Dayer, P. (1993) A major role of cytochrome P450TB (CYP2C subfamily) in the actions of non-steroidal antiinflammatory drugs. *Drugs exp. clin. Res.* **19**, 189–195

Leibold, E. & Schwarz, L.R. (1993) Inhibition of intercellular communication in rat hepatocytes by phenobarbital, 1,1,1-trichloro-2,2-bis(p-chlorophenyl)-ethane (DDT) and λ-hexachlorocyclohexane (lindane): Modification by antioxidants and inhibitors of cyclooxygenase. *Carcinogenesis*, **14**, 2377–2382

Levin, D.L., Mills, L.J., Parkey, M., Garriott, J. & Campbell, W. (1979) Constriction of the fetal ductus arteriosus after administration of indomethacin to the pregnant ewe. *J. Pediatr.*, **94**, 647–650

Lione, A. & Scialli, A.R. (1995) The developmental toxicity of indomethacin and sulindac. *Reprod. Toxicol.*, **9**, 7–20

Liss, R.H., Yesair, D.W., Watts, G.P., Cotton, F.A. & Kensler, C.J. (1968) Semiquantitative estimation of 14C-indomethacin radioactivity in whole-body sections of rats (Abstract 005). *Pharmacologist*, **10**, 154

Lobo, I.B. & Hoult, J.R.S. (1994) Groups I, II and III extracellular phospholipases A2: Selective inhibition of group II enzymes by indomethacin but not other NSAIDs. *Agents Actions*, **41**, 111–113

Löscher, W. & Blazaki, D. (1986) Effect of non-steroidal anti-inflammatory drugs on fertility of male rats. *J. Reprod. Fertil.*, **76**, 65–73

Lu, X.-J., Xie, W.-L., Reed, D., Bradshaw, W.S. & Simmons, D.L. (1995) Nonsteroidal antiinflammatory drugs cause apoptosis and induce cyclooxygenases in chicken embryo fibroblasts. *Proc. natl Acad. Sci. USA*, **92**, 7961–7965

Luk, G.D. & Baylin, S.B. (1984) Ornithine decarboxylase as a biologic marker in familial colonic polyposis. *New Engl. J. Med.*, **311**, 80–83

Major, C.A., Lewis, D.F., Harding, J.A. Port, M.A. & Garite, TJ. (1994) Tocolysis with indomethacin increases the incidence of necrotizing enterocolotis in the low-birth-weight neonate. *Am. J. Obstet. Gynecol.*, **170**, 102–106

Manaugh, L.C. & Novy, M.J. (1976) Effects of indomethacin on corpus luteum function and pregnancy in rhesus monkeys. *Fertil. Steril.*, **27**, 588–598

Marley, P.B. & Smith, C.C. (1974) The source and a possible function in fertility of seminal prostaglandin-like material, in the mouse. *Br. J. Pharmacol.*, **52**, 114

Martelli, A., Allavena, A., Campart Brambilla, G., Canonero, R., Ghia, M., Mattioli, F., Mereto, E., Robbiano, L. & Brambilla, G. (1995) In vitro and in vivo testing of hydralazine genotoxicity, *J. Pharmacol. exp. Ther.*, **273**, 113–120

Mason, R.W. & McQueen, E.G. (1974) Protein binding of indomethacin: Binding of indomethacin to human plasma albumin and its displacement from binding by ibuprofen, phenylbutazone and salicylate, *in vitro. Pharmacology*, **12**, 12–19

McArthur, J.N., Dawkins, P.D. & Smith, M.J.H. (1971) The binding of indomethacin, salicylate and phenobarbitone to human whole blood *in vitro. J. Pharm. Pharmacol.*, **23**, 32–36

McCormick, D.L. & Wilson, A.M. (1986) Combination chemoprevention of rat mammary carcinogenesis by indomethacin and butylated hydroxytoluene. *Cancer Res.*, **46**, 3907–3911

McCormick, D.L., Madigan, M.J. & Moon, R.C. (1985) Modulation of rat mammary carcinogenesis by indomethacin. *Cancer Res.*, **45**, 1803–1808

McDougall, C.J., Ngoi, S.S., Goldman, I.S., Godwin, T., Felix, J., DeCosse, J.J. & Rigas, B. (1990) Reduced expression of HLA class I and II antigens in colon cancer. *Cancer Res.*, **50**, 8023–8027

McElnay, J.C., Passmore, A.P., Crawford, V.L.S., McConnell, J.G., Taylor, I.C. & Walker, F.S. (1992) Steady state pharmacokinetic profile of indomethacin in elderly patients and young volunteers. *Eur. J. clin. Pharmacol.*, **43**, 77–80

McGeer, P.L., Schulzer, M. & McGeer, E.G. (1996) Arthritis and anti inflammatory agents as possible protective factors for Alzheimer's disease. A review of 17 epidemiologic studies. *Neurology*, **47**, 425-432

Mehta, R.G., Steele, V., Kelloff, G.J. & Moon, R.C. (1991) Influence of thiols and inhibitors of prostaglandin biosynthesis on the carcinogen-induced development of mammary lesions *in vitro. Anticancer Res.*, **11**, 587–592

Metzger, U., Meier, J., Uhlschmid, G. & Wheihe, H. (1984) Influence of various prostaglandin synthesis inhibitors on DMH-induced rat colon cancer. *Dis. Colon Rectum*, **27**, 366–369

Mingeot-Lerclercq, M.-P., Laurent, G. & Tulkens, P.M. (1988) Biochemical mechanism of aminoglycoside-induced inhibition of phosphatidylcholine hydrolysis by lysosomal phospholipases. *Biochem. Pharmacol.*, **37**, 591–599

Moise, K.J., Jr., Ou, C.-N., Kirshon, B., Cano, L.E., Rognerud, C. & Carpenter, R.J., Jr. (1990) Placental transfer of indomethacin in the human pregnancy. *Am. J. Obstet. Gynecol.*, **162**, 549–554

Momma, K. & Takao, A. (1987) *In vivo* constriction of the ductus arteriosus by nonsteroidal antiinflammatory drugs in near-term and preterm fetal rats. *Pediatr. Res.*, **22**, 567–572

Momma, K. & Takao, A. (1989) Right ventricular concentric hypertrophy and left ventricular dilatation by ductal constriction in fetal rats. *Circ. Res.*, **64**, 1137–1146

Montenegro, M.A. & Palomino, H. (1989) Inhibition of palatal fusion *in vitro* by indomethacin in two strains of mice with different H-2 backgrounds. *Arch. Oral Biol.*, **34**, 949–955

Montenegro, M.A. & Palomino, H. (1990) Induction of cleft palate in mice by inhibitors of prostaglandin synthesis. *J. Craniofac. Genet. dev. Biol.*, **10**, 83–94

Narisawa, T., Sato, M., Tani, M., Kudo, T., Takahashi, T. & Goto, A. (1981) Inhibition of development of methylnitrosourea-induced rat colon tumors by indomethacin treatment. *Cancer Res.*, **41**, 1954–1957

Narisawa, T., Sato, M., Sano, M., & Takahashi, T. (1982) Inhibition of development of methylnitrosourea-induced rat colonic tumors by peroral administration of indomethacin. *Gann.*, **73**, 3770–381

Narisawa, T., Satoh, M., Sano, M. & Takahashi, T. (1983) Inhibition of initiation and promotion by N-methylnitrosourea-induced colon carcinogenesis in rats by non-steroid anti-inflammatory agent indomethacin. *Carcinogenesis*, **4**, 1225–1227

Narisawa, T., Hermanek, P., Habs, M. & Schmähl, D. (1984) Reduction of acetoxymethyl-methyl nitrosamine induced large bowel cancer in rats by indomethacin. *Tohoku J. exp. Med.*, **144**, 237–243

Narisawa, T., Hosaka, S. & Niwa, M. (1985) Prostaglandin E2 counteracts the inhibition by indomethacin of rat colon ornithine decarboxylase induction by deoxycholic acid. *Jpn. J. Cancer Res.*, **76**, 338–344

Narisawa, T., Takahashi, M., Niwa, M., Fukaura, Y. & Wakizaka, A. (1987) Involvement of prostaglandin E2 in bile acid-caused promotion of colon carcinogenesis and anti-promotion by the cyclooxygenase inhibitor indomethacin. *Jpn. J. Cancer Res.*, **78**, 791–798

Niggli, B., Friederich, U., Hann, D. & Wurgler, F.E. (1986) Endogenous promutagen activation in the yeast *Saccharomyces cerevisiae*: Factors influencing aflatoxin B1 mutagenicity. *Mutat. Res.*, **75**, 223–229

Noguchi, M., Taniya, T., Koyasaki, N., Kumaki, T., Miyazaki, I. & Mizukami, Y. (1991) Effects of the prostaglandin synthetase inhibitor indomethacin on tumorigenesis, tumor proliferation, cell kinetics, and receptor contents of 7,12-dimethylbenz(a)anthra-cene-induced mammary carcinoma in Sprague-Dawley rats fed a high- or low-fat diet. *Cancer Res.*, **71**, 2683–2689

Nomura, M., Onodera, T., Kato, M., Yamada, A., Ogawa, H. & Akimoto, T. (1978) Acute, subacute and chronic toxicity of oxepinac. *Arzneimittel.-forsch.*, **28**, 445–451

Northover, B.J. (1977) Indomethacin – A calcium antagonist. *Gen. Pharmacol.*, **8**, 293–296

Norton, M.E., Merrill, J., Cooper, B.A., Kuller, J.A. & Clyman, R.I. (1993) Neonatal complications after the administration of indomethacin for premature labour. *New Engl J. Med.*, **329**, 1602–1607

Novy, M.J., Cook, M.J. & Manaugh, L. (1974) Indomethacin block of normal onset of parturition in primates. *Am. J. Obstet. Gynecol.*, **118**, 412–416

Oberto, G., Conz, A., Giachetti, C. & Galli, C.L. (1990) Evaluation of the toxicity of indomethacin in a 4-week study, by oral route, in the marmoset (*Callithrix jacchus*). *Fundam. appl. Toxicol.*, **15**, 800–813

O'Grady, J.P., Caldwell, B.V., Auletta, F.J. & Speroff, L. (1972) The effects of an inhibitor of prostaglandin synthesis (indomethacin) on ovulation, pregnancy and pseudopregnancy in the rabbit. *Prostaglandins*, **1**, 97

Olkkola, K.T., Maunuksela, E.L. & Korpela, R. (1989) Pharmacokinetics of postoperative intravenous indomethacin in children. *Pharmacol. Toxicol.*, **65**, 157–160

Orczyk, G.P. & Behrman, H.R. (1972) Ovulation blockade by aspirin or indomethacin — *In vivo* evidence for a role of prostaglandin in gonadotrophin secretion. *Prostaglandins*, **1**, 3–20

Ostensen, M. (1994) Optimisation of antirheumatic drug treatment in pregnancy. *Clin. Pharmacokinet.*, **27**, 486–503

Parks, B.R., Jordan, R.L., Rawson, J.E. & Douglas, B.H. (1977) Indomethacin: Studies of absorption and placental transfer. *Am. J. Obstet. Gynecol.*, **129**, 464–465

Pathak, D.N. & Roy, D. (1993) In vivo genotoxicity of sodium ortho-phenylphenol: Phenylbenzoquinone is one of the DNA-binding metabolite(s) of sodium ortho-phenylphenol. *Mutat. Res.*, **286**, 309–319

Pegg, A.E. & McCann, P.P. (1982) Polyamine metabolism and function. *Am. J. Physiol.*, **243**, C212–C221

Perkins, T, M, & Shklar, G. (1982) Delay in hamster buccal pouch carcinogenesis by aspirin and indomethacin. *Oral Surg.*, **53**, 170-178

Persaud, T.V.N. & Moore, K.L. (1974) Inhibitors of prostaglandin synthesis during pregnancy. 1. Embryopathic activity of indomethacin in mice. *Anat. Anz.*, **136**, 349–353

Peterson, H.I. (1986) Tumor angiogenesis inhibition by prostaglandin synthetase inhibitors. *Anticancer Res.*, **6**, 251–254

Petry, T.W., Eling, T.E., Chiu, A.L.H. & Josephy, P.D. (1988) Ram seminal vesicle microsome-catalyzed activation of benzidine and related compounds: Dissociation of mutagenesis from peroxidase-catalyzed formation of DNA-reactive material. *Carcinogenesis*, **9**, 51–57

Petry, T.W., Josephy, P.D., Pagano, D.A., Zeiger, E., Knecht, K.T. & Eling, T.E. (1989) Prostaglandin hydroperoxidase-dependent activation of heterocyclic aromatic amines. *Carcinogenesis*, **10**, 2201–2207

Phillips, C.A. & Poyser, N.L. (1981) Studies on the involvement of prostaglandins in implantation in the rat. *J. Reprod. Fert.*, **62**, 73–81

Phillips, M.W., Salyer, G. & Ray, R.S. (1980) Equine metabolism and pharmacokinetics of indomethacin. *Equine Pract.*, **2**, 48–49

Plescia, O.J. (1982) Does prostaglandin synthesis affect *in vivo* tumour growth by altering tumour/host balance? In: Powles, T.J., Bockman, R.S., Honn, K.V. & Ramwell, P., eds, *Prostaglandins and Cancer*, New York, Alan R. Liss, pp. 619–631

Plummer, S.M., Hall, M. & Faux, S.P. (1995) Oxidation and genotoxicity of fecapentaene-12 are potentiated by prostaglandin H synthase. *Carcinogenesis*, **16**, 1023–1028

Pollard, M. & Luckert, P.H. (1980) Indomethacin treatment of rats with dimethylhydrazine-induced intestinal tumors. *Cancer Treat. Rep.*, **64**, 1323–1327

Pollard, M. & Luckert, P.H. (1981a) Effect of indomethacin on intestinal tumors induced in rats by the acetate derivative of dimethylnitrosamine. *Science*, **214**, 558–559

Pollard, M. & Luckert, P.H. (1981b) Treatment of chemically-induced intestinal cancers with indomethacin. *Proc. Soc. exp. Biol. Med.*, **167**, 161–164

Pollard, M. & Luckert, P.H. (1983) Prolonged antitumor effect of indomethacin on autochthonous intestinal tumors in rats. *J. natl Cancer Inst.*, **70**, 1103–1105

Rane, A., Oelz, O., Frolich, J.C., Seyberth, H.W., Sweetman, B.J., Watson, J.T., Wilkinson, G.R. & Oates, J.A. (1978) Relation between plasma concentration of indomethacin and its effect on prostaglandin synthesis and platelet aggregation in man. *Clin. Pharmacol. Ther.*, **23**, 658–668

Rao, R. A. & Hussain, S.P. (1988) Modulation of methylcholanthrene-induced carcinogenesis in the uterine cervix of mouse by indomethacin. *Cancer Lett.*, **43**, 15–19

Rau, H.L., Aroor, A.R. & Rao, P.G. (1991) High-performance liquid-chromatographic determination of paracetamol and indomethacin in combined dosage forms. *Indian Drugs*, **29**, 48–50

Raveendran, R., Heybroek, W.M., Caulfield, M., Abrams, S.M.L., Wrigley, P.F.M., Slevin, M. & Turner, P. (1992) Protein binding of indomethacin, methotrexate and morphine in patients with cancer. *Int. J. clin. Pharmacol. Res.*, **12**, 117–122

Reynolds, J.E.F. & Prasad, A.B., eds (1982) *Martindale. The Extra Pharmacopoiea*, 28th Ed., London, Pharmaceutical Press, pp. 256–261

Rö, J., Sudmann, E. & Marton, P.F. (1976) Effect of indomethacin on fracture healing in rats. *Acta orthopaed. Scand.*, **47**, 588–599

Rogers, J., Kirby, L.C., Hempelman, S.R., Berry, D.L., McGeer, P.L., Kazniak, A.W., Zalinski, J., Cofield, M., Mansukhani, L. & Willson, P. (1993) Clinical trial of indomethacin in Alzheimer's disease. *Neurology*, **43**, 1609–1611

Rothermich, N.O. (1971) An extended study of indomethacin. I. Clinical pharmacology. *J. Am. med. Assoc.*, **195**, 123–128

Rowe, J.S. & Carless, J.E. (1982) Investigations on the *in vitro* dose-related metabolism of indomethacin in four laboratory species. *Eur. J. Drug Metab. Pharmacokinet.*, **7**, 159–163

Rubio, C.A. (1984) Antitumoral activity of indomethacin on experimental esophageal tumors. *J. natl Cancer Inst.*, **72**, 705–707

Rubio, C.A. (1986) Further studies on the therapeutic effect of indomethacin on esophageal tumors. *Cancer*, **58**, 1029–1031

Saito, Y., Okamoto, H., Mizusaki, S. & Yoshida, D. (1986) Inhibition of 12-O-tetradecanoylphorbol-13-acetate-induced induction of Epstein-Barr virus early antigen in raji cells by some inhibitors of tumor promotion. *Cancer Lett.*, **32**, 137–144

Saksena, S.K., Lau, I.-F. & Shaikh, A.A. (1974) Cyclic changes in the uterine tissue content of F-prostaglandins and the role of prostaglandins in ovulation in mice. *Fertil. Steril.*, **25**, 636–643

Salvemini, D., Misko, T.P., Masferrer, J.L., Seibert, K., Currie, M.G. & Needleman, P. (1993) Nitric oxide activates cyclooxygenase enzymes. *Proc. natl. Acad. Sci. USA.*, **90**, 7240–7244

Schlosser, M.J., Shurina, R.D. & Kalf, G.F. (1990) Prostaglandin H synthase catalyzed oxidation of hydroquinone to a sulfhydryl-binding and DNA-damaging metabolite. *Chem. Res. Toxicol.*, **3**, 333–339

Schoog, M., Laufen, H. & Dessain, P. (1981) A comparison of the pharmacokinetics of piroxicam with those of plain and slow release indomethacin. A crossover study. *Eur. J. Rheumatol. Inflamm.*, **4**, 298–302

Selby, J.V., Friedman, G.D., & Fireman B.H. (1989) Screening prescription drugs for possible carcinogenicity: Eleven to fifteen years of follow-up. *Cancer Res.*, **49**, 5736–5747

Semba, M. & Inui, N. (1990) Inhibition of 12-O-tetradecanoylphorbol-13-acetate-enhanced transformation *in vitro* by inhibitors of phospholipid metabolism. *Toxicology Lett.*, **51**, 1–6

Sevanian, A. & Peterson, H. (1989) Induction of cytotoxicity and mutagenesis is facilitated by fatty acid hydroperoxidase activity in Chinese hamster lung fibroblasts (V79 cells). *Mutat. Res.*, **224**, 185–196

Shacter, E., Lopez, R.L. & Pati, S. (1991) Inhibition of the myeloperoxidase-H_2O_2-Ci- system of neutrophils by indomethacin and other non-steroidal anti-inflammatory drugs. *Biochem. Pharmacol.*, **41**, 975–984

Shamon, L.A., Chen, C., Mehta, R.G., Steele, V., Moon, R.C. & Pezzuto, J.M. (1994) A correlative approach for the identification of antimutagens that demonstrate chemopreventive activity. *Anticancer Res.*, **14**, 1775–1778

Sharpe, G.L., Larsson, K.S. & Thalme, B. (1975) Studies on closure of the ductus arteriosus. XII. *In utero* effect of indomethacin and sodium salicylate in rats and rabbits. *Prostaglandins*, **9**, 585–596

Shen, T.Y. (1965) Synthesis and biological activity of some indomethacin analogs. *Excerpta Med. int. Congr. Ser.*, **82**, 13–20

Shen, T.-Y. & Winter, C.A. (1977) Chemical and biological studies on indomethacin, sulindac and their analogs. *Adv. Drug Res.*, **12**, 89–245

Shen, T.Y., Windholz, T.B., Rosegay, A., Witzel, B.E., Wilson, A.N., Willett, J.D., Holtz, W.J., Ellis, R.L., Matzuk, A.R., Lucas, S., Stammer, C.H., Holly, F.W., Sarett, L.H., Risley, E.A., Nuss, G.W. & Winter, C.A. (1963) Non-steroid anti-inflammatory agents. *J. Am. chem. Soc.*, **85**, 488–489

Shibata, M.A., Hasegawa, R., Imaida, K., Hagiwara, A., Ogawa, K., Hirose M., Ito N. & Shirai T. (1995) Chemoprevention by dehydroepiandrosterone and indomethacin in a rat multiorgan carcinogenesis model. *Cancer Res.*, **55**, 4870–4874

Shiff, S.J., Koutsos, M.I., Qiao, L. & Rigas, B. (1996) Nonsteroidal antiinflammatory drugs inhibit the proliferation of colon adenocarcinoma cells: Effects on cell cycle and apoptosis. *Exp. Cell Res., 222*, 179–188

Shobha Devi, P., & Polasa H. (1987) Evaluation of the anti-inflammatory drug indomethacin for its genotoxicity in mice. *Mutat. Res., 188*, 343–347

Shriver, D.A., Dove, P.A., White, C.B., Sandor, A. & Rosenthale, M.E. (1977) A profile of the gastrointestinal toxicity of aspirin, indomethacin, oxaprozin, phenylbutazone, and fentiazac in arthritic and Lewis normal rats. *Toxicol. appl. Pharmacol., 42*, 75–83

Shuster, S., Smith, H.S., Thor, A.D. & Sern R. (1993) Enhanced deposition of hyaluronan in the stroma of human breast cancer (Abstract 9). *Proc. Ann. Meet. Am. Assoc. Cancer Res., 34*, 2

Siegel, M.I., McConnell, R.T., Porter, N.A., Selph, J.L., Truax, J.F., Vinegar, R. & Cuatrecasas, P. (1980) Aspirin-like drugs inhibit arachidonic acid metabolism via lipoxygenase and cyclo-oxygenase in rat neutrophils from carrageenan pleural exudates. *Biochem. biophys. Res. Commun., 92*, 688–695

Singh, A.K., Hang, Y., Mishra, U. & Granley, K. (1991) Simultaneous analysis of flunixin, naproxen, ethacrynic acid, indomethacin, phenylbutazone, mefenamic acid and thiosalicylic acid in plasma and urine by high-performance liquid chromatography and gas chromatography–mass spectrometry. *J. Chromatogr. biomed. Appl., 106*, 351–361

Sjoholm, I., Kober, A., Odar-Cederlof, I. & Borga, O. (1976) Protein binding of drugs in uremic and normal serum: The role of endogenous binding inhibitors. *Biochem. Pharmacol., 25*, 1205–1213

Slaga, T.J. (1983) Overview of tumor promotion in animals. *Environ. Health Perspectives, 50*, 3–14

Smalley, W.E., Griffin, M.R., Fought, R.L. & Ray, W.A. (1996) Excess costs for gastrointestinal disease among nonsteroidal anti-inflammatory drug users. *J. Gen. Intern. Med., 11*, 461–469

Stepaniuk, G.I. & Stolyarchuk, A.A. (1985) [Effect of non-steroidal anti-inflammatory agents on the myocardial blood supply and oxygen regimen]. *Farmakol. Toksikol., 48*, 54–57 (in Russian)

Stewart, T.H.M., Hetenyi, C., Rowsell, H. & Orizaga, M. (1980) Ulcerative enterocolitis in dogs induced by drugs. *J. Pathol., 131*, 363–378

Sudmann, E. & Bang, G. (1979) Indomethacin-induced inhibition of haversian remodelling in rabbits. *Acta orthopaed. scand., 50*, 621–627

Swain, J.A., Heyndrickx, G.R., Boettcher, D.H. & Vatner S.F. (1975) Prostaglandin control of renal circulation in the unanesthetized dog and baboon. *Am. J. Physiol., 229*, 826–830

Szarka, C.E., Grana, G. & Engstrom, P. (1994) Chemoprevention of cancer. *Curr. Probl. Cancer, 18*, 6–78

Taffet, S.M. & Russell, S.W. (1981) Macrophage-mediated tumor cell killing: Regulation of expression of cytolytic activity by prostaglandin E. *J. Immunol., 126*, 424–427

Taggart, A.J., McElnay, J.C., Kerr, B. & Passmore, P. (1987) The chronopharmacokinetics of indomethacin suppositories in healthy volunteers. *Eur. J. clin. Pharmacol., 31*, 617–619

Takahashi, M., Furukawa, F., Toyoda, K., Sato, H., Hasegawa, R., Imaida, K. & Hayashi, Y. (1990) Effects of various prostaglandin synthesis inhibitors on pancreatic carcinogenesis in hamsters after initiation with N-nitrosobis(2-oxopropyl)amine. *Carcino-genesis., 11*, 393–395

Takeuchi, K., Furukawa, O., Okada, M. & Okabe, S. (1988) Duodenal ulcers induced by indomethacin plus histamine in the dog. Involvement of the impaired duodenal alkaline secretion in their pathogenesis. *Digestion, 39*, 230–240

Takyi, B.E. (1970) Excretion of drugs in human milk. *J. Hosp. Pharm., 28*, 317–325

Tanaka, T., Nishikawa, A., Mori, Y., Morishita, Y. & Mori H. (1989) Inhibitory effects of non-steroidal anti-inflammatory drugs, piroxicam and indomethacin on 4-nitroquinoline 1-oxide-induced tongue carcinogenesis in male ACI/N rats. *Cancer Letters., 48*, 177–182

Tanaka, T., Kojima, T., Yoshimi, N., Sugie, S. & Mori, H. (1991) Inhibitory effect of the non-steroidal anti-inflammatory drug, indomethacin on the naturally occurring carcinogen, 1-hydroxyanthraquinone in male ACI/N rats. *Carcinogenesis, 12*, 1949–1952

Tanaka, T., Kojima, T., Okumura, A., Sugie, S. & Mori, H. (1993) Inhibitory effect of the non-steroidal anti-inflammatory drugs, indomethacin and piroxicam on 2-acetylaminofluorene-induced hepatocarcinogenesis in male ACI/N rats. *Cancer Lett., 68*, 111–118

Tost, H., Kover, G. & Darvasi, A. (1995) Conjugate effects of saralasin and indomethacin on kidney function in anesthetized dog. *Acta physiol. hung., 83*, 63–77

Traeger, A., Noschel, H. & Zaumseil, J. (1973) Pharmacokinetics of indomethacin in pregnant and parturient women and in their newborn infants. *Zentralbl. Gynakol., 95*, 635–641

Tsioulias, G., Godwin, T.A., Goldstein, M.F., McDougall, C.J., Sing-Shang, N., DeCosse, J.J. & Rigas, B. (1992) Loss of colonic HLA antigens in familial adenomatous polyposis. *Cancer Res., 52*, 3449–3452 Tsioulias, G.J., Triadafilopoulos, G.,

Goldin, E., Papavassiliou, E.D., Rizos, S., Bassioukas, P. & Rigas, B. (1993) Expression of HLA class I antigens in sporadic adenomas and histologically normal mucosa of the colon. *Cancer Res.*, **53**, 2374–2378

Tsuji, Y., Kakegawa, H., Miyataka, H., Matsumoto, H. & Satoh, T. (1993) Pharmacological and pharmaceutical properties of freeze-dried formulations of egg albumin, indomethacin, olive oil or fatty acids. II. *Biol. pharm. Bull.*, **16**, 679–682

Tsukada, K., Church, J.M., Jagelman, D.G., Fazio, V.W., McGannon, E., George, C.R., Schroeder, T., Lavery, I. & Oakley, J. (1992) Noncytotoxic drug therapy for intra-abdominal desmoid tumor in patients with familial adenomatous polyposis. *Dis. Colon Rectum*, **35**, 29–33

Turakka, H. & Airaksinen, M.M. (1974) Biopharmaceutical assessment of phenylbutazone and indomethacin preparations. *Ann. clin. Res.*, **6**, 34–41

Vanderhoek, J.Y., Ekborg, S.L. & Bailey, J.M. (1984) Nonsteroidal anti-inflammatory drugs stimulate 15-lipoxygenase/leukotriene pathway in human polymorphonuclear leukocytes. *J. Allergy clin. Immunol.*, **74**, 412–417

Vane, J.R. (1971) Inhibition of prostaglandin synthesis as a mechanism of action for aspirin-like drugs. *Nature New Biol.*, **231**, 232–235

Veersema, D., de Jong P.A. & van Wijck, J.A. (1983) Indomethacin and the fetal renal nonfunction syndrome. *Eur. J. Obstet. Gynecol. Reprod. Biol.*, **16**, 113–21

Verma, A.K., Ashendel, C.L. & Boutwell, R.K. (1980) Inhibition by prostaglandin synthesis inhibitors of the induction of epidermal ornithine decarboxylase activity, the accumulation of prostaglandins, and tumor promotion caused by 12-O-tetradecanoylphorbol-13-acetate. *Cancer Res.*, **40**, 308–315

Vert, P., Bianchetti, G., Marchal, F., Monin, P. & Morselli, P.L. (1980) Effectiveness and pharmacokinetics of indomethacin in premature newborns with patent ductus arteriosus. *Eur. J. clin. Pharmacol.*, **18**, 83–88

Waddell, W.R. & Gerner, R.E. (1980) Indomethacin and ascorbate inhibit desmoid tumors. *J. surg. Oncol.*, **15**, 85–90

Waddell, W.R., Gerner, R.E. & Reich, M.P. (1983) Nonsteroidal antiinflammatory drugs and tamoxifen for desmoid tumors and carcinoma of the stomach. *J. Surg. Oncol.*, **22**, 197–211

Wallace, J.L., Arfors, K.E. & McKnight, G.W. (1991) A monoclonal antibody against the CD18 leukocyte adhesion molecule prevents indomethacin-induced gastric damage in the rabbit. *Gastroenterology*, **100**, 878–883

Wallach, E.E., de la Cruz, A., Hunt, J., Wright, K.H. & Stevens, V.C. (1975) The effect of indomethacin on HMG-HCG induced ovulation in the rhesus monkey. *Prostaglandins.*, **9**, 645–658

Waller, E.S. (1983) Evaluation of new indomethacin dosage forms. *Pharmacotherapy*, **3**, 324–333

Wallusch, W.W., Nowak, H., Leopold, G. & Netter, K.J. (1978) Comparative bioavailability: Influence of various diets on the bioavailability of indomethacin. *Int. J. Clin. Pharmacol. Biopharmacol.*, **16**, 40–44

Watanabe, K., Yakou, S., Takayama, K., Machida, Y., Isowa, K. & Nagai, T. (1993) Investigation on rectal absorption of indomethacin from sustained-release hydrogel suppositories prepared with water-soluble dietary fibers, xanthan gum and locust bean gum. *Biol. pharm. Bull.*, **16**, 391–394

Weitberg, A.B. (1988) Effects of arachidonic acid and inhibitors of arachidonic acid metabolism on phagocyte-induced sister chromatid exchanges..*Clin. Genet.*, **34**, 288–292

Whitehouse, M.W. (1964) Uncoupling of oxidative phosphorylation by some arylacetic acids (anti-inflammatory or hypercholesterolemic drugs). *Nature*, **201**, 629–630

Wichlinski, L.M., Pankowski, M., Marzec, A. & Krzysko, K. (1983) Influence of age on indomethacin clearance in humans. *Zentralbl. Pharm. Pharmakother. Laboratoriumsdiag.*, **122**, 731–733

Wild, D. & Degen, G.H. (1987) Prostaglandin H synthase-dependent mutagenic activation of heterocyclic aromatic amines of the IQ-type. *Carcinogenesis*, **8**, 541–545

Wilhelmi, G. (1974) Species differences in susceptibility to the gastro-ulcerogenic action of anti-inflammatory agents. *Pharmacology*, **11**, 220–230

Wu, C. & Mathews, K.P. (1983) Indomethacin inhibition of glutathione S-transferases. *Biochem. biophys. Res. Commun.*, **112**, 980–985

Yamada, I., Goda, T., Kawata, M., Shiotuki, T. & Ogawa, K. (1990) Gastric acidity-dependent bioavailability of commercial sustained release preparations of indomethacin, evaluated by gastric acidity-controlled beagle dogs. *Chem. pharm. Bull.*, **38**, 3112–3115

Yegnanarayan, R. & Joglekar, G.V. (1978) Anti-fertility effect of non-steroidal anti-inflammatory drugs. *Jpn. J. Pharmacol.*, **28**, 909–917

Yeh, K.C. (1985) Pharmacokinetic overview of indomethacin and sustained-release indomethacin. *Am. J. Med.*, **79**, 3–12

Yeh, K.C., Berger, E.T., Breault, G.O., Lei, B.W. & McMahon, F.G. (1982) Effect of sustained release on the pharmacokinetic profile of indomethacin in man. *Biopharm. Drug Disposition,* **3**, 219–230

Yesair, D.W., Callahan, M., Remington, L. & Kensler, C.J. (1970a) Role of the entero-hepatic cycle of indomethacin on its metabolism, distribution in tissues and its excretion by rats, dogs and monkeys. *Biochem. Pharmacol.,* **19**, 1579–1590

Yesair, D.W., Remington, L., Callahan, M. & Kensler, C.J. (1970b) Comparative effects of salicylic acid, phenylbutazone, probenecid and other anions on the metabolism, distribution and excretion of indomethacin by rats. *Biochem. Pharmacol.,* **19**, 1591–1600

Ziche, M., Jones, J. & Gullino, P.M. (1982) Role of prostaglandin E1 and copper in angiogenesis. *J. natl. Cancer Inst.,* **69**, 475–482

Zini, R., D'Athis, P., Barre, J. & Tillement, J.P. (1979) Binding of indomethacin to human serum albumin. Its non displacement by various agents, influence of free fatty acids and the unexpected effect of indomethacin on warfarin binding. *Biochem. Pharmacol.,* **28**, 2661–2665

Appendix 1

The concept of activity profiles of antimutagens

To facilitate an analysis of data from the open literature on antimutagenicity in short-term tests, we have applied the concept of activity profiles already used successfully for muta-genicity data (Waters *et al.*, 1988, 1990) to antimutagenicity data. The activity profiles display an overview of multi-test and multi-chemical information as an aid to the interpretation of the data. They can be organized in two general ways: for mutagens that have been tested in combination with a given antimutagen or for antimutagens that have been tested in combination with a given mutagen (Waters *et al.,* 1990). The profile presented here is an example of mutagens that have been tested in combination with a single antimutagen and they are arranged alphabetically by the names of the mutagens tested. These plots permit rapid visualization of considerable data and experimental parameters, including the inhibition as well as the enhancement of mutagenic activity. A data listing, arranged in the same order as the profile, is also given to summarize the short-term test used, the doses of mutagens and antimutagens, the response induced by the antimutagens, and the relevant publications.

The antimutagenicity profile graphically shows the doses for both the mutagen and antimutagen and the test response (either inhibition or enhancement) induced by the antimutagen. The resultant profiles are actually two parallel sets of bar graphs (Figure 1). The upper graph displays the mutagen dose and the range of antimutagen doses tested. The lower graph shows either the maximum percent inhibition represented by a bar directed upwards from the origin or the maximum percent enhancement of the genotoxic response, represented by a bar directed downwards. A short bar drawn across the origin on the lower graph indicates that no significant (generally < 20%) difference in the response was detected between the mutagen tested alone or the mutagen tested in combination with the antimutagen. Codes used to represent the short-term tests in the data listings have been reported previously (Waters *et al.*, 1988), and the subset of tests represented in this paper are shown in the Appendix.

In assembling the data base on antimutagens and presumptive anticarcinogens, the literature was surveyed for the availability of antimutagenicity data (Waters *et al.*, 1990), and publications were selected that presented original, quantitative data for any of the genotoxicity assays that are in the scope of the genetic activity profiles (Waters *et al.*, 1988).

The same short-term tests used to identify mutagens and potential carcinogens are being used to identify antimutagens and potential anticarcinogens. The tests are generally those for which standardized protocols have been developed and published. Many of these tests have been evaluated by the USEPA Gene-Tox Program (Waters, 1979; Green and Auletta, 1980; Waters and Auletta, 1981; Auletta *et al.*, 1991) or the National Toxicology Program (Tennant *et al.*, 1987; Ashby and Tennant, 1991) for their performance in detecting known carcinogens and noncarcinogens or known mutagens and nonmutagens (Upton *et al.*, 1984; Waters *et al.*, 1994).

It is not clear at the present time whether antimutagenicity observed in short-term tests is a reliable indicator of anticarcinogenicity since the available data are incomplete. Information on both antimutagenicity and anticarcinogenicity in vivo for a number of chemical classes is required before such a conclusion can be drawn. Clearly, antimutagenicity tests performed *in vitro* will not detect those compounds that act in a carcinogenicity bioassay *in vivo,* for example, to alter the activity of one or more enzyme systems not present *in vitro*. Rather, the in-vitro tests will detect only those compounds that inhibit the metabolism of the carcinogen directly, react directly with the mutagenic species to inactivate them or otherwise show an effect that is demonstrable *in vitro*. Thus, it is essential to confirm putative antimutagenic activity observed in vitro through the use of animal models. Indeed, the interpretation of antimutagenicity data from short-term tests must be subjected to all of the considerations that apply in the interpretation of mutagenicity test results. Moreover, the experimental variable of the antimutagens used must be considered in addition to the variables of the mutagens and short-term tests used. Obvious examples of parameters that must be considered in evaluating results from short-term tests *in vitro* are: (1) the endpoint of the test, (2) the presence or absence of an exogenous metabolic system, (3) the inducer that may have been used in conjunction with the preparation of the metabolic system, (4) the concentration of S9 or other metabolic system used and whether that concentration has been optimized for the mutagen under test, (5) the relative time and order of presentation of the mutagen and the antimutagen to the test system, (6) the concentration ratio of the mutagen relative to the antimutagen, (7) the duration of the treatment period, and (8) the outcome of the test, i.e. inhibition or enhancement of mutagenicity. Similar considerations apply to the evaluation of in vivo tests for antimutagenicity.

References

Ashby, J. & Tennant, R.W. (1991) Definitive relationships among chemical structure, carcino genicity and mutagenicity for 301 chemicals tested by the US NTP. *Mutat. Res.*, **257**, 229–306

Auletta, A.E., Brown, M., Wassom, J.S. & Cimino, M.C. (1991) Current status of the Gene-Tox program. *Environ. Health Perspectives*, **96**, 33–36

Green, S. & Auletta, A. (1980) Editorial introduction to the reports of 'The Gene-Tox Program': An evaluation of bioassays in *Genetic Toxicology*. *Mutat. Res.*, **76**, 165–168

Tennant, R.W., Margolin, B.H., Shelby, M.D., Zeiger, E., Haseman, J.K., Spalding, J., Caspary, W., Resnick, M., Stasiewicz, S., Anderson, B. & Minor, R. (1987) Prediction of chemical carcinogenicity in rodents from in vitro genetic toxicity assays. *Science*, **236**, 933–941

Upton, A.C., Clayson, D.B., Jansen, J.D., Rosenkranz, H.S. & Williams, G.M. (1984) Report of ICPEMC Task Group 5 on the differentiation between genotoxic and non-genotoxic carcinogens. *Mutat. Res.*, **133**, 1–49

Waters, M.D. (1979) Gene-Tox Program. In: Hsie, A.W., O'Neill, J.P. & McElheny, V.K., eds, *Mammalian Cell Mutagenesis: The Maturation of Test Systems* (Banbury Report 2), Cold Spring Harbor, NY, CSH Press, pp 451–466

Waters, M.D. & Auleta, A. (1981) The GENE-TOX program: Genetic activty evaluation. *J. chem. Inf. Computer Sci.*, **21**, 35–38

Waters, M.D., Stack, H.F., Brady, A.L., Lohman, P.H.M., Haroun, L. & Vainio, H. (1988) Use of computerized data listings and activity profiles of genetic and related effects in the review of 195 compounds. *Mutat. Res.*, **205**, 295–312

Waters, M.D., Brady, A.L., Stack, H.E. & Brockman, H.E. (1990) Antimutagenicity profiles for some model compounds. *Mutat. Res.*, **238**, 57–85

Waters, M.D., Stack, H.F., Jackson, M.A., Bridges, B.A. & Adler, I.-D. (1994) The performance of short-test tests in identifying potential germ cell mutagens: A qualitative and quantitative analysis. *Mutat. Res.*, **341**, 109–131

Figure 1. Schematic diagram of an antimutagenicity profile. Profiles are organized to display either the antimutagenic activity of various antimutagens in combination with a single mutagen or the activity of a single antimutagen with various mutagens. The upper bar graph displays the mutagen concentration and the range of antimutagen concentrations tested. The lower graph shows either the maximum percent inhibition, represented by a bar directed upwards from the origin, or the maximum percent enhancement of the genotoxic response, represented by a bar directed downwards. As illustrated in the lower graph, a bar across the origin indicates that no significant (< 20%) effect was detected (designated as 'negative data' in the text). Test codes are defined in Appendix 2.

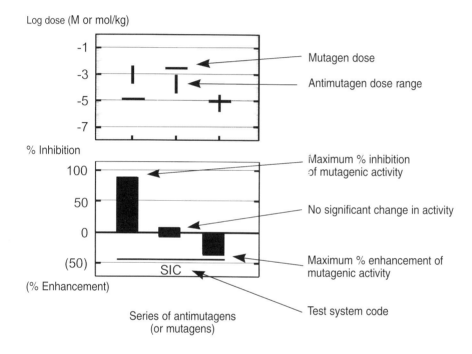

Appendix 2

Definitions of test codes

Test	Definition
AIA	Aneuploidy, animal cells *in vitro*
AIH	Aneuploidy, human cells *in vitro*
BID	Binding (covalent) to DNA *in vitro*
BSD	*Bacillus subtilis rec* strains, differential toxicity
CBA	Chromosomal aberrations, animal bone-marrow cells *in vivo*
CHF	Chromosomal aberrations, human fibroblasts *in vitro*
CHL	Chromosomal aberrations, human lymphocytes *in vitro*
CIC	Chromosomal aberrations, Chinese hamster cells *in vitro*
CVA	Chromosomal aberrations, other animal cells *in vivo*
DIH	DNA strand breaks, cross-links or related damage, human cells *in vitro*
DMX	*Drosophila melanogaster*, sex-linked recessive lethal mutation
ECK	*Escherichia coli* K12, mutation
G9H	Gene mutation *hprt* locus, Chinese hamster V79 cells *in vitro*
GIA	Gene mutation, other animal cells *in vitro*
HMM	Host mediated assay, microbial cells in animal hosts
MVM	Micronucleus formation, mice *in vivo*
SA0	*Salmonella typhimurium* TA100, reverse mutation
SA5	*Salmonella typhimurium* TA1535, reverse mutation
SA7	*Salmonella typhimurium* TA1537, reverse mutation
SA8	*Salmonella typhimurium* TA1538, reverse mutation
SA9	*Salmonella typhimurium* TA98, reverse mutation
SCG	*Saccharomyces cerevisiae*, gene conversion
SHL	Sister chromatid exchange, human lymphocytes *in vitro*
SHT	Sister chromatid exchange, transformed human cells *in vitro*
SIC	Sister chromatid exchange, Chinese hamster cells *in vitro*
SIM	Sister chromatid exchange, mouse cells *in vitro*
SIT	Sister chromatid exchange, transformed cells *in vitro*
SLH	Sister chromatid exchange, human lymphocytes *in vivo*
SPM	Sperm morphology, mouse
TCM	Cell transformation, C3H 10T1/2 mouse cells
URP	Unscheduled DNA synthesis, rat primary hepatocytes *in vitro*

IARC Monographs on the Evaluation of Carcinogenic Risks to Humans

IARC Scientific Publications

No. 25
Carcinogenic Risk: Strategies for Intervention
Edited by W. Davis and C. Rosenfeld
1979; 280 pages; ISBN 0 19 723025 3

No. 26
Directory of On-going Research in Cancer Epidemiology 1978
Edited by C.S. Muir and G. Wagner
1978; 550 pages; ISBN 0 19 723026 1
(out of print)

No. 27
Molecular and Cellular Aspects of Carcinogen Screening Tests
Edited by R. Montesano, H. Bartsch and L. Tomatis
1980; 372 pages; ISBN 0 19 723027 X

No. 28
Directory of On-going Research in Cancer Epidemiology 1979
Edited by C.S. Muir and G. Wagner
1979; 672 pages; ISBN 92 832 1128 6
(out of print)

No. 29
Environmental Carcinogens. Selected Methods of Analysis. Volume 3: Analysis of Polycyclic Aromatic Hydrocarbons in Environmental Samples
Editor-in-Chief: H. Egan
1979; 240 pages; ISBN 0 19 723028 8

No. 30
Biological Effects of Mineral Fibres
Editor-in-Chief: J.C. Wagner
1980; Two volumes, 494 pages & 513 pages; ISBN 0 19 723030 X

No. 31
N-Nitroso Compounds: Analysis, Formation and Occurrence
Edited by E.A. Walker, L. Griciute, M. Castegnaro and M. Börzsönyi
1980; 835 pages; ISBN 0 19 723031 8

No. 32
Statistical Methods in Cancer Research. Volume 1: The Analysis of Case-control Studies
By N.E. Breslow and N.E. Day
1980; 338 pages; ISBN 92 832 0132 9

No. 33
Handling Chemical Carcinogens in the Laboratory
Edited by R. Montesano, H. Bartsch, E. Boyland, G. Della Porta, L. Fishbein, R.A. Griesemer, A.B. Swan and L. Tomatis
1979; 32 pages; ISBN 0 19 723033 4
(out of print)

No. 34
Pathology of Tumours in Laboratory Animals. Volume III: Tumours of the Hamster
Editor-in-Chief: V.S. Turusov
1982; 461 pages; ISBN 0 19 723034 2

No. 35
Directory of On-going Research in Cancer Epidemiology 1980
Edited by C.S. Muir and G. Wagner
1980; 660 pages; ISBN 0 19 723035 0
(out of print)

No. 36
Cancer Mortality by Occupation and Social Class 1851–1971
Edited by W.P.D. Logan
1982; 253 pages; ISBN 0 19 723036 9

No. 37
Laboratory Decontamination and Destruction of Aflatoxins B1, B2, G1, G2 in Laboratory Wastes
Edited by M. Castegnaro, D.C. Hunt, E.B. Sansone, P.L. Schuller, M.G. Siriwardana, G.M. Telling, H.P. van Egmond and E.A. Walker
1980; 56 pages; ISBN 0 19 723037 7

No. 38
Directory of On-going Research in Cancer Epidemiology 1981
Edited by C.S. Muir and G. Wagner
1981; 696 pages; ISBN 0 19 723038 5
(out of print)

No. 39
Host Factors in Human Carcinogenesis
Edited by H. Bartsch and B. Armstrong
1982; 583 pages;
ISBN 0 19 723039 3

No. 40
Environmental Carcinogens: Selected Methods of Analysis. Volume 4: Some Aromatic Amines and Azo Dyes in the General and Industrial Environment
Edited by L. Fishbein, M. Castegnaro, I.K. O'Neill and H. Bartsch
1981; 347 pages; ISBN 0 19 723040 7

No. 41
N-Nitroso Compounds: Occurrence and Biological Effects
Edited by H. Bartsch, I.K. O'Neill, M. Castegnaro and M. Okada
982; 755 pages; ISBN 0 19 723041 5

No. 42
Cancer Incidence in Five Continents Volume IV

Edited by J. Waterhouse, C. Muir, K. Shanmugaratnam and J. Powell
1982; 811 pages; ISBN 0 19 723042 3

No. 43
Laboratory Decontamination and Destruction of Carcinogens in Laboratory Wastes: Some N-Nitrosamines
Edited by M. Castegnaro, G. Eisenbrand, G. Ellen, L. Keefer, D. Klein, E.B. Sansone, D. Spincer, G. Telling and K. Webb
1982; 73 pages; ISBN 0 19 723043 1

No. 44
Environmental Carcinogens: Selected Methods of Analysis.
Volume 5: Some Mycotoxins
Edited by L. Stoloff, M. Castegnaro, P. Scott, I.K. O'Neill and H. Bartsch
1983; 455 pages; ISBN 0 19 723044 X

No. 45
Environmental Carcinogens: Selected Methods of Analysis.
Volume 6: N-Nitroso Compounds
Edited by R. Preussmann, I.K. O'Neill, G. Eisenbrand, B. Spiegelhalder and H. Bartsch
1983; 508 pages; ISBN 0 19 723045 8

No. 46
Directory of On-going Research in Cancer Epidemiology 1982
Edited by C.S. Muir and G. Wagner
1982; 722 pages; ISBN 0 19 723046 6
(out of print)

No. 47
Cancer Incidence in Singapore 1968–1977
Edited by K. Shanmugaratnam, H.P. Lee and N.E. Day
1983; 171 pages; ISBN 0 19 723047 4

No. 48
Cancer Incidence in the USSR (2nd Revised Edition)
Edited by N.P. Napalkov, G.F. Tserkovny, V.M. Merabishvili, D.M. Parkin, M. Smans and C.S. Muir
1983; 75 pages; ISBN 0 19 723048 2

No. 49
Laboratory Decontamination and Destruction of Carcinogens in Laboratory Wastes: Some Polycyclic Aromatic Hydrocarbons
Edited by M. Castegnaro, G. Grimmer, O. Hutzinger, W. Karcher, H. Kunte, M. Lafontaine, H.C. Van der Plas, E.B. Sansone and S.P. Tucker
1983; 87 pages; ISBN 0 19 723049 0

No. 130
Directory of On-going Research in Cancer Epidemiology 1994
Edited by R. Sankaranarayanan, J. Wahrendorf and E. Démaret
1994; 800 pages; ISBN 92 832 2130 3

No. 132
Survival of Cancer Patients in Europe: The EUROCARE Study
Edited by F. Berrino, M. Sant, A. Verdecchia, R. Capocaccia, T. Hakulinen and J. Estève
1995; 463 pages; ISBN 92 832 2132 X

No. 134
Atlas of Cancer Mortality in Central Europe
W. Zatonski, J. Estéve, M. Smans, J. Tyczynski and P. Boyle
1996; 300 pages; ISBN 92 832 2134 6

No. 135
Methods for Investigating Localized Clustering of Disease
Edited by F.E. Alexander and P. Boyle
1996; 235 pages; ISBN 92 832 2135 4

No. 136
Chemoprevention in Cancer Control
Edited by M. Hakama, V. Beral, E. Buiatti, J. Faivre and D.M. Parkin
1996; 160 pages; ISBN 92 832 2136 2

No. 137
Directory of On-going Research in Cancer Epidemiology 1996
Edited by R. Sankaranarayan, J. Warendorf and E. Démaret
1996; 810 pages; ISBN 92 832 2137 0

No. 138
Social Inequalities and Cancer
Edited by M. Kogevinas, N. Pearce, M. Susser and P. Boffetta
1997; 412 pages; ISBN 92 832 2138 9

No. 139
Principles of Chemoprevention
Edited by B.W. Stewart, D. McGregor and P. Kleihues
1996; 358 pages; ISBN 92 832 2139 7

No. 140
Mechanisms of Fibre Carcinogenesis
Edited by A.B. Kane, P. Boffetta, R. Saracci and J.D. Wilbourn
1996; 135 pages; ISBN 92 832 2140 0

No. 142
Application of Biomarkers in Cancer Epidemiology
Edited by P. Toniolo, P. Boffetta, D.E.G. Shuker, N. Rothman, B. Hulka and N. Pearce
1997; 318 pages; ISBN 92 832 2142 7

IARC Technical Reports

No. 1
Cancer in Costa Rica
Edited by R. Sierra, R. Barrantes, G. Muñoz Leiva, D.M. Parkin, C.A. Bieber and N. Muñoz Calero
1988; 124 pages;
ISBN 92 832 1412 9

No. 2
SEARCH: A Computer Package to Assist the Statistical Analysis of Case-Control Studies
Edited by G.J. Macfarlane, P. Boyle and P. Maisonneuve
1991; 80 pages; ISBN 92 832 1413 7

No. 3
Cancer Registration in the European Economic Community
Edited by M.P. Coleman and E. Démaret
1988; 188 pages; ISBN 92 832 1414 5

No. 4
Diet, Hormones and Cancer: Methodological Issues for Prospective Studies
Edited by E. Riboli and R. Saracci
1988; 156 pages; ISBN 92 832 1415 3

No. 5
Cancer in the Philippines
Edited by A.V. Laudico, D. Esteban and D.M. Parkin
1989; 186 pages; ISBN 92 832 1416 1

No. 6
La genèse du Centre international de recherche sur le cancer
By R. Sohier and A.G.B. Sutherland
1990, 102 pages; ISBN 92 832 1418 8

No. 7
Epidémiologie du cancer dans les pays de langue latine
1990, 292 pages; ISBN 92 832 1419 6

No. 8
Comparative Study of Anti-smoking Legislation in Countries of the European Economic Community
By A. J. Sasco, P. Dalla-Vorgia and P. Van der Elst
1992; 82 pages; ISBN: 92 832 1421 8
Etude comparative des Législations de Contrôle du Tabagisme dans les Pays de la Communauté économique européenne
1995; 82 pages; ISBN 92 832 2402 7

No. 9
Epidémiologie du cancer dans les pays de langue latine
1991; 346 pages; ISBN 92 832 1423 4

No. 10
Manual for Cancer Registry Personnel
Edited by D. Esteban, S. Whelan, A. Laudico and D.M. Parkin
1995; 400 pages; ISBN 92 832 1424 2

No. 11
Nitroso Compounds: Biological Mechanisms, Exposures and Cancer Etiology
Edited by I. O'Neill and H. Bartsch
1992; 150 pages; ISBN 92 832 1425 X

No. 12
Epidémiologie du cancer dans les pays de langue latine
1992; 375 pages; ISBN 92 832 1426 9

No. 13
Health, Solar UV Radiation and Environmental Change
By A. Kricker, B.K. Armstrong, M.E. Jones and R.C. Burton
1993; 213 pages; ISBN 92 832 1427 7

No. 14
Epidémiologie du cancer dans les pays de langue latine
1993; 400 pages; ISBN 92 832 1428 5

No. 15
Cancer in the African Population of Bulawayo, Zimbabwe, 1963–1977
By M.E.G. Skinner, D.M. Parkin, A.P. Vizcaino and A. Ndhlovu
1993; 120 pages; ISBN 92 832 1429 3

IARC CancerBases

All IARC Publications are available directly from
IARCPress, 150 Cours Albert Thomas, F-69372 Lyon cedex 08, France (Fax: +33 4 72 73 83 02; E-mail:press@iarc.fr).

IARC Monographs and Technical Reports are also available from the
World Health Organization Distribution and Sales, CH-1211 Geneva 27 (Fax: +41 22 791 4857)
and from WHO Sales Agents worldwide.

IARC Scientific Publications, IARC Handbooks and IARC CancerBases are also available from
Oxford University Press, Walton Street, Oxford, UK OX2 6DP (Fax: +44 1865 267782).